Computer Applications for Augmenting the Management of Speech, Language, and Hearing Disorders

Computer Applications for Augmenting the Management of Speech, Language, and Hearing Disorders

Franklin H. Silverman
Marquette University
Medical College of Wisconsin

Allyn and Bacon
Boston • London • Toronto • Sydney • Tokyo • Singapore

Executive Editor: Stephen D. Dragin
Editorial Assistant: Christine Svitila
Editorial-Production Administrator: Joe Sweeney
Editorial-Production Service: Walsh & Associates, Inc.
Composition Buyer: Linda Cox
Manufacturing Buyer: Suzanne Lareau
Cover Administrator: Suzanne Harbison

A Viacom Company
160 Gould Street
Needham Heights, MA 02194

Internet: www.abacon.com
America Online: Keyword: College Online

Library of Congress Cataloging-in-Publication Data

Silverman, Franklin H.
Computer applications for augmenting the management of speech, language, and hearing disorders / Franklin H. Silverman.
p. cm.
Includes bibliographical references and index.
ISBN 0-13-124140-0
1. Communicative disorders—Data processing. I. Title.
RC423.S5184 1996
616.85'5'00285—dc20 96-9411
CIP

Printed in the United States of America
10 9 8 7 6 5 4 3 2 1 01 00 99 98 97 96

Contents

Preface

Speech-language pathologists and audiologists are expected by their employers to be able to use microcomputers for a number of applications including report writing, record keeping, billing, appointment making, administering diagnostic tests, analyzing data (e.g., language samples), decision making, administering language stimulation and other types of drills, augmentative communication, literature searching, controlling instrumentation, and professional education. The growing importance of microcomputers to speech-language pathologists and audiologists is evinced by the existence of hundreds of convention papers, articles, books, and book chapters describing microcomputer applications in the management of speech, language, and hearing disorders (see Appendix A).

There are also several related technologies, sometimes referred to as *new technologies*, with which employers are beginning to expect speech-language pathologists and audiologists to be familiar. These technologies—all of which are microcomputer based—include interactive videodisks, virtual reality, personal digital assistants, and electronic organizers.

This book introduces you to microcomputers and related new technologies and the variety of ways that you can use them to facilitate your clinical activities. It also provides you with a "tool"—a comprehensive bibliography—to facilitate your search for additional information about the applications described and the hardware and software needed for doing them. No previous knowledge of computers or an "objective attitude" toward them is assumed. If you resist using microcomputers for certain applications because you lack confidence in your ability to understand or learn them, perhaps the information in this book will give you the confidence to try using them. If you presently use a sophisticated word-processing program such as WordPerfect or Microsoft Word, you probably have the ability to understand and learn to use any application described in this book!

Much of the information that we have about microcomputer applications in speech-language pathology and audiology comes from convention presentations, particularly those at annual meetings of the American Speech-Language-Hearing Association. I have included references to abstracts of them in the bibliography. Further information is usually available from presenters. If they are ASHA members, their addresses and telephone numbers will be in the Association's membership directory.

Microcomputer hardware and software are upgraded periodically. Most manufacturers and publishers tend to do so at least once a year. Consequently, specific computer models and software versions that were available while this book was being written are unlikely to be available when it is published. Fortunately, while computer models and software versions are constantly changing, their basic features are not. Most, if not all, of the commands that are essential for report writing could be issued by the sophisticated word processing programs available during the early 1980s, such as WordStar. And the basic hardware components of microcomputers during the early 1980s are essentially the same as those today. Both hardware and software, of course, have greater capabilities today than they did during the early 1980s: Contemporary computers, for example, have much more random access memory (RAM) and contemporary word processing programs have far more sophisticated desktop publishing capabilities. The basics, however, remain the same. Consequently, the focus of this book is on them rather than on the platforms (computers) and software that were being marketed while this book was being written.

Just as the basic features of computer hardware and software have not changed since the early 1980s, neither have the basic tasks that can be done with them. Any application that was possible with obsolete hardware and software is also possible with that available now. My primary goal in this book is to alert you to ways that a computer can enable you to perform professional tasks better or more efficiently. Consequently, I have included papers in which the author(s) utilized hardware or software that is obsolete.

Computer Applications for Augmenting the Management of Speech, Language, and Hearing Disorders is divided into two parts. The first part (Chapters 1, 2, and 3) describes what microcomputers can do clinically for speech-language pathologists and audiologists and provides the essential information about microcomputer and related new technology hardware and software required for understanding the literature dealing with their clinical application. The second part (Chapters 4 through 15) provides information—including a review of the literature—about specific ways that microcomputers and related new technologies can be, have been, and could be used directly or indirectly for promoting the welfare of persons who have a communicative disorder. The "could be" discussion is based on reports in the literatures of other health- and education-related fields.

The application chapters (Chapters 4 through 15) can be understood by students who have not read previous ones and consequently, they can be read in any order. The order in which they appear here is the one in which I decided, somewhat arbitrarily, to discuss them in my "Computer Applications in Communicative Disorders" course. One prepublication reviewer of the manuscript, incidentally, indicated that the following ordering of these chapters would relate better to his course syllabus: 7, 9, 10, 14, 6, 8, 11, 4, 12, 5, 13, and 15.

The review of the literature includes discussions of ways that microcomputers that are now obsolete have been used clinically. While neither the hardware nor software used for these applications is of current interest, this isn't the case for the applications themselves. All can be done with any IBM-compatible or Macintosh microcomputer available now!

This book can serve as a tool for *networking* as well as for becoming acquainted with the literature on computer applications in speech, language, and hearing. Most of the papers cited are relatively recent and their authors are still both active professionally and members of ASHA. Consequently, you can find current addresses for them in the ASHA Membership Directory. The majority would be more than willing to share their clinical experience with computer applications with you (see Krupke, 1990).

It is impossible to give credit to the many sources from which the concepts presented in this book have been drawn. The book is the result of years of teaching about, reading about, and interacting with microcomputers (both as a user and programmer) as well as hundreds of hours of conversations with students and colleagues about microcomputer and related technology applications in speech-language pathology, audiology, and other education and health related fields. Thus, I cannot credit this or that concept to a specific person, but I can say thank you to all who have helped, particularly the undergraduate and graduate students who have taken my computer course at Marquette University, whose questions and challenges through the years have helped me to clarify my ideas.

▶ 1

Computers and Clinicians

Speech-language pathologists and audiologists have incorporated new technologies (e.g., the audiometer and videotape recorder) into their clinical practice when they felt that doing so would be likely to benefit their clients—that is, when they felt that their incorporation had the potential to increase the efficiency with which clinical services could be dispensed and/or make possible clinical services that it would be impossible or impractical to offer otherwise. The microcomputer has been shown to be a technology that has this kind of potential (Fitch, 1983a, 1985f, 1989b; Fox, 1990; Garrett, 1989; Gelatt, 1987; Gelatt & Minghetti, 1989; Mills, 1985).

Why is it reasonable to believe that microcomputer technology can be helpful clinically to speech-language pathologists and audiologists? There are several reasons. First, there have been hundreds of reports published in American Speech-Language-Hearing Association (ASHA) and other professional journals and presented at ASHA conventions (see References and Bibliography list in the back of the book) that indicate it can increase the efficiency with which clinical services are dispensed and expand the clinician's repertoire of assessment and intervention strategies. A second reason is that surveys indicate many speech-language pathologists and audiologists are using them for doing clinical tasks, both in the United States (Fein, 1983, 1984; Flahive, Nasir, & Watson, 1995; Harding & Tidball, 1982; Rose & Waldron, 1984; Shewan, 1988, 1989; Wolfman & Silverman, 1985) and in other countries (Kaasgaard & Lauritsen, 1995). A third reason is the introduction of computer literacy courses in speech-language pathology and audiology training programs (Cochran, Masterson, Long, Katz, Seaton, Wynne, Lieberth, & Martin, 1993; Cooper, 1985). And finally, a search of the Medline and PsyLIT databases indicates that practitioners in other education- and health-related fields are routinely using microcomputers for some of the same tasks done by speech-language pathologists and audiologists.

My two main objectives in this chapter are to give you an overview of computer technology and its clinical applications and to help you develop an "objective attitude" toward the clinical use of microcomputers and related new technologies if you don't already have one. I begin by operationally defining the term "computer" and indicating how microcomputers differ from the other two types—minicomputers and mainframes. Next, I present an overview of how speech-language pathologists and audiologists have used microcomputers clinically. And, finally, I discuss sources of resistance to and types of information and experience needed for using a microcomputer maximally to promote the welfare of persons served professionally.

WHAT IS A COMPUTER?

Computers are *appliances*. Like all appliances, they utilize technology—the practical application of scientific knowledge. For computers, this knowledge comes, in part, from the branch of physics dealing with electricity and magnetism. Computers differ from appliances like microwave ovens and washing machines in that they can be used for doing more than one task. They do *some* tasks better and/or more efficiently than alternative approaches.

What functions do computers perform? They are four of them: *accepting* information, *storing* information, *processing* information, and *giving out* processed information. An overview of each is presented here and a detailed description is found in Chapter 2.

Accepting Information

Information accepted by a computer usually is entered in *alphanumeric* form (i.e., through the use of a character set that contains letters, digits, punctuation marks, and special symbols) by means of a keyboard. It also can be entered in other ways. A number of devices that can be used to input information are described in Chapter 2.

Storing Information

The memory unit stores the information accepted by the computer—both programs and data. It also stores the information processed by the computer prior to its being displayed or otherwise utilized. The type of memory in which such information is stored is known as *random access memory* or *RAM*. It is referred to as random access memory because any information stored in it can be directly accessed, or located. A computer's RAM can be viewed as a filing cabinet (or system) to which file folders can be added or deleted and the information in individual file folders can be modified. If the folders in such a filing system were in alphabetical order, a given folder could be accessed by going directly to its location in the alphabetical sequence.

RAM is regarded as temporary memory. There are two reasons. First, information that is stored in RAM can be changed. And second, the information stored in RAM is "lost" when the power to the RAM chips is turned off. With the exception of a few computers and related devices such as personal digital assistants and electronic organizers (see Chapter 15) that use a battery to power the RAM chips, this occurs whenever the computer is turned off.

All computers also have a second type of memory that is referred to as *read only memory* or *ROM*. Some of the programs that a computer needs to operate regardless of the application for which it is being used usually are stored in ROM. ROM is permanent memory: The information stored in it cannot be changed and it is not lost when the computer is turned off.

Some computers contain a special type of ROM chip known as a *PROM* or *EPROM*. Like RAM chips, user programs can be stored in them. And like ROM chips, programs are not lost when the computer is turned off. They can be used for programming microcomputer-based augmentative communication devices (e.g., Korabic, Silverman, & Rosera, 1987).

Processing Information

The *central processing unit (CPU)* carries out the instructions in the programs stored in the memory unit. The CPU is the "brain" of the computer. It "reads" the contents of ROM, RAM, and disks and can store ("write") the information that it processes in RAM and/or on disks. It can also control input and output devices. The role played by a computer's CPU is discussed further in Chapter 2.

Displaying or Otherwise Utilizing Processed Information

The output unit displays or otherwise utilizes some or all of the processed information stored in RAM. For example, it may cause information to be displayed on a monitor screen or it may use it to control an instrument such as an audiometer (see Chapter 12). The software being used determines both what information is utilized and how it is utilized. The software controls the CPU, which, in turn, controls the output device or devices. Several output devices can be used simultaneously (e.g., a monitor and a printer).

TYPES OF COMPUTERS

There are three types of computers: mainframes, minicomputers, and microcomputers. While they all perform the four basic functions described in the preceeding section, they differ in some significant ways. These are discussed here.

Mainframe Computers

These are the largest and most expensive computers. The most powerful of them—supercomputers—cost millions of dollars. Historically, mainframe computers were the first type developed. The first generation of mainframes (built between 1942 and 1959) utilized vacuum tubes, were huge (their components filled a room), and cost hundreds of thousands of dollars. However, they were much slower and had much less RAM than the least expensive Macintosh or IBM-compatible computer available now. The second generation mainframes (built between 1959 and 1965) were smaller than the first because they used transistors instead of vacuum tubes. And the third generation, built after 1965, used integrated circuits instead of transistors or vacuum tubes and were smaller, faster, and contained more RAM than those of previous generations.

Mainframe computers are accessed using a *terminal*. A number of terminals (possibly hundreds) can access and utilize a mainframe computer simultaneously. Doing so is referred to as operating in a *time-shared conversational mode*. Terminals contain keyboards and computer-type video monitors and are connected to a mainframe by a *network* or a t*elephone line and modem* (see Chapter 11). A modem is a device that enables computers to communicate with each other over telephone lines. Terminals function as both input and output devices and can be located thousands of miles from the mainframe computer they are accessing. Microcomputers can be programmed to function as terminals.

A mainframe computer when it is functioning in a *conversational mode* processes each piece of information it receives from a terminal almost immediately and responds to it on the terminal's monitor screen. Travel agents usually "converse" with a computer in this manner while making airline reservations for their clients.

Minicomputers

These tend to be smaller and less expensive than mainframe computers. While they can do most of the tasks that can be done with mainframe computers, they usually have less memory and can support fewer terminals in a time-sharing conversational mode. If more terminal capacity is needed, several minicomputers can be linked together. Speech-language pathologists and audiologists may be required to use their institutions' minicomputers for such applications as appointment making, billing, and maintaining client records.

The use of minicomputers for applications *other than networking* has reduced during the past twenty years. Microcomputers (see next section) have become more powerful during this period and consequently, they can now do applications that previously required a minicomputer. Since microcomputers are smaller, cheaper, and more "user friendly" than minicomputers, it is not particularly surprising that they have replaced minicomputers for many applications.

Microcomputers

These are the smallest and least expensive computers. Speech-language pathologists and audiologists use this type most often. Ones that are relatively large and cannot be powered by batteries may be referred to as desktop computers, personal computers, or PCs. And ones that are relatively small and can be powered by batteries may be referred to as laptop computers, notebook computers, palmtop computers, or personal digital assistants (see Chapter 15 and LaPine, 1990). The two most popular brands of microcomputers when this chapter was written were the Macintosh and the IBM-compatible (MS-DOS). A third, the Apple II, remained popular in the public schools even though it was no longer being manufactured.

Microcomputers usually have less RAM than mainframes and minicomputers and most cannot be used in a time-sharing conversational mode. They can, however, be programmed to function as "dummy" terminals for minicomputers, mainframes, and other microcomputers when they are functioning in networks as file servers for shared applications (see Chapter 11). Incidentally, while you are using the Internet, America On Line, Compuserve, or another computer network, your computer is functioning as a dummy terminal.

Devices that are microcomputers may not be labeled as such. Examples are electronic calculators (see Chapter 15), telecommunication devices for the deaf (see Chapter 15), virtual reality devices (see Chapter 15), electronic organizers (see Chapter 15), electronic measuring instruments (see Chapter 12), speech-generating augmentative communication aids (see Chapter 5), video game devices, and fax machines. These are all *dedicated* microcomputers—ones that are designed and programmed for (i.e., dedicated to) a single application. A standard microcomputer can be programmed to simulate all of them—even a fax machine (see Chapter 11).

The emphasis in this book is on microcomputer applications in speech-language pathology and audiology because microcomputers are the type that clinicians have used the most and there is more general access to them than to minicomputers or mainframes. However, most of the tasks that are mentioned in the book can be done with a minicomputer or mainframe if the cliniciain doesn't have access to a microcomputer but does have access to one of these.

MICROCOMPUTER USE BY SPEECH-LANGUAGE PATHOLOGISTS AND AUDIOLOGISTS

Speech-language pathologists and audiologists have used microcomputers clinically in three general ways. The first is to *facilitate doing administrative tasks*. Microcomputers make it possible for speech-language pathologists and audiologists to do these tasks better and/or more efficiently. Such tasks include writing evaluation and progress reports, writing IEPs, letter writing (including individually addressed form letters), preparing inservice presentations, preparing materials for marketing programs (e.g., announcements and flyers), maintaining client records, clinic scheduling, managing budgets, billing, check writing, completing insurance forms, maintaining employee records, inventory control (e.g., stock of hearing aids), and gathering and analyzing statistical information for end-of-the-year reports (Magilen, 1991; Merson, Rolnick, & Weiner, 1995; Wynne, Seaton, & Allen, 1993).

The second is to *facilitate doing clinical tasks*. Microcomputers make it possible for speech-language pathologists and audiologists to do tasks associated with evaluation and therapy better and/or more efficiently. Such tasks include taking case histories, administering and scoring tests, analyzing speech and language samples, making decisions regarding etiology, defining goals, motivating clients, creating materials for use by clients, fitting hearing aids, administering therapy (e.g., language stimulation drills), and literature searching.

The third of these is to *provide unique services*. Such applications do not use microcomputers merely as labor-saving devices; they use them to provide clients with a service that they could not be provided otherwise. An example would be programming a microcomputer to function as an augmentative communication device (Mizuko, 1993; Montgomery, 1989; Morris & Ray, 1991). Microcomputer utilization for this purpose is described in Chapter 5.

Speech-language pathologists and audiologists have also used microcomputers for research and professional education. Research-related tasks for which they have been used them include literature searching, data analysis and management, control of instrumentation, preparation of research reports, and creation of models that either simulate the functioning of aspects of the speech and hearing mechanisms or simulate devices—such as hearing aids—that are used to manage disorders affecting them (e.g., Egolf, 1978; Eilers, Miskiel, Ozdamar, Urbano, & Widen, 1991; Eilers, Widen, Urbano, Hudson, & Gonzalez, 1991; Engebretson & Miller, 1982; Fausti, Olson, Frey, & Schaffer, 1991). And for *professional education*—undergraduate, graduate, and continuing—they have used microcomputers for preparing presentations and teaching materials, doing literature searches, sharing information with other clinicians (e.g., through the use of bulletin boards on the Internet—see Chapter 11 and Appendix B), and learning to do tasks such as administering audiometric tests (Levitt, Slosberg, Hawie, Mazor, & Rosenstein, 1978).

Detailed descriptions of the applications described in this section are included in Chapters 4 through 15.

WHY DO CLINICIANS RESIST USING MICROCOMPUTERS?

Many clinicians who have access to and could use a microcomputer to promote the welfare of the persons whom they serve professionally resist using one. They may resist using a microcomputer for all clinical applications, or only a few. Periodic membership surveys conducted by the American Speech-Language-Hearing Association indicate that the majority of speech-language pathologists and audiologists are using microcomputers for report writing but not for the other clinical applications. Possible reasons for clinicians' underutilization of this technology will be explored in this section.

People tend to both fear and resist innovations (Larson & Whiteside, 1986). They fear that they will be unable to cope with a new situation or circumstance and/or it will somehow have a detrimental effect on them. They also tend to resist trying new ways to do a task, particularly if they have an approach they're satisfied with.

The introduction of computers into the workplace has been met with considerable fear and resistance, particularly among persons who did not learn to feel comfortable with them in school. Many clinicians who are currently employed in educational or medical settings graduated before microcomputer labs were common in schools and did not have the opportunity to become comfortable with them. Fear of computers is so common that it has been given a name—computerphobia (Rosen & Weil, 1995). Blue- and white-collar workers as well as professionals (including clinicians) manifest this fear.

There are several reasons why clinicians may resist using computers, including the following:

- They may feel that it is a threat to their job security—that is, they will be replaced by a computer.
- They are comfortable doing things the way they have been, particularly if they have been doing them in a particular way for a number of years. They don't see any reason to "fix what isn't broken." This is particularly likely to be a source of resistance in clinicians over the age of forty.
- They lack confidence in their ability to learn to use a computer. They may assume, for example, that they are too old—they may assume that "You can't teach an old dog new tricks." Or they may lack confidence in their ability to learn to use almost any electronic device competently.
- They may feel that the time it takes to learn to use a computer for certain clinical applications is not a good investment of this valuable resource.
- They may feel that having clients interact with computers somehow dehumanizes the clinical process.
- They may feel that the software available for clinical use is unlikely to contribute much to helping their clients achieve their goals.
- They may feel that the high level of interest at present in the clinical use of microcomputers is merely a fad.
- They may believe that a computer isn't the best tool for doing some clinical tasks for which software is available. They may doubt, for example, that this sophisticated and expensive a tool is needed for doing a particular task and, consequently, they would believe that using it for the purpose would be somewhat similar to using a sledge hammer to pound thumb tacks.

Both the validity and implications of each of these reasons for not using a computer clinically are considered in the paragraphs that follow.

Concern about Job Security

One reason why some persons resist the introduction of computers into the workplace is a concern about job security (Pentz, 1987a). This is particularly apt to be a concern now because of the high level of interest in reducing the cost of health care. The fear is that if employers learn that some types of therapy can be administered by a computer, they will use them to replace some clinicians. While this certainly could happen to speech-language pathologists and audiologists, it doesn't appear to have happened to them very often judging by the absence of reports about it occurring in ASHA publications.

Comfort Level

It is easy to greet a new thing with despair at losing the familiar, compounded by fear of the unknown. Perhaps one of the main reasons why some people over the age of forty tend to resist using computers is that they are both comfortable and satisfied with the status quo—that is, with the ways they have been doing tasks—and find the thought of changing how they do them anxiety arousing. Their assumption ("certainty") appears to be that using a computer for doing tasks is unlikely to result in their being done better or the doing of them becoming more enjoyable.

When microcomputers with word processing software became affordable during the early 1980s, many clinicians—including myself—initially resisted using them for report writing because we were comfortable drafting reports with a typewriter and found the thought of drafting them with a computer to be anxiety arousing. However, after we were "forced" by our employers or peer pressure to try drafting reports with a computer, most of us found that our "certainty" was wrong—we found it was both more efficient and enjoyable to complete reports with a computer than with a typewriter. Few clinicians today would choose to use a typewriter for report writing!

While most speech-language pathologists and audiologists are using computers for report writing (Fein, 1983, 1984; Harding & Tidball, 1982; Robins, 1996; Rose & Waldron, 1984; Shewan, 1988, 1989; Wolfman & Silverman, 1985), this does not appear to be true for some clinical tasks for which software is available. In some cases the reason for this lack of use is that the clinician does not have access to the software needed to do the tasks. However, I suspect that in a significant number of cases, the reason is that the clinician is comfortable with the ways that he or she is currently doing tasks (i.e., being comfortable with the status quo) or that the clinician finding the idea of using a computer for these tasks to be anxiety arousing.

Everyone obviously wants to behave in a rational manner. To determine whether a "certainty" that is keeping you from using a computer for doing a particular task is rational, you should test it. You test a "certainty" by trying to do the task with a computer. If the evidence supports your "certainty," it obviously would be sensible to continue doing the task the way you have been doing it. On the other hand, if the evidence indicates that the task could be done better and/or more efficiently with a computer, it probably would make sense to begin doing it with one.

Lack of Confidence

Some clinicians avoid using computers for doing certain tasks because they lack confidence in their ability to learn to do them with one. Their "certainty" appears to be: "If I try to learn to do the task with a computer, I will fail because I don't know enough about computers." While it would be sensible for them to continue doing a task as they have been if this "certainty" is true, it would not be if they were capable of learning to do it with a computer and a computer could enable them to do it better and/or more efficiently.

One of the main reasons why clinicians may lack confidence in their ability to learn to use a computer is that they lack confidence in their ability to learn to use almost any kind of electronic instrumentation. They do not consider themselves to have an "engineering mentality." Microcomputers are no more difficult to learn to use than some other instruments with which speech-language pathologists and audiologists have been successful in learning to cope, including audiometers and videotape recorders.

One of the best ways to test this "certainty" is to have a few hours of hands-on experience with a program that you don't think you are capable of learning to use. If the program comes with a tutorial, you might want to try working through it. In fact, if you have been able to learn to use a sophisticated word processing program such as WordPerfect or Microsoft Word, you are likely to find that this program is no more difficult to learn to use—perhaps even easier.

Time Investment Too Great

Clinicians may assume that learning to use a computer for other clinical applications—not just word processing—would require a time investment they cannot afford. This is unlikely to be the case. There is no software described in this book—with the possible exception of HyperCard—that requires a time investment to learn as great as does word processing software like WordPerfect or Microsoft Word. In fact, the basics of almost all the software described in this book can be mastered in a few hours. Even those of HyperCard programming can be mastered in a weekend.

Dehumanization of the Clinical Process

Some clinicians object to having clients interact with computers during diagnosis and therapy because they feel that it dehumanizes the clinical process—that is, it results in clients interacting with machines rather than people (Minifie, 1984). For this argument to be cogent, it would be necessary to demonstrate that such interaction adversely affects the client-clinician relationship. There has been considerable research on this question in clinical psychology and other health-related fields and the preponderance of evidence indicates that this is highly unlikely to occur. A clinician, of course, could use such technology to avoid interacting with clients—doing so would be reprehensible. Most technologies can be misused. Fire, for example, can be helpful, but it can also cause harm.

It can be argued that the use of computers can enhance the client-clinician relationship by releasing clinicians from routine tasks, thereby providing them with more time to get to know their clients (and significant others) and provide supportive services (Minifie, 1984). For example, a clinician could counsel an aphasic's spouse while he or she is in another room doing language stimulation drills with a computer—possibly under the supervision of a volunteer or a paraprofessional. Supervising computer-administered drills, incidentally, is a task that many such persons can do competently.

Poor Software

Some clinicians resist using computers for diagnosis and therapy because they have heard that the software available for these purposes does not make the delivery of services better or more efficient. While some programs that are intended to facilitate these activities appear to be of little or no value (judging by reviews), this is not the case for all of them. Reviews of some of these programs (see References and Bibliography) suggest that they can be quite helpful.

There is a potential danger in using clinical software. You can be tempted to work toward the goals the software is designed to achieve rather than ones clients need to achieve (Cochran, 1989). You are particularly likely to be tempted to do so if you enjoy having clients use a computer during therapy sessions and you don't have software that can help them achieve their goals.

The approach you would use to select software for achieving clinical goals is no different than the one you would use to select other materials for achieving them. Regardless of the nature of the material, the choices are unlikely to all be of equal quality. To separate "the sheep from the goats," you would both read the reviews and other literature on materials you are considering and talk with colleagues who have used them. Reviews of software intended for clinical use are published in *Asha* and *Asha Leader*. If what you have learned about a program suggests that the activity might help clients achieve a goal, it may be worth trying with a client or two.

Computers as a Fad

The current high level of interest in microcomputers is still regarded by at least a few clinicians as being a fad (see Menosky, 1984 for an early expression of this viewpoint). They believe that clinicians will lose interest in them when they fail to meet their unrealistically high expectations.

While some clinicians undoubtedly will become disillusioned with computers for certain applications when they fail to meet their expectations, interest in the clinical application of computers is unlikely to cease. Computers have precipitated a major technological revolution, comparable to those that were precipitated by television, the automobile, and the telephone. Many children who in future years will major in speech-language pathology and audiology are becoming computer literate and undoubtedly will search for ways to apply their knowledge professionally. And many persons who will be their clients are also becoming computer literate and would be highly motivated to use a computer to facilitate their rehabilitation. Furthermore, more and more software with the potential to assist in the management of communication disorders is becoming available (see References and Bibliography), and the cost of microcomputers is now so low that any facility that offers speech, language, or hearing services can afford to purchase at least one. Finally, the American Speech-Language-Hearing Association has committed itself to making both students in training and practicing clinicians computer literate (see Robins, 1996).

Inappropriate Tool

A clinician may resist using a microcomputer for doing a particular task because he or she does not regard it as the best tool for the purpose. The clinician may feel that the computer would not do it as well as some other tool or that there are simpler, more cost-effective, and/or more efficient ways of doing it. Resistance on this basis is justifiable. A microcomputer is merely a tool, and it only makes sense to use one if it is advantageous to do so. As Fulton, Larson, and Worthy (1983, p. 572) have pointed out in a somewhat different context:

> The role of technology is to implement and support conceptualization. It should never be the role of conceptualization to modify itself to adapt to technology.

Not being the best tool, incidentally, is probably the main reason why most persons who have a computer do not use a personal checkbook program—computers are less portable than checkbooks and consequently, are less convenient to use (Chial, 1989).

KNOWLEDGE AND EXPERIENCE NEEDED TO USE A MICROCOMPUTER

What knowledge and experience do you need to use a microcomputer effectively? There are several types, including the following:

- You need to understand the terminology associated with microcomputer hardware, at least on an intuitive level, to understand manuals and other literature in which microcomputers and their components are discussed as well as to make intelligent decisions when purchasing them. This terminology is discussed in Chapter 2.

- You need to be acquainted with the terminology ("jargon") associated with computer software. This terminology is discussed in Chapters 3 through 15.
- You need to become acquainted with how microcomputers have been used by speech-language pathologists, audiologists, and others in health- and education-related fields. Some human service professionals have developed applications that have not been reported by practitioners in our field. Information about specific microcomputer applications is presented in Chapters 4 through 15. Furthermore, the References and Bibliography section contains more than 1500 papers that provide such information.
- You have to know how to evaluate hardware and software for its ability to facilitate achieving a goal in a manner that is *cost-effective.* A relatively inexpensive component or program may be as likely to facilitate your achieving a particular goal as a relatively expensive one. Information that is needed to do such an evaluation is presented throughout the book.
- Finally, you need hands-on experience doing clinical tasks with a microcomputer. You cannot identify tasks for which a microcomputer can augment your ability to promote the welfare of the persons you serve professionally merely by reading reports by other clinicians!

2

Microcomputer Components and Terminology: Hardware

This chapter will acquaint you with the basic hardware components of microcomputers and the terminology associated with them. No previous knowledge of either has been assumed.

While microcomputer manufacturers tend to introduce new models every six months or so and the new models tend to be faster and have more features than the ones they replace, the five basic hardware components they contain remain the same. In fact, all of them have been components of microcomputers—in less developed form—since the late 1970s. Consequently, my focus in this chapter will be on these components rather than on the features of the microcomputers that were being sold when this chapter was written. If I had focused on the latter, some of the content of this chapter would have been obsolete even before the book was published.

The five hardware components (or units) of a microcomputer and their interrelationships are diagrammed in Figure 2.1. The *input unit* (which usually includes a keyboard) accepts information and sends it by way of the *central processing unit* (*CPU*) to the *memory unit* where it is stored. The information put into the memory unit consists of both data and instructions for processing it (i.e., programs). Information stored in memory is sent to the central processing unit, which processes it in the manner dictated by the instructions contained in the software being used. The processed information is sent to the memory unit for storage and then to the *output unit* (by way of the central processing unit) where it is stored, displayed, and/or used for controlling a device (e.g., an audiometer). The *power source* supplies electrical energy to the other units. These same hardware components are also found in minicomputers and mainframes. Detailed descriptions of the contribution of each component follow.

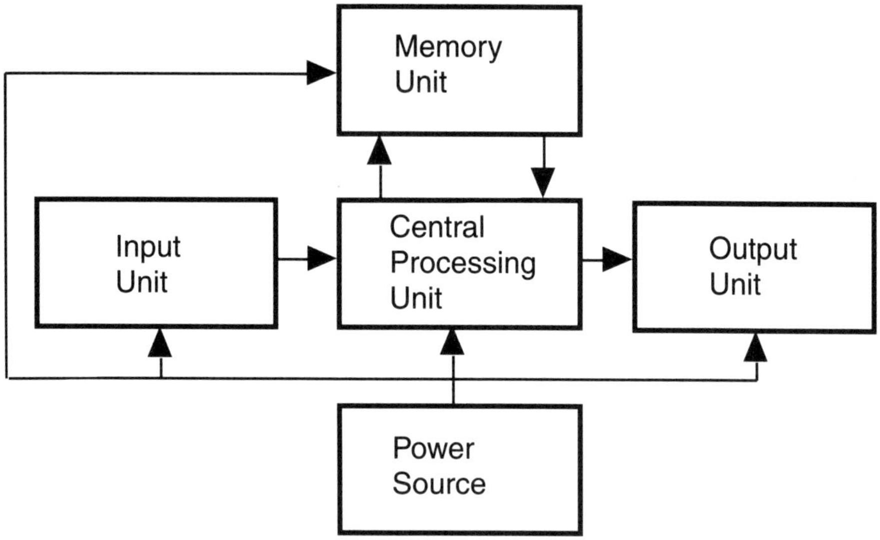

FIGURE 2.1 **The five hardware components of a microcomputer.**

THE INPUT UNIT

The input unit consists of one or more devices that put information into the computer. Input devices translate information into a form that the central processing unit can interpret. This unit interfaces the user with the computer; that is, it provides the communication channel through which the user lets the computer know what he or she wants it to do.

Input devices sometimes are referred to as *I/O* (input/output) *devices*. They are designated as such, in part, because some (e.g., modems) can function as output devices as well as input ones. Input devices are also referred to as *peripheral equipment*, or *peripherals*. Any hardware component of a microcomputer system other than its central processing unit or power source can be classified as a peripheral. At least some of the peripherals in a microcomputer system usually are not mounted in the same enclosure (case) as the central processing unit. These are connected to the CPU with electrical cables.

All of the peripherals attached to a microcomputer may not be manufactured and/or marketed by the company that manufactured the CPU. Some companies manufacture peripheral equipment rather than entire systems. It is often possible to purchase a peripheral (e.g., a hard drive) from such a manufacturer at a significantly lower price than from the manufacturer of the CPU. It may, in fact, be the same device. Computer manufacturers often purchase peripherals, such as hard drives, from other companies and retail them under their names at a higher price. In addition to the price being lower, a peripheral purchased from such a manufacturer may be warranted for longer than one purchased from the manufacturer of the computer. This was the case when this chapter was written for hard drives for Macintosh computers.

Because all of the input devices and other peripherals you will need are unlikely to be packaged with a computer when you purchase it, you will have to plan carefully so that you will get the best total package for your money. If you are a computer novice, you are likely to feel lost when you have to do such planning. Your minimum requirements for peripherals will be determined by the software you want the computer to run and the tasks that you want to do with the software. Your word processing program, for example, may be capable of printing in color, but you may have no need to print in any color but black. Consequently, you would not need a color printer. If you don't determine your actual software and task requirements before purchasing peripherals, you are likely to be encouraged to purchase ones that will have greater capability and be more expensive than those you need. Furthermore, if you don't do such planning prior to purchasing a computer, you may find that it lacks the capacity to do what you want to do with it. Of course, if you make a mistake when purchasing a peripheral, you can replace it. However, doing so can get expensive.

Input devices are connected to the CPU through the use of an *interface*. Output devices are connected to the CPU by one as well. The interface "translates" the data generated by the device into the form that the CPU can process—that is, digital form (see Chapter 3). The interface also adjusts for any differences in speed of data transmission between the input device and the CPU. The rate at which an input device transmits information to a CPU must be within the range the CPU can accept. It may be necessary, for example, for the interface on a keyboard to perform this function if the user sometimes types at a faster rate than the CPU is able to accept.

There are two types of interfaces that are used for connecting input and output devices to the CPU: *serial* and *parallel*. Parallel interfaces tend to transmit data at a faster rate than serial ones. This difference in rate of data transmission would be significant for some applications, but not for others. Parallel interfaces are usually used for interfacing keyboards to the CPU. Serial interfaces are used for connecting modems to it. And parallel interfaces are used to connect printers to the CPU on IBM-compatible computers and serial interfaces are used to do so on Macintosh ones.

A number of input devices are described in this section. They are not the only ones that are used with microcomputers. However, they are the ones that you are most likely to use for doing clinical tasks.

Keyboards

Almost all microcomputers have keyboards (Figure 2.2). The keys on them are push switches: There usually are at least five rows. On most keyboards, each switch is topped with a plastic cap. Computer keyboards are similar to those on electric typewriters except that they have more keys.

There are two types of keys on computer keyboards: character-generating ones

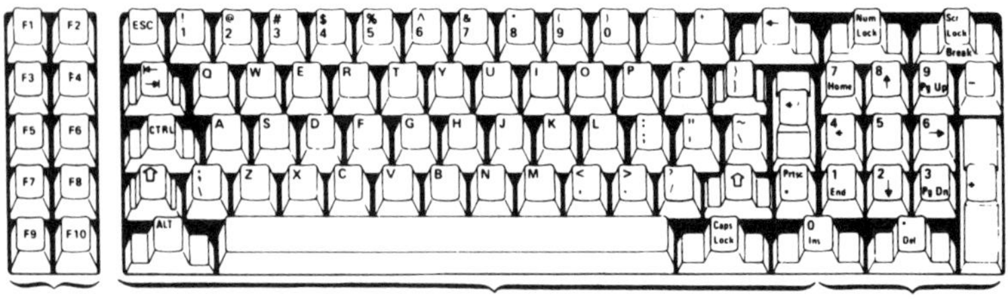

FIGURE 2.2 **Keyboard with function keys and a numeric keypad.**

and function ones (Figure 2.2). Character-generating keys produce letters, numbers, and marks of punctuation. On most microcomputers they can be programmed to generate special symbols (or components thereof) such as Blissymbols (Wertz, 1983), the International Phonetic Alphabet (Ashbaugh, 1988; Barratt & Bakker, 1994; Filter, Powell, & Campbell, 1994; Larson & Thornton, 1991; Miltich & Miltich, 1994; Shriberg, 1985, 1986), or *pixels* in various configurations. Pixels are tiny dots (or squares) that are used for drawing graphs and other figures on a monitor screen (see Chapter 6). Furthermore, the keys on most microcomputers can be programmed to generate speech segments (keyboards are often programmed in this way for augmentative communication—see Chapter 5).

Function keys control the operation of the computer, including how characters generated by the other keys are displayed. Some have the same function as those on typewriter keyboards (e.g., SHIFT, SPACE, and RETURN). Others have functions similar to those on calculators (e.g., + and –). And still others have functions that are unique. An example of such a function is *cursor* control. Four keys usually are used for this purpose. Each usually has an arrow on it pointing in a different direction—up, down, left, and right. These keys move the cursor (which can be a square, line, or other symbol) on the monitor screen. The location of the cursor determines where the next character will be displayed, deleted, or otherwise manipulated.

Most of the alphanumeric keys on a microcomputer keyboard can be programmed to do more than one thing. A key, for example, can be programmed to both generate the capital and lower-case versions of a letter and issue one or more commands. Changing the function of a key may require you to perform a shift-key-type operation—that is, holding down one or two control keys while pressing one or two alphanumeric ones.

Some application programs (e.g., word processing ones) automatically program the keyboard so that pressing certain keys or key combinations will issue commands to perform certain operations (e.g., SAVE or PRINT). If the software you are using does not program the keyboard to issue a command that you would like it to be capable of issuing, you can program the keyboard to issue it by using *macro* generating software (see Chapter 3).

Many keyboards have special sets of keys for making certain operations more efficient. One such set is known as a *numeric keypad* (Figure 2.2). This is a compact grouping of number keys that makes entering numerical data more efficient. Another is a set of *programmable function keys* (Figure 2.2). Such keys enable you to issue commands by pressing a single key that it would otherwise take a number key presses and/or mouse manipulations to issue. Some programs—including many word processing ones—automatically program these keys. They can also be programmed with macro generating software (see Chapter 3).

Microcomputer keyboards differ in ways other than those mentioned in the preceding paragraphs. Some of the more important of these are described below.

Type of Key. The desirable type for most applications is the same size and shape as those used on office-model electric typewriters. The tops of such keys usually are *sculpted* (slightly concave), which makes it easier for your fingers to remain where they should be during touch typing. In addition, the D and K keys usually have small bumps on them that help you to orient your fingers while they are in the "ASDF" row.

The keys on the keyboards of some portable microcomputers—for example, ones that are known as electronic organizers (see Chapter 15)—are smaller than those on typewriter keyboards (Figure 2.3). Such keys sometimes are referred to as *calculator-style* ones. While keyboards with calculator-style keys are adequate for some applications (see Chapter 15), they are not recommended for word processing—other than writing short notes—because they are so small.

The least desirable type of keyboard for most applications is one that has *membrane* keys (Figure 2.4). Membrane keyboards are flat. You press the keyboard where the key you wish to activate is printed. (These types of keys are used for setting cooking times on many microwave ovens.) Membrane keyboards obviously are not practical for word processing other than writing short notes. They do, however,

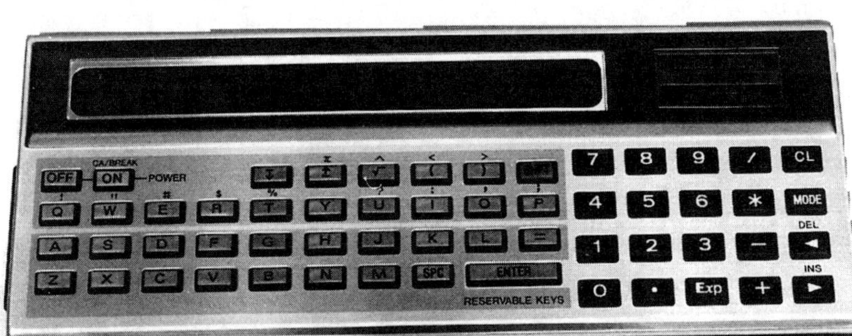

FIGURE 2.3 **A calculator-style keyboard.**

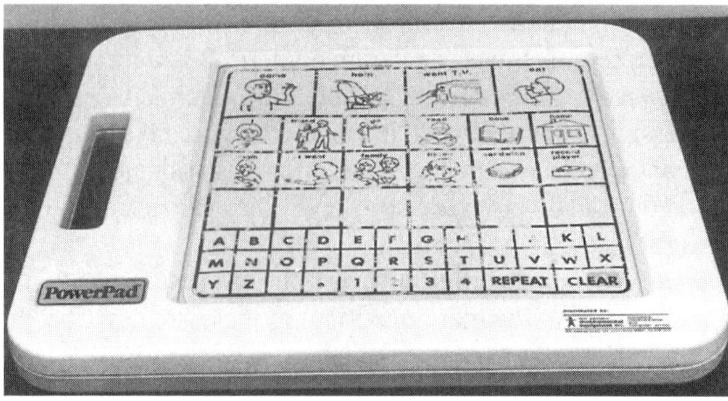

FIGURE 2.4 **A membrane keyboard used for augmentative communication.**

have one advantage over other types. They usually aren't damaged if liquids are spilled on them. This can make then desirable for use with microcomputer-based augmentative communication devices (see Chapter 5).

These types of keys are not the only ones that can be used. Stassen, Soede, and Bakker (1982), for example, have designed light-spot keyboards (Figure 2.5). These are intended to be used by people who are paralyzed from the neck down. Each key is activated by a photoelectric cell that the user directly or indirectly shines a light on. The light is attached to his or her forehead.

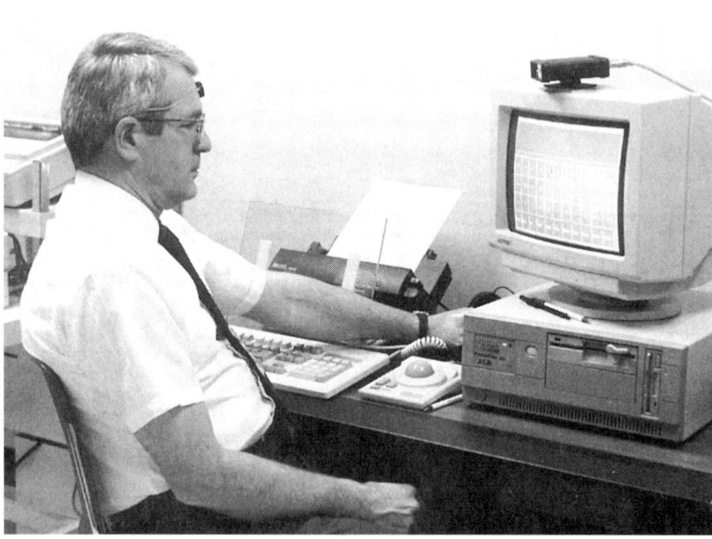

FIGURE 2.5 **A light-spot operated keyboard.**

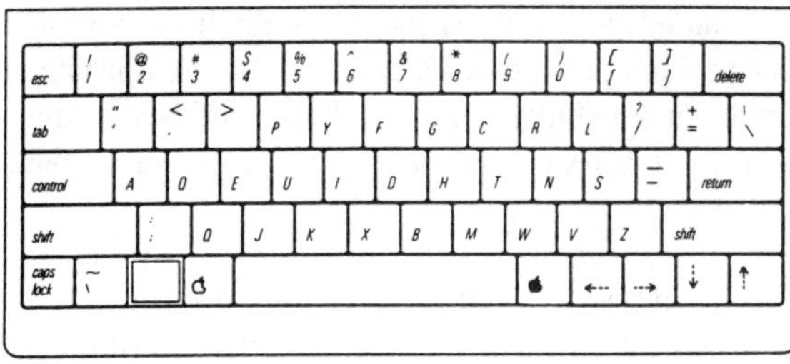

FIGURE 2.6 **The Devorak arrangement of alphanumeric keys.**

Arrangement of Alphanumeric Keys. The alphanumeric keys on most computer keyboards are arranged in the sequence used on standard typewriters. This is known as the "QWERTY" arrangement. Most can be programmed for an alternative one, the *Devorak* (Figure 2.6), which some advocates claim is easier to learn and faster to use.

Attachment of the Keyboard to the CPU. Keyboards for portable computers—for example, "laptop" ones (Figure 2.7)—usually are mounted in the same case as the CPU and those for others in a separate enclosure. The latter are attached to the CPU by a cable. It can be advantageous for the keyboard to be detachable from the CPU. There are more options for how you can position yourself while using the computer. If the cable is sufficiently long, you can even sit with the keyboard in your lap!

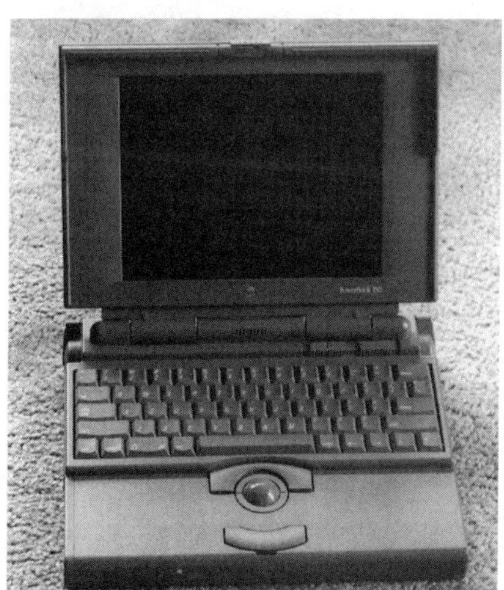

FIGURE 2.7 **A laptop computer.**

Rollover. Keyboards intended for high-speed data entry must have a feature called rollover. If you press a key and then press a second key before releasing the first key, a keyboard without rollover capability will miss the second key entirely. Rapid typists continuously overlap keystrokes and, therefore, are severely handicapped by keyboards without rollover.

Keyboard Buffers. A keyboard buffer is a storage medium (i.e., memory) for characters waiting to be transmitted to the CPU. The presence of the buffer reduces keyboard error by giving the CPU more time to handle characters.

Magnetic Storage Devices

These devices, which record information on a magnetic medium, can store both programs and data. They enable you to input the programs and data that are stored on them into your microcomputer's CPU by way of its memory unit (Figure 2.1).

The two main types of magnetic storage media are diskettes and hard disks. These two types of disks and the devices that are used for recording information on them are described in the paragraphs that follow.

Diskettes ("Floppy" Disks). Most microcomputers can store information on diskettes (Figure 2.8). These are thin plastic disks that are coated with a magnetic material and enclosed in a protective "envelope." These protective envelopes have openings through which the disk in them is accessed—that is, "written on" and "read". Diskettes are available in two diameters: 5.25 inch and 3.5 inch. Newer computers use only the 3.5 inch ones. The 5.25 inch diskettes are referred to as "floppy"

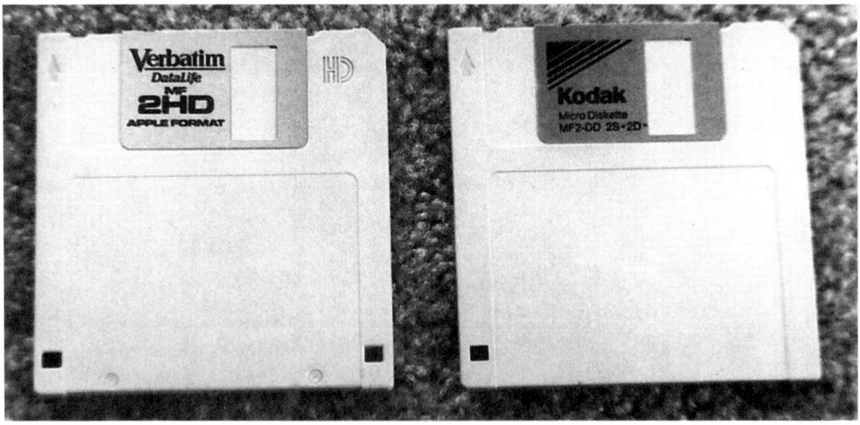

FIGURE 2.8 **Two types of 3.5 inch diskettes. The one on the left can store almost twice as much information as the one on the right.**

because they are flexible. However, under no circumstances should they be bent: doing so is likely to damage them sufficiently to make it impossible to retrieve the information stored on them.

The amount that can be stored on a diskette is determined by its diameter, the particular computer on which it is being used, and the density of its magnetic coating. A 3.5 inch diskette can store much more information than 5.25 inch one—for some computers more than six times as much. A Macintosh computer can store a 800 kilobytes of information on a double-sided, double-density 3.5 inch diskette and a Windows (IBM-compatible) computer can store 720 kilobytes of information on one. The difference is due to the way in which the two types of computers store information on such a diskette.

The density of the magnetic coating on a diskette also makes a difference. The coating on some 3.5 inch diskettes allows them to store about twice as much information as the double-sided, double-density diskettes, regardless of the computer in which they are used. The storage capacity of these diskettes—referred to as high density (HD)—is about 1.44 megabytes. The entire manuscript for this book can be stored on one (with room left over)!

The magnetic recording and playback device for diskettes is referred to as a disk drive. Some disk drives are internal (their circuitry is inside the computer) and others are external (their circuitry is in a plastic or metal case that is connected to the computer by a cable). Disk drives intended for high-density 3.5 inch diskettes can be used with double-sided, double-density ones, but the reverse is not true.

Diskettes are inserted into an opening (slot) on the front of the device. When a disk drive is functioning (i.e., "saving" or "loading" information), an indicator light on the drive is lit. You should never turn off your computer or attempt to remove a diskette while this light is lit!

Most microcomputers using diskettes for storage have either one or two disk drives. The disk drives used on a Macintosh computer will all be for 3.5 inch diskettes and those used on an IBM-compatible (or Apple II) computer could be for either 5.25 or 3.5 inch ones. Newer IBM-compatible computers have only 3.5 inch disk drives.

You should use copies of program diskettes, rather than originals. Doing so both reduces wear and tear on them and provides a backup if they are damaged.

You should make at least one backup copy of each diskette on which you have important information and possibly store it at a different location. Diskettes can be damaged (e.g., coffee can be spilled on them) or accidentally erased. Also, the information on them can be modified by being in close proximity to a magnetic field (such as that generated by a ringing telephone). Furthermore, they can just wear out.

Hard Disks. These devices, also known as *Winchester* disks, are currently the most popular of the magnetic storage media. Almost all users of IBM-compatible and Macintosh computers store both programs and data on them. They function in much the same way as diskettes except that they are made of metal, are usually permanently mounted in a disk drive, can store much more information (possibly more than 1000 times as much), and can process information more rapidly. They may be mounted inside the computer or in a case that is connected to it by a cable.

Hard disk drives are more complex mechanically than diskette drives and, consequently, they are more likely to malfunction. Since hard disks can store much more information that diskettes, the potential consequences of a malfunction can be far more serious. It is important, therefore, that you make frequent backup copies of data files that you save on your hard drive. You can make them on diskettes, another hard drive, or on tape using a special tape recorder that is intended for this purpose.

CD ROM Drives

CD ROM (Compact Disk Read Only Memory) drives are quite similar to those used for playing music compact disks. In fact, some of them can play music CDs. The compact disks they access (which are the same as those used for recording music) can store huge amounts of information, such as the contents of an entire set of encyclopedias.

Unlike hard disks and diskette drives, not all can record information. Some can only "read" it. When this chapter was written, affordable CD ROM drives were becoming available that could "write" approximately 650 MB of data on a disk. These could have a number of clinical applications including archival storage of clinic records (a disk or two could store as much as a four-drawer filing cabinet) and creating multimedia clinical materials—ones containing text, graphics, sound, and/or videos (see Chapter 8).

An older microcomputer-controlled technology that can be used for some of the same multimedia applications as the CD ROM one is the interactive videodisc technology. Videodiscs can store sound, text, and graphics (including videotape segments). They have been used for teaching speechreading and language skills to persons who have communicative disorders (Brawley & Peterson, 1983; Cochran, Bull, & Allen, 1988; Kopra, Dunlop, Kopra, & Abrahamson, 1985; Kopra, Kopra, Abrahamson, & Dunlop, 1987; Mahshie, 1987; Miller, Slike, Bailey, & Hobbis, 1987; Ott-Rose & Cochran, 1992; Printz, 1991; Tye-Murray, 1992; Tye-Murray & Tyler, 1988; Tye-Murray, Tyler, Bong, & Nares, 1988; Tye-Murray, Tyler, & Lowder, 1987).

Modems

A modem is a device that enables computers to communicate with each other via telephone lines. It can both transmit and receive information. Consequently, it can function as both an input and an output device.

Some modems are acoustic coupled to telephone lines and others are directly connected to them. An *acoustic coupled modem* is interfaced with a telephone line by pressing the handpiece of a standard telephone into rubber cups on the modem (the TDD in Figure 15.3 has this type of modem). Sound waves generated by the modem of the computer from which information is being sent is transmitted to the modem of the other computer (via telephone lines). The modem on a computer from which information is being sent *transduces* electrical energy into acoustical energy and that on the other computer *transduces* acoustical energy into electrical energy. Computers that are communicating in this manner may be separated by thousands of miles.

Direct-connect modems are now much more popular than acoustic coupled ones. They function similarly to acoustic coupled modems except that they do not use a telephone to interface the computer with a telephone line. The modem circuit in the computer (or in a case connected to the computer) is attached directly to the telephone line by means of a cable. The end of the modem cable is inserted into a wall receptacle that is intended for a telephone cable. Electrical signals generated by the modem circuit in the computer from which information is being transmitted is sent via telephone lines to the other computer (which could have either a direct-connect or acoustic coupled modem).

The word modem is a contraction of *MOdulator/DEModulator*. Computers and telephones use different languages—the modem is the translator. The modem attached to the computer from which data are sent *modulates*, or translates, the data into a form telephone lines can carry (i.e., electrical, or analog). And the modem attached to the computer receiving the data *demodulates*, or translates, the signals carried to it by the telephone lines into a form the computer can understand (i.e., digital).

The speed at which a modem can transmit and receive information is known as its *baud rate*. Baud rates are specified in *bits per second* (BPS). The higher the baud rate, the faster information can be transmitted and received. The four most frequently used baud rates for microcomputers when this chapter was written were 2,400 BPS, 9,600 BPS, 14,400 BPS, and 28,800 BPS. Others used less frequently were 300 BPS, 1,200 BPS, and 4,800 BPS. Four times as many characters can be transfered per second at 9,600 BPS than at 2,400 BPS. Almost all modems can operate at baud rates slower than their maximum; they have to be able to reduce their speed if the modem on the other computer is operating at a slower rate. Modems on both sending and receiving computers must be set at the same baud rate.

Almost all contemporary modems will operate in either a *half-duplex mode* or a *full-duplex mode*. The half-duplex mode handles communication in only one direction at a time. Consequently, information you are transmitting to another computer is not displayed on your monitor screen. The full-duplex mode enables computers to communicate in both directions at once. Consequently, information you are transmitting is displayed on your monitor screen. A full-duplex mode is essential when you are transmitting messages that you are entering with a keyboard on-line—for example, while you are writing e-mail messages or using a telecommunication relay service (see Chapter 11).

For further information about modems and what you can do with them, see Chapter 11 and Appendix B.

Mouse Cursor Control Devices

These, like keyboards, come with almost all desktop microcomputers. They are utilized for most of the applications described in this book.

A *mouse* (Figure 2.9) is a small box-like device that fits under your hand. It is attached to the computer by a cable. When you move it on a flat surface, such as a foam rubber mouse pad, it causes the rubber ball on the bottom (Figure 2.9B) to move and the position of the cursor to change on the monitor screen. Moving the mouse to the right, for example, will cause the cursor to move to the right. For some applications, it is easier and/or faster to control cursor movement with a mouse than with a keyboard. An example of such an application would be drawing. A mouse would be moved when making such a drawing in the same manner as a pen or pencil.

When the cursor is pointing to an instruction you want the computer to execute or when the cursor is at a location where you want an instruction executed, you push a button on the top of the mouse (Figure 2.9A). To execute some instructions it is only necessary for the button to be depressed for a fraction of a second. To execute others, it is necessary for the button to be depressed several times rapidly or continuously for a period of time.

Instructions on the monitor screen that are executed with a mouse may be in the form of a pictogram (e.g., a drawing of a file cabinet), words that indicate some action (e.g., "save file"), or a combination of the two. Pictograms that are used for this purpose are referred to as *icons* (Figure 2.10).

Pad Cursor-Control Devices

These function like mice. They are small pads (usually less than two inches square) that you *move your finger on* to control the cursor. They were used mainly on laptop computers when this chapter was written.

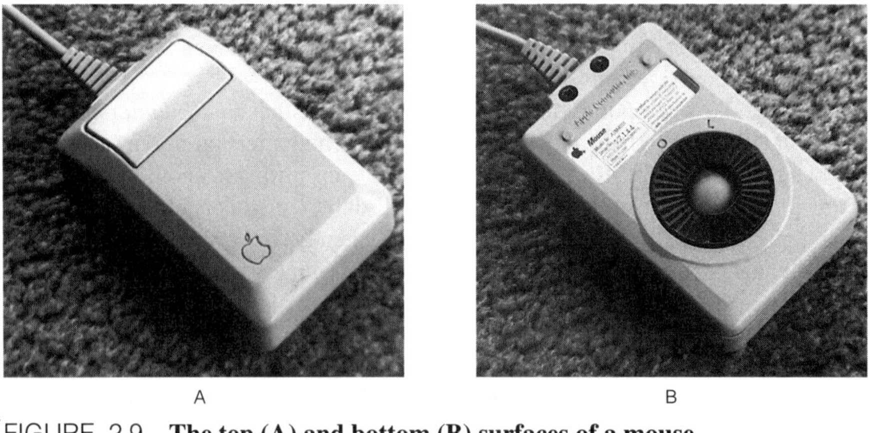

A B

FIGURE 2.9 **The top (A) and bottom (B) surfaces of a mouse.**

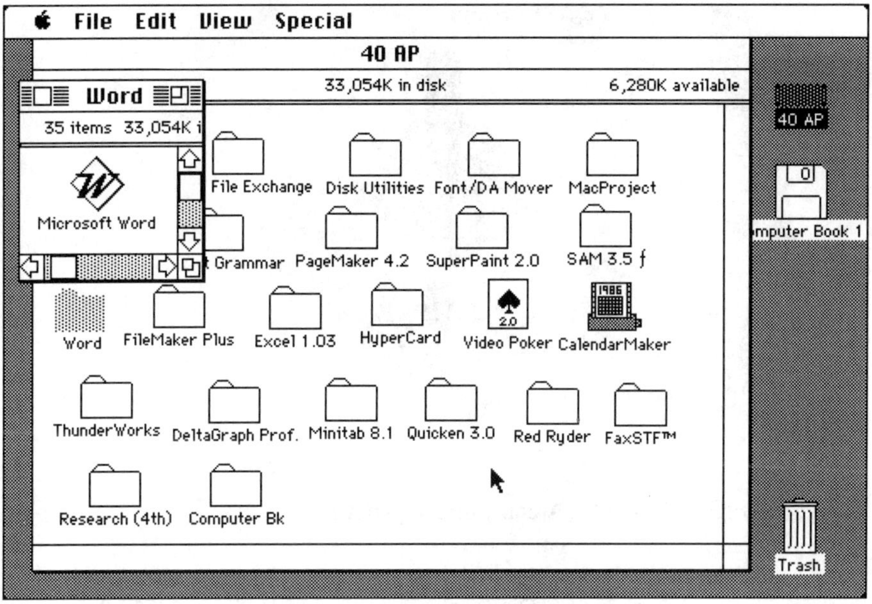

FIGURE 2.10 **A monitor screen containing icons on which the cursor can be controlled—that is, commands can be issued—with a mouse.**

Trackball Cursor-Control Devices

A trackball functions in the same manner as the ball on the bottom of a mouse (Figure 2.9B). However, while the ball with a mouse is moved *indirectly* by pushing it on a flat surface, with a trackball it is moved *directly* with the hand. One advantage of a trackball over a mouse is that it requires less desk space to operate (a mouse requires an area at least 4 inches by 6 inches). Some laptop computers use a trackball for cursor control (Figure 2.7).

Joysticks

Joysticks (Figure 2.11) are devices for activating a number of switches (usually four) by pushing a vertical shaft (stick) in a particular direction. They are the most common type of control device used on videogames. One type that is used with microcomputers contains four switches that can be activated by pushing the shaft forward, back, left, or right. Speech-language pathologists have used joysticks to interface clients with microcomputer-based augmentative communication devices (see Chapter 5).

Another type that is used with microcomputers is referred to as a *proportional joystick*. With this type of joystick, the distance that the shaft is pushed in a particular direction has an effect; it could, for example, control the speed that an action

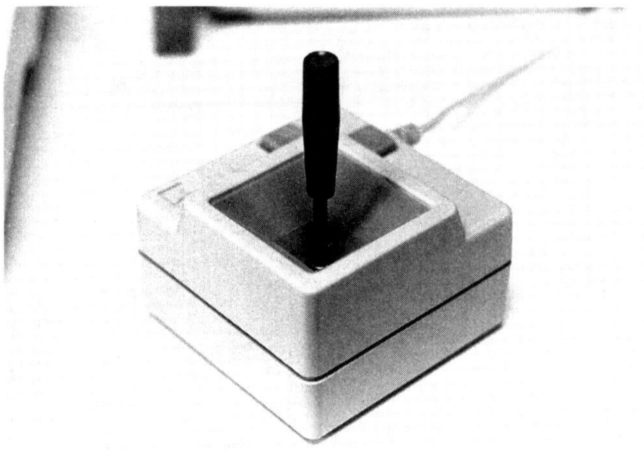

FIGURE 2.11 **A computer joystick.**

(e.g., cursor movement) occurs. Obviously, this type of joystick requires the user to be more intact motorically than does the type described in the preceding paragraph.

Scanners

These devices enable you to load printed material (including drawings and photographs) into your computer. After you load such material and save it on a disk, you can modify (edit) and/or print it. The most common type of scanner is the *flatbed* one (Figure 2.12). Some flatbed scanners can handle color as well as black-and-white material.

You are particularly likely to benefit from having a scanner if you regard yourself as having little, or no, ability to draw and you have to produce materials for your clients that contain drawings—such as communication boards and sheets of stimulus pictures for eliciting target phonemes from nonreaders. You would scan drawings that could serve your purpose from books, magazines, or other sources into your computer, simplify ("erase" unwanted detail) and change their size if necessary, and then place them at the appropriate location in the material you are creating. If drawings that you want to use are copyrighted, you may need to get the permission of the copyright owner to use them—it depends on how much of a drawing you will be using, whether the drawing is "generic," and whether the way that you plan to use it would be regarded as "fair use" (see Chapter 8 in Silverman, 1992a).

There is another way that you may be able to use a scanner—to create files from printed text documents (e.g., clinical reports and manuscripts) that can be stored on disk and edited with word-processing software. An *OCR (Optical Character Recognition)* program is used to do this. Some of the more advanced of these programs can be "taught" to recognize hand printing and cursive writing.

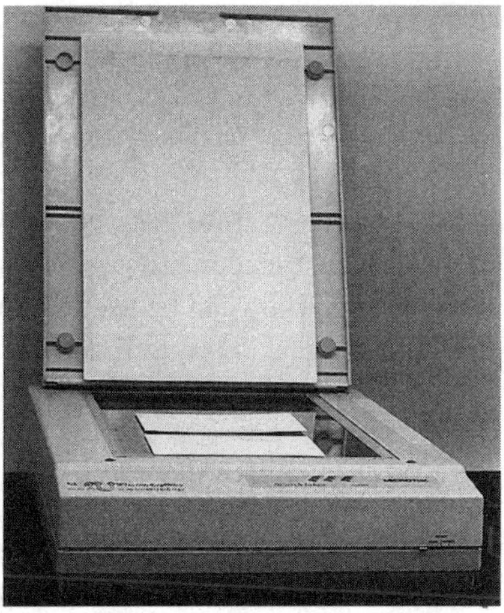

FIGURE 2.12 **A flatbed scanner.**

Single Switches

Almost any type of switch can be programmed to perform the function of any key on a keyboard. The switch usually is interfaced with the computer by a cable. Many motor impaired persons who do not have the ability to use a standard keyboard can control a computer with such a switch. The types of switches that have been used for this purpose include large push switches, suck-blow switches, photoelectric switches, tip-tilt switches, voice-actuated switches, and myoelectric switches. These and other types are described in Chapter 5 and in Silverman (1995).

Incidentally, you can program a microcomputer keyboard to function as a single switch. When this is done, all of the keys have the same function. Some motor impaired persons can do single-switch tasks with a keyboard programmed in this manner. They could, for example, use it to control a single-switch scanning program for augmentative communication (see Chapter 5).

Voice (Speech) Recognition Devices

These devices allow you to input information into and control a computer by talking into a microphone (Bickley, Hunnicutt, & Lamel, 1993; Bryant, Tonkovich, Horowitz, & Tan, 1992; Fitch, 1989a; Fried-Oken, 1984, 1985b; LaRiviere & Sherblom, 1986; Macurik, 1981). The computer recognizes what you say and does what it is told to do, at least theoretically. These devices can enable some severely dysarthric or mentally retarded clients to control a computer with word approximations and/or vocalizations (Brown, Cavalier, Sauer, & Wyatt, 1992; Carlson & Bernstein, 1987; Coleman & Meyers, 1991; Doyle, Leeper, Katler, & Thomas-Stonell, 1993; Ferrier, Jarrell,

Carpenter, & Shane, 1991, 1992; Fried-Oken, 1989; Huckle, Haaf, & Doyle, 1995; Kotler & Thomas-Stonell, 1993; Lee, Blackstone, & Poock, 1987).

Measuring Instruments

These devices can put any type of information that is in an electrical signal or a signal that can be transduced into an electrical one (e.g., an acoustic signal) into a computer for measurement and analysis. They can be used to abstract information from both physiological and acoustical signals. For further information about them, see Chapter 12.

Digitizers (Including Graphics Tablets)

A digitizer is a device that translates nondigital information into digital form. Information must be in this form before it can be processed by a computer.

One type of digitizer translates distance measurements into digital form. There are several devices that can be used for this purpose. One is a pair of *calipers*. The distance between the two points is translated into digits and entered into the computer. This type of digitizer has been used by speech-language pathologists for measuring the distance between the upper surface of the soft palate and the posterior pharyngeal wall in X-ray studies of persons who have cleft palates.

Another type of digitizer is a *graphics tablet*. This is a pressure-sensitive surface that has the same x-y coordinates as a monitor screen. An image drawn on the tablet with a penlike device is translated into digital form, processed by the computer, and displayed on the monitor screen. One way that speech-language pathologists and audiologists have used graphics tablets is for making drawings for diagnostic and therapy materials. They also use them entering information with "personal assistant" devices, such as the Apple Newton MessagePad (See Chapter 15).

A third type of digitizer is a *speech digitizer*. These devices translate electrical (analog) information that is abstracted by microphones from speech signals into digital form. They are a component of all voice/speech measurement devices that utilize a computer (microprocessor), including the Visipitch. Speech digitizers are discussed further in Chapter 12.

Touch Screens

These devices are pressure-sensitive surfaces like graphics tablets. They are transparent and are mounted over (overlaid on) computer monitor screens. Electronically, they consist of a matrix of cells, each about a half an inch square to accommodate the end of a person's finger. The program displays options on the screen (e.g., four drawings for a "which of these things doesn't belong with the others" task) and the user selects one by touching the location on the screen where the option appears. They have been used with young children for language stimulation drills (Brown, 1989; Wilson & Fox, 1992d).

Light Pens

A *light pen* can be used for drawing or making choices on a monitor screen. The device, which is penlike and sensitive to light, can detect and control the x-y coordinates of the cursor on the monitor screen when placed in close proximity to it. The cursor can be automatically locked on to the position of the pen—that is, the location of the cursor at any moment can be the location of the pen tip. The device can be used to create or modify images directly on the screen that can be stored and processed by the computer. The device also can be used for selecting options from a *menu* on a monitor screen. A menu is a list of options. To select an option with a light pen you would point the tip of the device at it and press a button. A related clinical application would be to have clients use one for responding to items on multiple-choice format, drill/practice language stimulation programs. This is a more direct and easily understood way to respond than pressing a particular key on a keyboard.

THE OUTPUT UNIT

The output unit consists of one or more devices that put information out. When these devices receive information from the central processing unit, they translate it into a form that communicates a message (e.g., one in written or spoken English) or manipulates something (e.g., a control device—see Chapter 12).

Output devices are similar to input devices in several ways. Like them, they are referred to as I/O devices, peripheral equipment, and peripherals, and the same types of interfaces (parallel and series) are used to connect them to the central processing unit. Furthermore, some of them (e.g., modems and disk drives) also function as input devices.

This section describes number of output devices that can be used for clinical tasks. These, of course, are not the only ones that are available for microcomputers.

Monitors

The appearance of a computer monitor for a desktop computer is similar to that of a television set. The image on it may be monochrome (black and white, green, or amber) or in color. Most color monitors can generate a monochrome image; however, the quality (sharpness) of the image may not be quite as good as on a monochrome monitor.

Some monochrome monitors have a *gray scale* capability. They can display graphics in various shades of gray (like black and white photographs). Those that have this capability tend to be more expensive than those that don't.

Some laptop computers have monochrome monitors and some have color ones. The monochrome monitors usually have at least a little gray scale capability. Two types of color monitors are used on them: passive color matrix and active color matrix. While laptops having the active matrix type of color monitor tend to display higher quality images than do those that have the passive matrix type, they were considerably more expensive when this chapter was written. Perhaps the additional expense for one with an active matrix display would be most justifiable if the computer is to be used for making presentations (see Chapter 8), augmentative communication (see Chapter 5), and/or for administering diagnostic tasks and drills to clients (see Chapter 4).

Monitors used for microcomputers come in a number of sizes. Most have screens with a diagonal measurement between 3 inches and 21 inches. The most popular size for desk-top units when this chapter was written was in the 12- to 14-inch range; that for portable (laptop) computers was a little smaller. Larger screens can display more material at one time than smaller ones and tend to cause less eye-strain. Screens larger than 14 inches are particularly useful for applications such as word processing and desktop publishing because they can display entire pages the size they will be when they are printed.

Printers

All microcomputers that will be used administratively, such as for word processing, have a printer. And most that are intended for clinical use (e.g., augmentative communication or administering language-stimulation drills) also have one. Printers enable you to make *hard copies* of the material (graphics and/or text) that is displayed on your monitor screen.

There are four types of printers that you may encounter at a clinical facility: *dot-matrix, ink jet, laser*, and *daisywheel*. The latter, although no longer manufactured, are still being used. All four are described in this section.

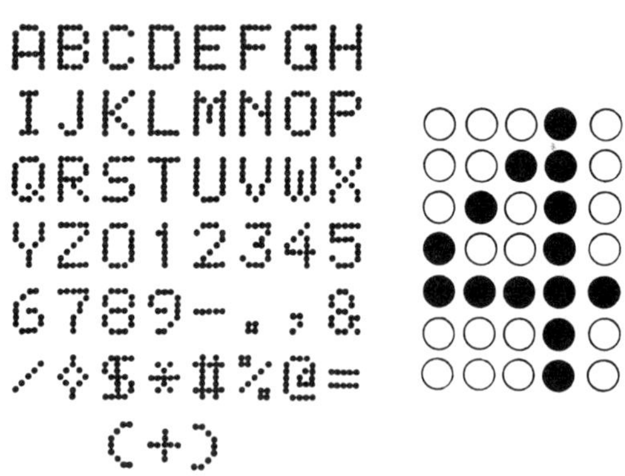

FIGURE 2.13 **Letters, numerals, and symbols reproduced by a 7 × 5 dot-matrix printer.**

Dot-Matrix Printers. These printers form characters from a matrix of dots. The dots may be round or square. The manner in which characters are formed with a 7 × 5 matrix is illustrated in Figure 2.13. Some of them use larger matrices to form characters. Larger matrices tend to produce characters that look more solid (i.e., have a less obvious dot pattern) than do smaller ones.

The printhead of a dot-matrix printer may print characters in one of several ways. The most common printhead in printers used with microcomputers has a matrix of needles (i.e., styli) that *impact* on a typewriter-like ribbon that is in contact with the paper during the actual printing of characters (Figure 2.14). The particular needles that impact on the ribbon during the printing of a character are those that are used for forming the character.

All dot-matrix printers have a pressure (friction) feed mechanism. Some also come with a tractor- or pin-feed mechanism or have one available as an accessory. A pressure-feed mechanism is all you need if you do your printing on single sheets of paper. While relatively long documents obviously can be printed in this manner (manually inserting a new sheet after each page is printed), it is more time-consuming than using a tractor- or pin-feed mechanism that loads paper in fan-fold strips (Figure 2.15). Fan-fold paper, incidentally, is available in different weights, cotton contents, and colors.

Almost all dot-matrix printers can print a standard 8.5-inch-wide page and some can print wider ones. In addition, most can print narrower pages—such as, strips of mailing labels.

Dot-matrix printers can print characters in several sizes, and some offer *proportional* as well as fixed spacing between characters. With proportional spacing, the widths of the spacings between characters are the same regardless of their widths—e.g., the width of the spacing between an **i** and the letter that precedes and follows it is the same as that for a **w** (Figure 2.16). Proportional spacing of characters, incidentally, is used throughout this text. Dot-matrix printers can also be used for printing graphs and other types of drawings.

Daisywheel Printers. These, like typewriters, print characters that are solid—that is, not composed of dots. The impression of a character embossed on a metal or plas-

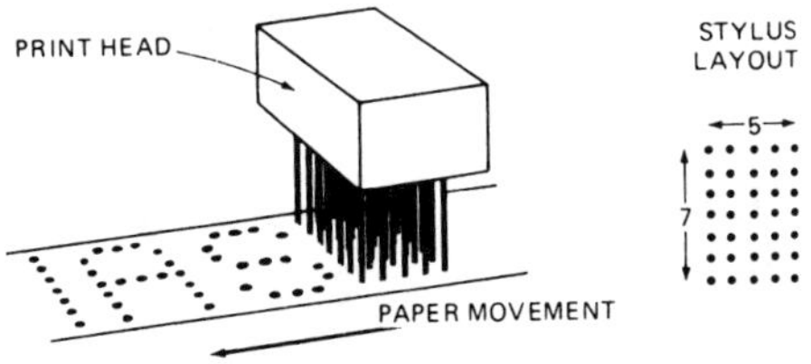

FIGURE 2.14 **Print head (7 × 5) from a dot-matrix printer.**

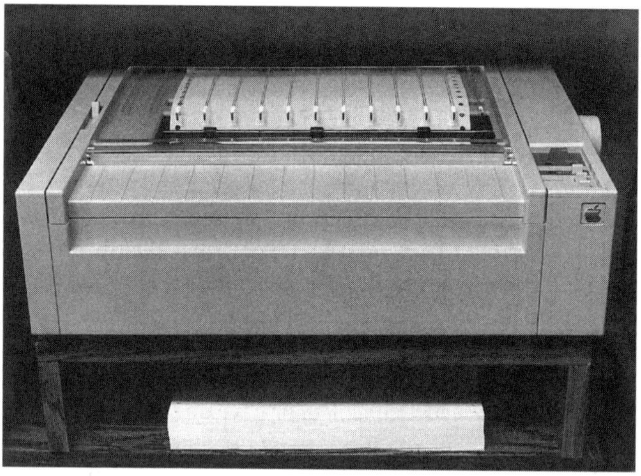

FIGURE 2.15 **A dot-matrix printer with a pin-feed mechanism and utilizing fan-fold paper.**

tic print element—known as a daisywheel (Figure 2.17)—impacts against a typewriter-style ribbon in contact with a sheet of paper. These sometimes are referred to as letter-quality printers because their print quality is comparable to that from an office model electric typewriter, such as an IBM Selectric. They are no longer popular, in large part, because of the availability of inexpensive laser and inkjet printers.

Laser Printers. Laser printers (Figure 2.18) produce an extremely high quality output. The quality is so good that many documents appear to have been typeset. Most facilities that employ speech-language pathologists and audiologists have at least one laser printer available for printing correspondence and reports.

Laser printers are actually a type of dot-matrix printer. The least expensive laser printers form alphanumeric characters and graphics from dots arranged in a matrix in which there are 300 rows and 300 columns per inch—referred to as 300 dpi (dots per

```
This is fixed character
spacing [A]
```

This is proportional character
spacing [B]

FIGURE 2.16 **A sentence printed with fixed (A) and proportional (B) character spacing. Note particularly the distance between the letter** i **and the letter preceding and following it with each type of spacing.**

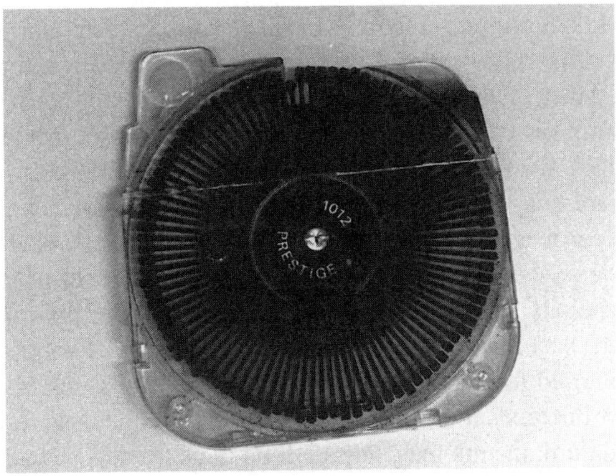

FIGURE 2.17 **A daisywheel print element.**

inch). More expensive ones form such characters and graphics from a matrix containing up to 2400 dpi. The difference in quality between the output of a 300 dpi and a 2400 dpi laser printer is greater for graphics (particularly photographs) than for text.

Laser printers differ in ways other than the number of dots they can print per inch. One is maximum paper size. While all can print pages up to legal size ($8^{1}/_{2}$ by 14 inches), some can print pages as large as 11 by 17 inches. Another is the number of pages they can print per minute. Less expensive ones tend to print fewer pages per minute than more expensive ones. A third difference is the colors they can print. Some can print text and graphics in ones other than black and white.

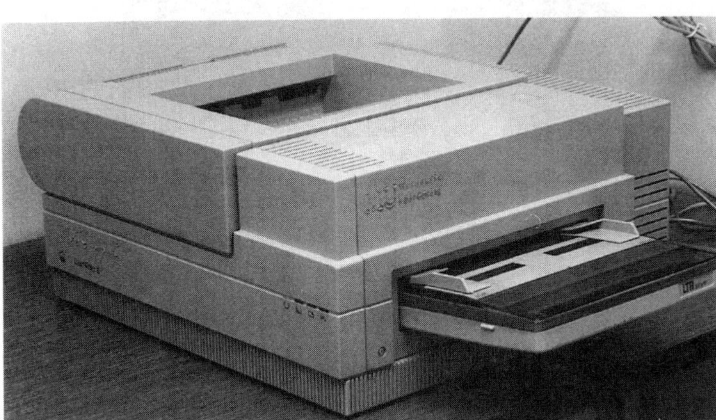

FIGURE 2.18 **A 300 dpi laser printer with a "loaded" sheet feeder.**

Inkjet Printers. Inkjet printers (Figure 2.19) have a mechanism that sprays dots of one or more colors of ink onto paper. Like laser printers, they are actually a type of dot-matrix printer. Most of them can produce between 300 dpi and 360 dpi. The quality of their printing is comparable to that of a 300 dpi laser printer. Some will print text and graphics in color as well as black and white.

Inkjet printers are quite popular because they can be purchased for about half as much as the least expensive laser printer and for a little less than most dot-matrix printers. They do, however, have several limitations. First, the number of pages per minute they can print is generally fewer than for either laser printers or dot-matrix printers. Most, however, have sheet feeders for paper and can print in *the background*—that is, the computer can be used for another purpose while pages are being printed Second, the cost per page for ink tends to be a little higher than for either laser printers or dot-matrix printers. And third, the ink may smear a little if a page gets wet accidentally.

Plotters

Clinicians now use plotters mainly for graphing data from physiological and acoustical measurement processes (see Chapter 12). Some have only one pen and others have several. The advantage of having a plotter that has several pens simultaneously is that several processes can be monitored (graphed) simultaneously.

There are several types of plotters. The type that speech-language pathologists and audiologists are most likely to encounter is the *flatbed*, or *X-Y,* type (Figure 2.20).

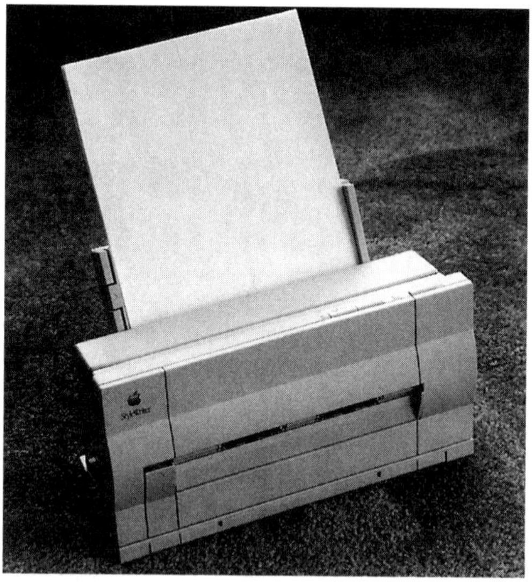

FIGURE 2.19 **A 360 dpi inkjet printer with a "loaded" sheet feeder.**

The paper is held flat on the bed of the device. The pens are moved in small steps by two motors: One moves them horizontally (*X* direction) and the other vertically (*Y* direction). A "drawing" is produced by the computer moving the pens in the appropriate directions. X-Y plotters vary with regard to the largest sheet of paper (or acetate) they can accommodate, the speed at which pens move, and the smallest changes possible in a given direction. The smaller this change, the more detail it is possible for drawings to have. A tympanogram is an example of a drawing created by an X-Y plotter.

Speech Synthesizers

Computers with speech synthesizers can be programmed to say almost anything. While most of the utterances they generate are usually intelligible, their quality is likely to deviate somewhat from that of normal speech (Keating, Evans, Wyper, & Cunningham, 1986; Reynolds, Fucci, Bettagere, & Gonzales, 1995; Sevcik & Romski, 1985). The extent to which they deviate will be partially a function of the strategy (algorithm) that the synthesizer uses to generate them. There are three main strategies: formant synthesis, linear-predictive coding, and waveform digitization. The quality of speech from synthesizers using waveform digitization is generally regarded as being the best and that from formant synthesis the poorest. Synthesizers using waveform digitization, however, tend to be more expensive than those using formant synthesis.

Speech-language pathologists and audiologists have used computer-synthesized speech in a number of ways (Chial, 1985; Cohen & Palin, 1986; Egolf, 1983; Fried-

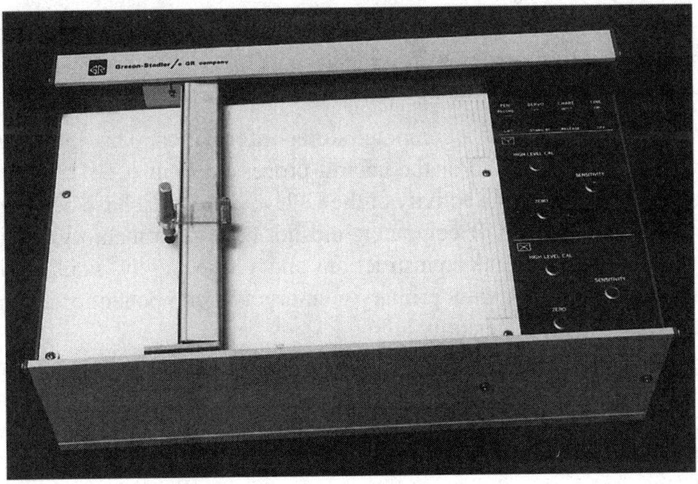

FIGURE 2.20 **A flatbed plotter.**

Oken, 1985a; Klatt, 1985; Klatt, Tetschner, Tiao, & Pisoni, 1984; LaRiviere & Sherblom, 1986; Massey, 1988; Rentschler, 1985; Rimac, 1991; Sevcik & Romski, 1985). They have utilized it, for example, in diagnostic and therapy programs—directions, prompts, and verbal reinforcers are spoken rather than (or in addition to) being printed on the monitor screen (see Chapter 4). They have also utilized it for augmentative communication (see Chapter 5).

Modems

Telephone modems are described in the section on input devices. They also function as output devices. They translate digital information from the computer's central processing unit (CPU) into an analog (electrical) form that can be transmitted by telephone lines.

Magnetic Storage Devices

Magnetic storage media (including diskettes and hard disks) are described in the section on input devices. Like modems, they also function as output devices. They can *load* information stored on them into a computer's CPU for further processing.

Control Mechanisms

These peripherals allow you to use a computer for controlling electronic devices. With one, for example, you could control the frequency and loudness of pure tones delivered by an audiometer during a self-administered hearing test. These devices are described in Chapter 12.

THE PRIMARY MEMORY UNIT

The primary memory unit of a computer stores information. This information can originate in the input unit and/or the central processing unit (CPU). It consists of both *programs* that control the activity of the CPU and *data* that have been and/or are about to be processed by it. If computers did not have such memory, their central processing units would receive no instructions and, consequently, would do nothing. Some authors, incidentally, view primary memory as a component of a computer's CPU rather than as a separate entity.

Some input and output devices—including modems and printers—have their own (usually small) primary memory units. These memory units enable the input and output devices to perform their function without tying up the computer.

Microcomputers also have a *secondary* memory unit—magnetic storage devices (see the discussions in this chapter of input and output devices). They *save* programs and data that are stored in the primary memory unit.

Information is stored in a microcomputer's primary memory unit in a binary digital code that consists of the presence or absence of electrical charges at particular locations (cell addresses) on small silicon wafers, or chips. The memory chips in most microcomputers contain more than a million cells, each of which can store an electrical charge. One *bit* (element) of code is recorded in each cell as the presence or absence of an electrical charge. The code computers use is similar to Morse code in that it is *binary*—that is, it has only two elements. Instead of dots and dashes, it uses 1s and 0s. If a cell contains an electrical charge, it is interpreted by the computer as a 1. And if a cell does not contain a charge, it is interpreted by the computer as a 0.

A 1 or 0 (i.e., a bit) by itself does not convey meaningful information. However, by grouping bits it is possible to do so. A grouping of eight bits that stands for a letter or other referent is known as a byte.

The manner in which bits are grouped into bytes is illustrated in Table 2.1. This table contains the standard *ASCII* (American Standard Code for Information Exchange) eight-bit, byte code for each capital letter. Note that the byte code for each character consists of a different pattern of 1s and 0s. There are 256 possible patterns for an eight-bit byte. Each upper- and lower-case letter, each number from 0 to 9, and each commonly used punctuation mark has its own unique eight-bit code. Numerous instructions (e.g., space) also have their unique codes.

The primary memory units of all microcomputers contain two types of memory chips: *ROM* and *RAM*. They also may contain two other types of memory chips: *PROM* and *EPROM*.

ROM is *read-only memory*. A computer can "read" the bytes of information stored in ROM, but it cannot add to or alter them. Programs are stored in a computer's ROM chip when it is manufactured. ROM is used for storing information that

TABLE 2.1 **The Eight-Bit ASCII Code for Each of the Capital Letters.**

A	11000001	N	11001110
B	11000010	O	11001111
C	11000011	P	11010000
D	11000100	Q	11010001
E	11000101	R	11010010
F	11000110	S	11010011
G	11000111	T	11010100
H	11001000	U	11010101
I	11001001	V	11010110
J	11001010	W	11010111
K	11001011	X	11011000
L	11001100	Y	11011001
M	11001101	Z	11011010

it is not necessary to change, such as instructions the computer needs to function and/or to understand programs written in a particular language (e.g., machine language—see Chapter 3). ROM is *nonvolatile*—its contents are not lost when the power to the memory unit is turned off.

RAM is *random access memory*. A computer can both "read" information stored in RAM and "write" information in it. All information (data and programs) put in a computer is stored in RAM. The contents of RAM can be selectively added to or deleted. During word processing, for example, words can be selectively added to or deleted from a document stored in RAM. The length of time it takes the CPU to locate specific information stored in RAM generally ranges from a few *nanoseconds* (billionths of a second) to one *microsecond* (millionth of a second). RAM is *volatile*—its contents are lost when the power to the memory unit is turned off. Some portable microcomputers have a battery-powered backup system for their RAM chips so that the contents of RAM are not lost when the computer is turned off.

PROM stands for *programmable read-only memory*. A PROM chip functions similarly to a ROM chip after a program has been recorded, or *burned*, on it by a device intended for the purpose. Once a program has been burned onto a PROM chip it cannot be modified because these chips cannot be erased. If a program is changed, it has to be burned onto a new PROM chip.

PROMs are nonvolatile—the programs they contain are not lost when the electrical power to the computer is turned off. PROM chips (along with the circuitry needed for them to function) may be mounted in a plastic cartridge (case) and plugged into a special input on the computer. The cartridges that some videogames use contain PROMs.

EPROM stands for *erasable programmable read-only memory*. These chips function the same as PROMs except that they can be erased and reused. EPROM chips are erased by exposing them to an ultraviolet light.

How many bytes can a memory chip store? Chips are available with various storage capacities. The storage capacity of a memory chip may be specified in *kilobytes* (the abbreviation for which is K), in *megabytes* (the abbreviation for which is *M* or *MG*), or in *gigabytes* (the abbreviation for which is *Gb*). One kilobyte is equal to 1,024 bytes, one megabyte is equal to 1,048,576 bytes and one gigabyte is equal to 1,073,741,824 bytes. (Although memory chips with gigabyte capacity were not available for microcomputers when this chapter was written, they may be in the future.) Consequently, a computer that has 2MB of RAM chips can store a maximum of 2,097,152 ($2 \times 1{,}048{,}576$) bytes of programs and data at a time in RAM.

The amount of ROM in microcomputers is determined by the number and types of programs the manufacturer puts in it and is not something about which users have to be concerned.

The amount of RAM now installed in microcomputers ranges from 1MB to more than 30MB. The most common amount that was installed by manufacturers when this chapter was written was 8MB. The amount of RAM in most microcomputers can be increased, sometimes substantially.

The larger a computer's RAM, the more sophisticated the programs it will be capable of running and the more programs it will be capable of running simultaneously. A microcomputer that has 16MB of RAM would be able to run more programs simultaneously than one that has 4MB of RAM.

CENTRAL PROCESSING UNIT

The central processing unit (CPU) is the "brain" of a computer—that is, its control center. It processes the data put into it in the manner specified by the programs being used and sends the processed data to RAM.

The central processing unit has two subunits: the control unit and the arithmetic/logic unit. The *control unit* controls and coordinates the activities of the computer. It acts like a police officer directing traffic. It sends information that has been put into the computer to RAM to be stored. It takes information from RAM that is to be processed and sends it to the arithmetic/logic unit. It sends processed information to output devices. These and other functions of the control unit are diagrammed in Figure 2.21.

The *arithmetic/logic unit* (ALU) is the one that actually processes information. This unit has many capabilities including performing arithmetic operations (e.g., adding), transferring data from one location in storage to another, editing data, and decision making. The ALU can perform such functions in a millionth or sometimes even a few billionths of a second.

The CPU in a microcomputer is known as a *microprocessor*. Microprocessor chips may be designated by a name or a number. Microprocessors used in IBM-

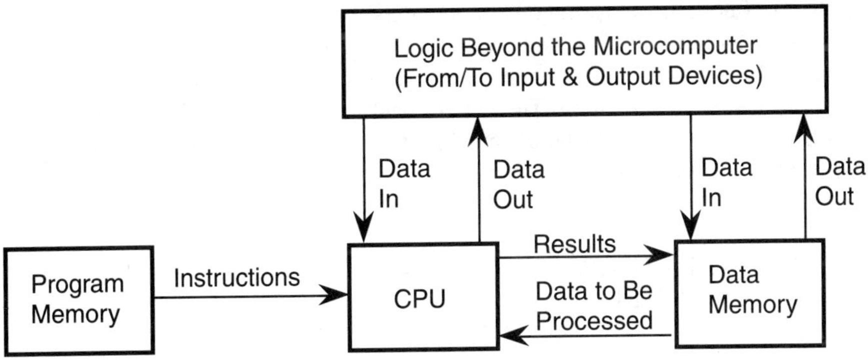

FIGURE 2.21 **The logical functioning of a microcomputer.**

compatible (Windows) computers, for example, include the 386, the 486, and the pentium. Microprocessors differ with regard to the number of bits they can handle at one time and consequently, the speed at which they can process information. The three most common bit-values for microprocessors are 8, 16, and 32. A 32-bit microprocessor can process information faster than an 8-bit one.

Microprocessor chips vary in ways other than the number of bits they can handle at one time. One is their speed aside from the number of bits they can process at at one time—for example, a pentium microprocessor chip can enable information to be processed faster than a 386 one. A second way is the maximum amount of RAM they can support—a pentium chip can support more RAM than a 386. And a third is the set of instructions that the chip will understand. These vary from microprocessor to microprocessor and are one of the main reasons why programs will only run on certain computers. If all computers had microprocessors that understood the same instruction set, there would be fewer problems with software compatibility.

POWER SUPPLY

A microcomputer needs electricity to function. Not all of its components require the same amount (i.e., voltage). The primary function of a microcomputer's power supply is to provide its components with the voltages they need *at a constant level*. The voltages must be at a constant level because a *ripple* (an occasional voltage higher or lower than that required) can cause the computer to malfunction—or behave in an erratic manner.

One type of voltage variation that can affect a computer is a power line glitch. This is a very brief spike of high voltage that causes programs that were running perfectly to suddenly run amok. They can be kept from affecting a computer by plugging its components into a device known as a *surge protector* rather than directly into a power line. The surge protector is plugged into a power line.

Most, if not all, laptop and other computers that are intended to be portable can be powered by household current and alkaline or rechargable batteries. Powering a computer by a battery pack is convenient because you can then use it anywhere. However, there is a limitation. The battery pack is likely to run down after you've used the computer for a few hours, making it unusable unless you have a spare battery pack or access to household current.

SELECTING HARDWARE FOR MICROCOMPUTERS

The process that I recommend for selecting microcomputer hardware is a two-step one. The *first step* is identifying the microcomputers and peripherals that could meet your needs. The *second step* is selecting from those microcomputers and peripherals the ones that would best meet your needs, considering available funding and the tasks you want to do now and in the future. Among the factors you should consider are the following:

- The features offered by each alternative from the perspective of the tasks you want to do
- The reliability of each alternative—how well its mechanism is likely to hold up under the type of use you plan to give it
- The ease with which each alternative can be serviced—for example, whether it can be serviced locally
- The clarity of the manuals
- The cost—that is, if the alternatives would be equally likely to meet your needs, the least expensive probably would be the best choice
- The amount of support offered by the dealer from whom each alternative would be purchased
- The software that you have available—it may run on only some alternatives
- The other computers that you will be using and the computers used by persons with whom you will be sharing document files—for example, it may be desirable that the computer you use at home be compatible with the one you are purchasing for the office or vice versa.

Where can you find information you need to undertake this selection process? In addition to the information presented in this chapter, a second source is publications dealing with the use of microcomputers in speech-language pathology and audiology (see the References and Bibliography list). A third source is hardware reviews in microcomputer magazines. These can be found in both general microcomputer magazines (e.g., *Byte*) and ones that limit their coverage to specific microcomputers (e.g., *MacUser*).

Other professionals (particularly other speech-language pathologists or audiologists) who have used microcomputers for doing the same tasks for which you want to use them are another potential source of information and advice. Still another is persons who sell microcomputers. While the majority of salespersons employed by microcomputer dealers are *not* highly knowledgeable about available hardware and software, most large dealers employ at least one person who knows a great deal. Such a person can recommend components, answer questions about their operation, and possibly arrange for some hands-on experience with them. It is desirable to have hands-on experience with components before purchasing them. This is the only way that you can really be certain the ones you select will do the job(s) that you want them to do.

If possible, discuss your needs with knowledgeable consultants from several dealers. If their recommendations are similar and intuitively make sense to you, you are probably selecting appropriate components. It's also a good idea to comparison shop for another reason. Microcomputer hardware and software are often sold for less than list price and, consequently, it is possible to save money by getting bids on them from several dealers. You may also be able to save money by purchasing them from a mail-order house.

Another way that you may be able to save some money is by purchasing hardware (and software) that is not state-of-the-art. Computer technology changes rapidly. No matter how good a particular computer, peripheral, or program may be, an updated version will probably be available in a year or less. However, the ones you use will not become obsolete if they enable you to do what you want to do (Chial, 1986b). Much of this book, in fact, was written with a Macintosh Plus computer from 1986 and an older version of Microsoft Word.

▶ 3

Microcomputer Components and Terminology: Software

Without software, a computer cannot do anything. It cannot store or process information, nor can it display or otherwise utilize it. A computer has to be told how to do a task *step by step* each time it does it, even if it has done it thousands of times. The instructions that a computer needs to do tasks are provided by its software, or programs.

Software controls your computer. You get your computer to do a task, in part, by "running" a program that can issue the commands (instructions) needed for doing it. The words "in part" were used because your computer gets instructions for doing tasks from software other than the program you are running, including its *operating system* (which probably is MS-DOS—with or without the *Windows* extension—if you have an IBM compatible computer). Operating system software is described elsewhere in this chapter.

WHAT IS A PROGRAM?

The software used by a microcomputer to do tasks consists of a set of programs. The user runs some of them, the computer runs the rest. The ones that the computer runs include programs in its ROM and/or RAM that together make up its operating system.

Microcomputer programs vary considerably in length. Some can be stored in less than 1K of memory and others require more than 4MB. The more tasks a program can do and the more options there are for doing each, the larger the set of instructions that is needed and, consequently, the longer the program.

What a computer does while running a program is somewhat similar to what you do while following a recipe in a cookbook. In both, a process is broken down into small steps; if the instructions for each step are followed, the process will be completed successfully. This process can be communicated by a diagram known as a *pro-*

gram flowchart, a diagram containing geometric symbols that are interconnected in various ways. Figure 3.1 is a program flowchart for making a three-egg omelet. Two geometric symbols are used in this flowchart: Rectangles symbolize operations and diamonds symbolize points at which decisions have to be made. The decision in this flowchart is whether a total of three eggs have been cracked and placed in the bowl. A *do loop* occurs on the left side of the flowchart. The process of cracking eggs and adding them to the bowl is *repeated* until there are a total of three eggs in the bowl.

Computer programmers are likely to construct a flowchart for a program prior to writing it in a computer language, particularly if the program is a complex one. This flowchart graphically depicts the logical design of the program (i.e., the process by which the program does the tasks it is intended to do) in a very concise manner. Programmers use flowcharts for *consumer documentation* as well as for guides. It is almost always easier for a user to understand the logic of a program by studying a flowchart than by studying lines of computer code.

Each instruction in a program is written in a language that the computer can understand ("read"). There are more than 100 such languages. Several of them are described elsewhere in this chapter.

Computer languages, like spoken languages, have dialects. Different dialects of a computer language do not have identical vocabularies (commands) and specific

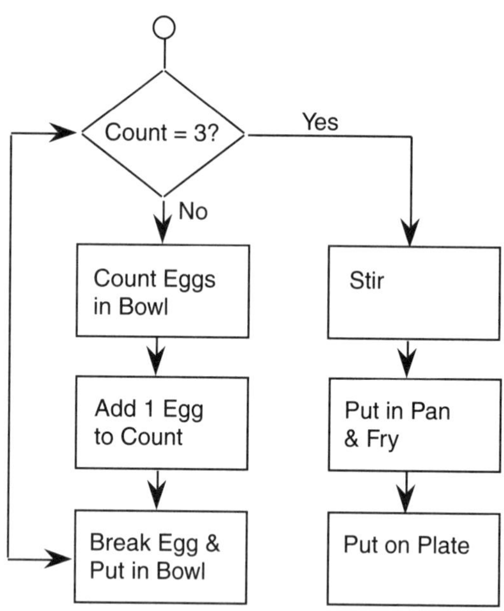

FIGURE 3.1 **A program flowchart for making a three-egg omelet.**

commands may not have the same meaning in different dialects. The dialect of a language that an IBM-compatible computer can understand is unlikely to be identical to one that an Apple Macintosh computer can understand. Consequently, the programs that would be written for these two computers in a particular language from the same flowchart would be different.

Computer languages, like spoken ones, have a linguistic structure. They can be analyzed semantically, syntactically, and pragmatically.

A *semantic* analysis of a computer language would consider its vocabulary. All computer languages have a finite vocabulary. It may consist of English-like words, combinations of letters, and/or combinations of digits. The size of the vocabulary would be relatively small compared to that of a spoken language—there may be fewer than 100 "words." The meanings of words in computer languages are unambiguous (i.e., each only has one meaning).

A *syntactic* analysis of a computer language would consider the rules it uses for arranging, or ordering, symbols. All programming languages have such rules. There tend to be fewer of them then there are in spoken languages.

A *pragmatic* analysis of a computer language would consider how it is used for doing particular tasks. The focus here would not be on the vocabulary items or the rules used for ordering them, but on what specific statements cause the computer to do.

The program in Figure 3.2 illustrates the semantic, syntactic, and pragmatic aspects of a computer language. It is written in a dialect of BASIC used by the Apple II computer. I developed it to demonstrate how a single-switch, scanning augmentative communication aid works. The program segments the monitor screen into four cells and causes the cursor to move from cell to cell every few seconds; the user signals a "message" by activating the switch when the cursor is in the cell containing it. The four messages are laid out for printing on a sheet of overhead transparency material in such a way that one would be in each cell when the transparency was mounted on the monitor screen.

The vocabulary in this program (Figure 3.2) consists of eighteen English-like words: FOR, GET, GOTO (go to), GOSUB (go subroutine), HOME, IF, INVERSE, NEXT, NORMAL, PDL (paddle), PEEK, POKE, PRINT, REM (reminder), RETURN, THEN, TO, and VTAB (vertical tab). Punctuation marks and mathematical symbols (e.g., =) also function as vocabulary in this program.

The arrangement of the vocabulary words within statements as well as the ordering of statements in the program was determined by a number of syntactic rules. One states that all statements must be numbered in a manner that indicates the order in which they are to be executed. Another states that each statement should begin with a vocabulary word.

Analyzing this program pragmatically would involve determining how I got the computer to do what I wanted it to do. It would be necessary for you to answer questions such as: How does the computer divide the screen into four cells? How is the cursor make to move from cell to cell? How is the rate of cursor movement controlled? How is the cursor made to stop when the switch is activated?

```
200  HOME : VTAB 5: POKE 32,7: PRINT : PRINT "**************************"

210  PRINT "*                        *"
220  PRINT "*  PRESS SWITCH WHEN     *"
230  PRINT "*  THE CURSOR IS IN      *"
240  PRINT "*  THE CELL CONTAINING   *"
250  PRINT "*  THE RESPONSE YOU      *"
260  PRINT "*  WANT TO COMMUNICATE.  *"
270  PRINT "*                        *"
280  PRINT "**************************"
290  POKE 32,0: PRINT : VTAB 22: PRINT "PRESS ANY KEY TO CONTINUE: ";: GET
   A$: PRINT : GOTO 320
300  PRINT  PDL (0): REM   ACTIVATES EXTERNAL SWITCH
310  HOME
320  HOME : VTAB 1: POKE 32,0: PRINT
330  PRINT "                  *                    "
340  PRINT "                  *                    "
350  PRINT "                  *                    "
360  PRINT "                  *                    "
370  PRINT "                  *                    "
380  PRINT "                  *                    "
390  PRINT "                  *                    "
400  PRINT "                  *                    "
410  PRINT "                  *                    "
420  PRINT "                  *                    "
430  PRINT "**************************************"
440  PRINT "                  *                    "
450  PRINT "                  *                    "
460  PRINT "                  *                    "
470  PRINT "                  *                    "
480  PRINT "                  *                    "
490  PRINT "                  *                    "
500  PRINT "                  *                    "
510  PRINT "                  *                    "
520  PRINT "                  *                    "
600  REM  MOVE CURSOR
610  VTAB 1: POKE 32,0
620  INVERSE
630  PRINT : PRINT "XX"
640  NORMAL
650  FOR T = 1 TO 2000
660  NEXT T
665  IF  PEEK ( - 16287) > 127 THEN  GOSUB 1000
670  VTAB 1: POKE 32,0
680  PRINT : PRINT "  "
690  VTAB 1: POKE 32,36
700  INVERSE
710  PRINT : PRINT "XX"
720  NORMAL
730  FOR T = 1 TO 2000
740  NEXT T
745  IF  PEEK ( - 16287) > 127 THEN  GOSUB 1000
750  VTAB 1: POKE 32,36
760  PRINT : PRINT "  "
770  VTAB 22: POKE 32,0
780  INVERSE
790  PRINT : PRINT "XX"
800  NORMAL
810  FOR T = 1 TO 2000
820  NEXT T
825  IF  PEEK ( - 16287) > 127 THEN  GOSUB 1000
830  VTAB 22: POKE 32,0
840  PRINT : PRINT "  "
850  VTAB 22: POKE 32,36
860  INVERSE
870  PRINT : PRINT "XX"
880  NORMAL
890  FOR T = 1 TO 2000
900  NEXT T
905  IF  PEEK ( - 16287) > 127 THEN  GOSUB 1000
910  VTAB 22: POKE 32,36
920  PRINT : PRINT "  "
930  GOTO 610
1000  REM   CURSOR DELAY SUBROUTINE
1010  FOR T = 1 TO 5000
1020  NEXT T
1030  RETURN
```

FIGURE 3.2 **A four-cell scanning program for augmentative communication.**

MICROCOMPUTER PROGRAMMING LANGUAGES

There are many programming languages. Each can be classified as being either *high level* or *low level* (Figure 3.3). These designations refer to their level of abstraction (Johnson, 1946)—that is, their degree of closeness to the *machine language* computers actually use for processing information. Programs written in a language other than machine language have to be translated into it before they can be processed.

The *high level-low level* designation is not a dichotomous one. Programming languages are on a continuum with respect to level of abstraction. The lowest level language on this continuum is machine language. The others are ordered on the basis of the number of instructions needed to have the computer perform the same tasks as machine language programs (which requires the most instructions). The fewer this number, the higher the level of abstraction of the language.

Low Level Languages

The two computer languages at the lowest level on the abstraction continuum are machine language and assembly language. Both are used for programming all types of computers.

Machine Language. Computers use a binary code consisting of 1s and 0s for storing and processing information. Machine language programs are written in this code. The standard ASCII eight-digit binary codes for the capital letters are presented in Table 2.1.

Machine language is the most difficult and time-consuming one in which to write programs, in part because instructions have to be written in *binary number codes*. Each instruction causes the computer to perform one operation; many operations may be needed for even a simple task like adding two numbers.

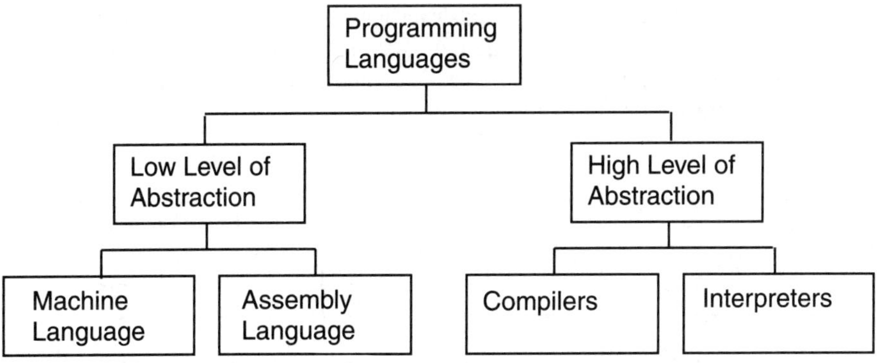

FIGURE 3.3 **Types of languages used for programming computers.**

Assembly Language. This language is one step up the abstraction ladder from machine language. Like machine language, it tells the computer not only what to do but how to do it. Instead of assigning a binary number code to each machine instruction, assembly language assigns it a two- or three-letter word or abbreviation (e.g., ADD or MVI). This word or abbreviation is called a *mnemonic*. Assembly code has a one-to-one relationship with machine code. Each instruction in machine code has a mnemonic.

Why would it be advantageous to write programs in assembly language rather than machine language? The main reason is that it is easier to remember mnemonics than binary digit codes.

Programs written in assembly language have to be translated into machine language before they can be executed. Assembly language programs are translated into machine language programs by means of a utility program known as an *assembler* (Figure 3.4). The assembly language program is referred to as the *source program* and the machine language output from the assembler is referred to as the *object code*.

All microcomputers do not use the same dialect of assembly language. The one they use is determined by their microprocessor chip. Theoretically, two microcomputers that have the same chip could use the same dialect of assembly language.

High Level Languages

Programming in either machine language or assembly language requires some knowledge of how the microprocessor functions. Computer languages that are higher on the abstraction ladder than these are easier to use because they do not require such knowledge.

The instructions in higher-level languages are *task* centered rather than *computer* centered. They tell the computer to process information in a particular manner, but they do not tell the computer how to do it. Instructions in low-level languages, on the other hand, tell the computer to perform certain operations, which will result in it processing information in a particular manner. Suppose, for example, you wanted the computer to add 2 and 2. In a high-level language you would simply give the computer the instruction for "add" and it would perform the task. In a low-level language, on the other hand, you would give the computer a series of instructions that it has to execute for the addition process to occur.

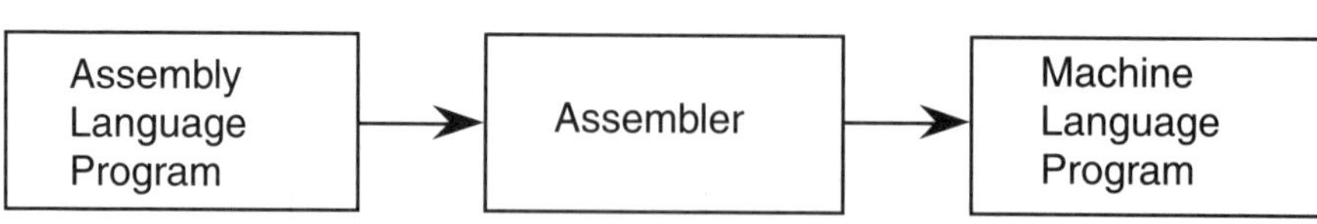

FIGURE 3.4 **An assembler translates assembly language programs into machine language programs.**

The main advantage of high-level languages is that they speed up and simplify the programming process. Familiarity with how the microprocessor processes data is not necessary. It is only necessary to learn how to use the language to tell the computer to perform certain tasks in a particular sequence. The tasks the computer would have to perform and the sequence in which it would have to perform them for a particular program could be specified in a flowchart.

High-level language programs, like assembly language programs, have to be translated into machine language before they can be executed. There are two types of utility programs that are used for this purpose: compilers and interpreters.

The *compiler*, like the assembler, translates a source program into a machine language object program (Figure 3.5). After a program has been translated into machine code, it can be executed without the compiler program. The compiler is not needed to run the program, only to translate it.

Interpreters are similar to compilers and assemblers in that they generate a machine language program from a high-level language program. However, the way they do it is different (Figure 3.6). Rather than translating the source program into a machine language object program, they examine each instruction in the source program and then perform the operation specified in it by selecting an appropriate *machine language subroutine* from among those present in the interpreter program. There is a machine language subroutine in this program for each instruction in the programming language. Hence, interpreters do not generate machine code, but select segments of such code (i.e., subroutines) from the interpreter program. Unlike compilers, interpreters are needed for running programs.

One advantage that interpreter languages have over other languages is that they are totally *interactive*. They allow you to interact, or converse, with the computer. When you enter an instruction using a keyboard, the interpreter selects the appropriate machine language subroutine (program) from those in it and enters this subroutine into the computer. The computer can be made to execute this subroutine (alone or in conjunction with others) and display information about the results on the monitor screen. The user may then respond to this information, thereby entering into a dialogue with the computer. This type of interaction between user and computer is sometimes referred to as being in a *conversational mode*. It is not possible to do this with assembler or compiler languages because programs written in such languages cannot be run until they have been translated into machine language. If you change

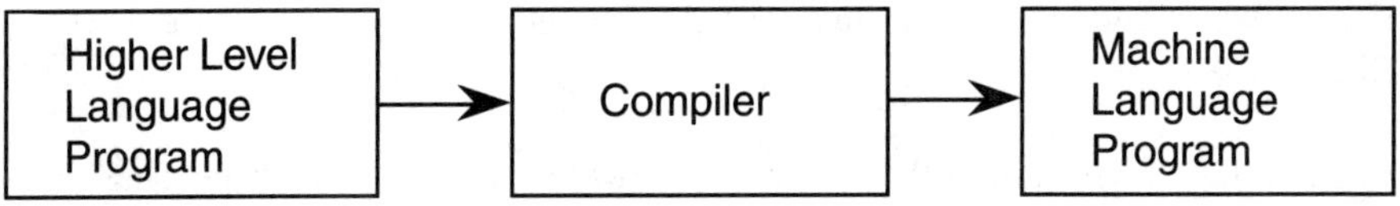

FIGURE 3.5 **A compiler translates higher level language programs into machine language programs.**

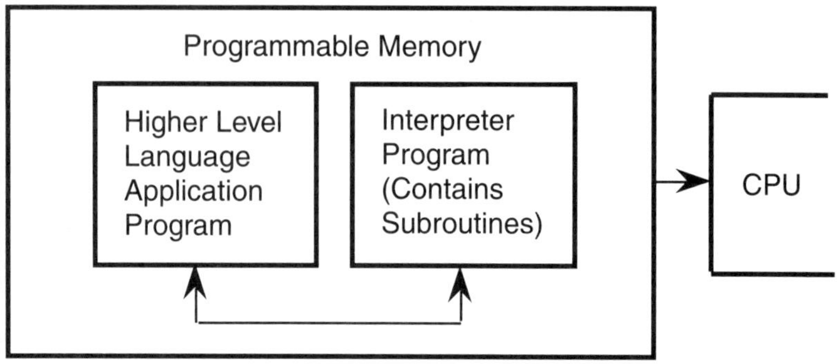

FIGURE 3.6 **An interpreter translates higher-level language programs into subroutines (one statement at a time) that it causes the computer to perform.**

even one character in an assembly language or high-level compiled language program, you have to translate the entire program again into machine language before it can be executed. Consequently, it is far less time-consuming to modify a program written in an interpreter language than in a compiler one.

There are more than 100 high-level languages. Judging by reports in the literature (see References and Bibliography) list, the two that speech-language pathologists and audiologists are likely to use are BASIC and Macintosh HyperTalk. Both are described below.

BASIC. BASIC, which stands for *Beginners All-Purpose Symbolic Instruction Code*, was developed at Dartmouth College in the 1960s primarily for teaching beginners the fundamentals of computer languages and programming. However, because of the ease with which programs can be written in BASIC, it has been widely implemented. BASICs can be either compilers or interpreters; most are interpreters.

There are a number of dialects of BASIC. All of them use a limited number of straightforward English-like commands, algebraic-like expressions, and simple punctuation (Figure 3.2). It has been used by speech-language pathologists and audiologists to develop programs for clinical use (e.g., Bull, 1983; Chial, 1986c; Esterreicher, 1985; Harlan, Larimore, & Smith, 1984; Horii, 1986; Hughes & Low, 1990; Katz, 1985a; Korabic & Silverman, 1983; Korabic, Silverman, & Rosera, 1987; Oshrin, 1985).

HyperTalk. HyperTalk is the language used with HyperCard, an "authoring" program for the Macintosh computer (Winkler & Kamins, 1990). It consists of a large number of subroutines, or procedures, that when assembled (combined) "erector set" fashion can generate software for many types of applications, including tutorials and drill/practice activities. The resulting programs—known as *HyperCard stacks*—can generate sound (including synthesized speech) as well as text and graphics in color or black and white on a monitor screen. It has been used extensively by both speech-language pathologists and audiologists for creating *augmentative communication devices* (e.g., Harlan, 1988; Mizuko & Hornstadt, 1992b; Mizuko, Hornstadt, & Erickson, 1993), *tutorials* (e.g., Anderson, Kneil, & Burk, 1991; Bernstorf, Kneil, & Burk, 1991; Clarke & Kneil, 1990; Cuda & Wynne, 1991; Cuda, Wynne, & Sawyer, 1992; de Jonge, 1992; Kneil, 1991, 1992a, 1992b; Kneil, Gordon, & Hodson, 1991; Leeper, 1991a, 1991b, 1992c; Leeper & Stuart, 1993; Martin & Lieberth, 1991, 1992a, 1992b, 1993; Palmer, 1992; Parish, Waynne, & Kneil, 1993; Pickering, 1992; Wiepsuj, Xue, & Savage, 1992) and *drill/practice activities for clients* (e.g., Bless, Canfield, Emerich, Leddy, Poburka, & Ramos, 1992; Bluestone, 1991, 1992a; Dressler, 1992; Fischer, 1991a, 1992a, 1992b, 1993; Leeper, 1992a; Lieberth, 1992; Lieberth & Martin, 1992).

There are comparable authoring programs for computers other than the Macintosh. Those for the Apple IIGS include HyperStudio and HyperCard IIGS (see Leeper, 1992c). And those for IBM-compatible computers include Plus, Linkway, and Audio-Visual Connection (Pickering, 1992).

HyperCard-type authoring program are discussed further in Chapter 13.

Two other high-level languages that have been used clinically by speech-language pathologists and audiologists are Pascal and Logo (Bull & Cochran, 1985a, 1985b; Gsell, 1990).

TYPES OF SOFTWARE

A number of types of software are needed for the applications described in this book. Since there is at least one program of each type available commercially for IBM-compatible, Macintosh, and Apple II computers, you do not have to know how to write computer programs to do them. You may, however, want to know how to use an authoring program such as HyperCard so that you can create language stimulation and other drill/practice software that is tailored to the specific needs of clients.

There are two general types of computer software: application and system. *Application programs* enable you to do clinical tasks such as word processing and analyzing language samples. Programs for these and other tasks that could facilitate your clinical activities are described in Chapters 4 through 15.

System software consists of programs that a microcomputer needs to function regardless of the application for which it is being used. System software is responsible for performing a computer's "housekeeping" functions. When a computer is turned on, for example, an *initialization program* readies all system components for processing information. System programs can be located in ROM and/or RAM.

Types of System Software

There are two general types of system software: disk operating systems and programming languages. Both require or can be enhanced by utility programs.

The *disk operating system* (DOS) has been called the software "soul" of the computer and the "boss" of the computer. It functions like a traffic cop, directing information to the proper place, and it contains the first program executed when a computer is turned on and the last one executed when it is turned off. It is a computer's most important software since without it the computer can't do anything.

To illustrate the supervisory role played by a computer's disk operating system, let's consider what happens when a key on a keyboard is pressed.

> By itself, a computer isn't capable of recognizing that a key has been pressed, much less deciding what it means. But the operating system instructs the computer to periodically check to see if a key has been pressed and tells the computer what to do about it. The operating system routine will instruct the machine on how to decode the signal produced by the key-press and, most of the time, tell the computer to display the appropriate character on the video screen. (Cook, 1984, p. 112)

While many disk operating systems have been developed for microcomputers, only the eight listed below were being used by significant numbers of speech-language pathologists and audiologists when this chapter was written.

- *DOS 3.3.* One of the 8-bit disk operating systems for the Apple II and compatible computers. Since the Apple II was one of the most popular microcomputers during the late-1970s and 1980s, it is not particularly surprising that tens of thousands of programs were written using DOS 3.3. Much of the clinical software intended for speech-language pathologists and audiologists that was published during the 1980s used this disk operating system.
- *Macintosh.* The 32-bit disk operating system used on Apple's Macintosh computers. The current version when this chapter was written was 7.5. It is designed to make life easy for the user. Rather than having to manipulate the disk operating system with written commands, a mouse is used to point to icons (see Chapter 2). This makes microcomputers with this disk operating system somewhat easier to use than those with the other systems mentioned in this section, with the exception of Windows and ProDOS 16. Both of these issue commands the same way as Macintosh DOS.
- *MS-DOS.* (MicroSoft Disk Operating System). More 16-bit microcomputers use MS-DOS as their operating system than any other. Its popularity now is due, in part, to the fact that IBM had been offering it as an operating system for its microcomputers since they were introduced in the early 1980s. Its popularity originally was partially due to its commands being similar to those of an 8-bit

disk operating system that was very popular during the late 1970s and early 1980s—that is, CP/M. The most recent versions of MS-DOS contain the Windows extension (see the discussion of Windows below).

- *OS/2*. A highly sophisticated 32-bit disk operating system for some top-of-the-line IBM microcomputers. While it has its own applications, it is compatible with both *MS-DOS* and *Windows*.
- *ProDOS*. Another 8-bit disk operating system for the Apple II and compatible computers. It is actually an updated version of Apple *DOS 3.3*.
- *ProDOS 16*. The 16-bit disk operating system for the Apple IIGS. This computer, which like the other Apple II models is no longer being manufactured, can also run programs that use the 8-bit *ProDOS* and Apple *DOS 3.3* disk operating systems.
- Unix. An operating system originally developed by Bell Laboratories for use with multiuser minicomputer systems. It is more complicated and more powerful than any of the other operating systems that have been discussed. Some authorities predict that Unix will be the standard operating system on larger microcomputers in the years to come. Because Unix is written in a high-level language, it does not have the hardware restrictions of MS-DOS. In particular, it does not require that the computer use one of a certain family of microprocessors.
- *Windows*. An extension of the MS-DOS disk operating system. It provides users of IBM-compatible computers with a desktop environment similar but not identical to the Macintosh. The current version when this chapter was written was *Windows 95*.

It is possible to enhance (add features to) a microcomputer's disk operating system (DOS). Programs that are used for doing so—known as *utility programs*—can enhance a microcomputer's DOS in a number of ways, including the following:

- *Add macro capability*. A macro is a *recording* of a series of keystrokes and/or mouse movements that you can store on your hard disk and execute by pressing two or three keys. You can create large numbers of macros; each would be executed by a different key combination. Macros can contain a large number of keystrokes or mouse movements. The keystrokes can be for characters, commands, or both. Macros enable you to do tasks (particularly ones that you do often) more efficiently, with fewer keystrokes and/or mouse movements. An example of such a task would be "copying" the inside address from a business letter, "pasting" it in a mailing label file, and printing it on a mailing label.
- *Protect the monitor screen*. Screen saver programs prevent what is on the monitor screen from being "burnt into" it if the computer is kept on but not used for a period of time. If an image is burnt into a monitor screen, it will be visible whenever the monitor is being used. The simplest programs of this type will darken the image on the screen if there hasn't been a keystroke or a mouse

movement for a predetermined number of minutes or if an instruction is issued to do so (e.g., by placing the cursor at a specified location on the screen); the screen automatically brightens again when a key is pressed or the mouse is moved. Others put a constantly changing image, such as fireworks or goldfish swimming on the screen—the latter also enable you to keep what you are working on confidential when you are away from your computer.

- *Increase disk storage capacity.* File compression programs enable you to store more and/or longer files on a diskette or hard disk than would ordinarily be possible. The use of such a program could make it possible for an 80MB hard disk to hold as much information as an 160MB one. Some automatically compress everything stored on a disk and others allow you to do so selectively. Their main disadvantage is that files stored in compressed form have to be decompressed before they are used. This means that programs that are compressed or are using data files that are compressed will do tasks a little slower than they would otherwise.
- *Recover data.* Data recorded on diskettes and hard disks can be damaged or accidentally erased. These programs often make it possible to at least partially recover such data.
- *Detect viruses.* A virus is a program that is used to "infect" a computer. It is buried within an existing program, and once the program is loaded into the computer and saved on its hard disk, it infects the other programs on it. The "symptoms" of a virus can range from a strange message that pops up on the screen out of the blue to the actual destruction of programs and data. Virus detection programs can be used to either screen programs being loaded into a computer or those already on a hard disk for known viruses. Some can "kill" (remove) viruses that are found.
- *Reduce hard disk file fragmentation.* It takes a computer a certain amount of time to locate files on a hard disk. This time is likely to increase as the drive ages because new files are not usually recorded on it in a way that is optimal for retrieving them. They may, for example, be *fragmented*—that is, parts of them may be recorded at different locations on the hard disk. These programs reorganize the files on a hard disk in a way that minimizes the time needed to retrieve them.
- *Increase the number of fonts.* All disk operating systems come with at least a few fonts of alphanumeric characters. There are thousands available—for English and other languages—that can be added.
- *Convert data files created with other DOSs and programs to formats that are compatible with your application programs.* These enable files that were created with one program and/or disk operating system to be "read" and edited by another. They enable you, for example, to read and edit word processor files that were created with a Macintosh computer with an IBM-compatible one and vice versa.

These are not the only types of utility programs, but these are the ones that you are likely to find most useful.

Application Software

Many types of application software have been used clinically by speech-language pathologists and audiologists (see References and Bibliography). Some of them are general business productivity programs, such as word processing, drawing, telecommunications, spreadsheets, and databases (Bull & Cochran, 1985). These as well as programs that were created specifically for practitioners in our field are described in Chapters 4 through 15.

SELECTING AND EVALUATING SOFTWARE

The amount that you are likely to benefit from having a microcomputer will be determined largely by the software it can run. If a microcomputer can run software that enables you to do a least a few tasks better and/or more efficiently than you could have done them otherwise, you are likely to benefit significantly from having one available. On the other hand, if there is no such software, a microcomputer would be of questionable value to you.

There are three general types of software: copyrighted software sold by vendors, copyrighted shareware, and public domain software. The first is the type with which you are probably most familiar. It is published by a firm rather than its author and you purchase it from a local store or a mail-order house. Because it is copyrighted, the publisher can place restrictions on its use that a court will enforce. This may be done through a *licensing agreement*. The purchaser "signs" the agreement by breaking the seal on the envelope containing the program disks. Restrictions include the number of computers on which the program can be installed. This is usually one unless the purchaser has a *site license*. Many school systems, hospitals, universities, and other institutions purchase site licenses for programs that are used by many of their employees, such as word-processing ones. Restrictions also include the number of back-up copies that can legally be made of the program. Making other copies and giving or selling them to others (known as "pirating") can result in a suit for copyright infringment and a fine of $25,000 or more!

Shareware is published by its author and you obtain a copy from him or her or from a telecommunication network (see Chapter 11). Although the program is copyrighted, you are permitted to use it without paying a fee for a short period of time. If you continue to use it after that period, you are expected to send a check to the author. The amount that you were expected to pay for most shareware programs when this chapter was written was less than $50—for some it was as little as $5. Programs that are distributed as shareware are almost always less expensive than comparable ones published by commercial firms and they are often as good as (or even superior to) them. A high percentage of them are utility programs.

Public domain software (freeware), like shareware, is published by its author and usually distributed by him or her on telecommunication networks. It is not copyrighted and consequently, no fee has to be paid to use it. The quality of such software ranges from worthless to extremely high. Some clinical programs (i.e., "stacks") created with HyperCard (see Chapter 13) are not copyrighted and distributed by their authors as public domain software.

Selecting Software

The first step in the software selection process is identifying the tasks you want the microcomputer to do. You may find it helpful to answer the following questions:

1. Do I want to use the microcomputer for administrative (clerical) tasks such as appointment making, report writing, maintaining client records, and billing? If "yes," for what tasks?
2. Do I want to use the microcomputer for administering tests (e.g., audiometric ones) and other types of assessment tasks (e.g., case histories) to clients and/or for analyzing test and other diagnostically relevant data (e.g., language samples)? If "yes," for administering what tasks and analyzing what data?
3. Do I want to use the microcomputer as a tool for teaching, stimulating, and/or motivating clients? If "yes," with what clients and for what purposes?
4. Do I want to use the microcomputer for analyzing statistical and other numerical data? If "yes," what types of data?
5. Do I want to use the microcomputer for augmentative communication? If "yes," in what ways?
6. Do I want to use the microcomputer to make measurements or control instrumentation for either clinical or research purposes? If "yes," what measurements and/or what instrumentation?
7. Do I want to use the microcomputer for telecommunication applications such as sending and receiving faxes and searching literature databases? If "yes," what applications?
8. Do I want to use the microcomputer for desktop publishing or for preparing overheads, slides, and/or handouts for inservice or other types of presentations? If "yes," what specifically do I want it to do?

Once you have identified the task or tasks for which you want to use the microcomputer, you can begin the software selection process. For each task, you identify the programs that could be used for doing it that are compatible with your computer. Unfortunately, some of the programs that could be used may not be compatible with it (see Rosenblum, 1991) After you have identified this subset of programs, your next task is to select from this group the program (or combination of programs) that would best meet your needs. There is a set of criteria for evaluating programs in the next section. You, of course, may conclude that none of them would allow you to do the tasks better and/or more efficiently than the approach you are currently using.

Evaluating Software

What criteria should you consider when evaluating microcomputer software? The ASHA Committee on Educational Technology suggested some a number of years ago (*Asha*, May, 1984, p. 67) that are still applicable. These criteria are listed below along with some questions you should attempt to answer when evaluating programs for them.

1. Program Description
   A. Is the purpose of the program clearly defined?
   B. Is the manner in which the program works clearly described?
   C. Are the instructions for getting started with the program clearly described?
   D. Are the instructions for storing and retrieving data clearly described?
   E. Are the hardware requirements clearly stated?

2. Program Effectiveness
   A. Is the software program logical and reasonable?
   B. Will the program produce consistent results in various settings under various conditions?
   C. Is there a reprint of an article, a technical report or other information describing the results of a study(ies) of effectiveness?

3. User Friendliness
   A. Is the program easy to enter?
   B. Is the program easy to exit?
   C. Are the instructions displayed on the screen easy to understand and complete?
   D. Are the input responses to the machine familiar (such as "Y" for "yes" and "N" for "no")?
   E. Are program options displayed as "menus"?
   F. What does the program do if the user strikes a wrong key (does it give a prompt reminding the user of the correct options and disregard the error)?
   G. Can input errors be easily corrected?
   H. Are data outputs easily retrieved?
   I. Are data outputs complete and attractively formatted?

4. Support/Documentation
   A. Is the documentation complete (does it tell you everything you need to know)?
   B. Is the documentation concise (does it tell you more than you want to know)?
   C. Is the documentation written in terms you can understand?
   D. Is the documentation well organized (can you find answers to specific problems by referring to an index or table of contents)?
   E. Does it adequately describe the hardware needed and any special instructions for its use?
   F. Are the hardware and software options clearly explained?

G. Is there a source for help (someone to call or write if you have a question)?
H. Are back-up copies provided (if not, are instructions for making back-up copies included)?
I. Can the program be returned if the user decides that it is not appropriate for his setting?
J. Can replacement copies be obtained at a reduced rate if the originals become damaged?
K. Can updated program revisions be obtained at a reduced rate?

Where can you get the information you need to answer these questions? There are several sources from which may be able to obtain it. The first is the author or publisher of a program. Information that you obtain from this source can tell you what the program is *intended* to do. If the information that you obtain suggests that the program is unlikely to meet your needs, you would go no further. However, if this information indicates that it might meet your needs, you would attempt to determine if it would perform the task well for which you would be using it. You can do this by communicating with persons who have used the program and/or by reading critical reviews. Reviews of programs that are intended for practitioners in our field are published in *Asha* and *Asha Leader* (see the reference section for reviews of particular programs). Reviews of programs that are not intended specifically for practitioners in our field (e.g., reviews of word processing programs) are published in computer magazines. Since most of these reviews are indexed, a librarian should be able to help you locate those for specific programs.

Of course, the best way to find out whether a program will meet your needs is to try it. Some software vendors will allow you to try out programs. Also, *demonstration versions* of some programs (both those that are and are not intended for practitioners in our field) are available for free or for a nominal charge. These are versions of programs that have been "crippled" in some way—for example, you may not be able to save the documents or drawings that you create. You can find out about the availability of demonstration versions of programs by contacting their publishers.

For further information about software selection, see Amerine (1991), Chial (1986a), Gardner (1991), Rushakoff (1984b), and Scherz (1993a).

The remainder of the book—Chapters 4 through 15—contains descriptions of computer applications that clinicians are likely to find useful. The software available for doing them is not all of equal quality. The criteria presented in this section can help you to "separate the wheat from the chaff."

▶ 4

Evaluation, Therapy, and Clinical Decision Making

The programs discussed in this chapter and the next are the only ones considered in this book intended solely (or almost solely) for practitioners who treat communicative disorders. These programs are supposed to help you manage your client's communicative disorders. While some are both conceptually sound and executed well, others have serious limitations. Fortunately, there are reviews in professional journals that can help you to separate the wheat from the chaff.

My primary objective in this chapter is to alert you to ways in which you may be able to use computers when working with clients. There are brief descriptions of how computers have been used with clients and references to papers in which the various applications are described, sometimes in considerable detail. Many of the papers cited are American Speech-Language-Hearing Association (ASHA) Convention presentations. There are bibliographical data for locating abstracts in the reference list. Copies (and sometimes related software) often can be obtained from presenters. The *ASHA Membership Directory* is useful for obtaining current addresses.

The items cited in this chapter include clinical software and reviews of it. Some of the programs cited are no longer being marketed, but they were included for two reasons. First, many of them are still being used. And second, the focus of this chapter (as well as the remaining ones) is on how computers can be used—that is, their *potential*—for facilitating the clinical process. Software that is no longer available can sometimes be simulated by someone who has little or no knowledge of computer programming with an authoring program such as HyperCard (see Chapter 13).

Because the focus of this chapter is on clinical tasks that can be facilitated by using a computer rather than on programs that are currently being marketed for doing them, chapter content has been influenced in another way. Information is presented on how some of these tasks might be done with software other than that specifically dedicated to (being marketed for) doing it. Particular attention is given to the possibility of using general-purpose word-processing, database, spreadsheet, and authoring software. These four types of software are described elsewhere in the book. Some attention also is given to the possibility of using educational software to perform these tasks. Some educational drill/practice programs can be adopted fairly easily for use in clinical activities (Scherz & Lieberth, 1995).

While my focus in this chapter is not on the clinical programs that were being marketed while this book was being written, I did feel some obligation to make you aware of both them and those that are currently being marketed. There is information about some of the former in the chapter. Furthermore, all of the clinical programs of which I was aware when the book was being written as well as reviews of them are included in the References and Bibliography. In addition, I included a directory of publishers of clinical software for managing communicative disorders (see Appendix C); information about the clinical programs they are currently marketing can be obtained from them. Also, I recommend that you check the software advertisements and reviews in recent issues of *Asha* and *Asha Leader* since publishers may have entered the communicative disorders market after December 1995—the month that the manuscript for this book was completed.

We will begin with a discussion of potential applications for microcomputers in the diagnostic (assessment) process, followed by a discussion of potential microcomputer applications in the therapy (intervention) process. The chapter will conclude with a discussion of considerations for evaluating and designing software intended to be used by clients alone or together with clinicians.

DIAGNOSTIC (ASSESSMENT) SOFTWARE

A computer can enable you to perform evaluations more efficiently by making it possible for you to do certain tasks quicker, and consequently, for less cost. The assumption is being made here that these are tasks you usually do—not ones that you are doing just because you have a program for doing them. For example, a program that analyzes language samples in ways that you do not ordinarily analyze them would not reduce costs. However, if such analyses would be helpful for planning therapy and are not too expensive (i.e., too time-consuming) to do with a computer, making them in this way could be justified on the basis that doing so makes them affordable.

Seven types of tasks for which microcomputers can be used in the diagnostic or assessment process are described in this section: history taking, test selection, test administration, test scoring, speech/language sample analysis, decision making, and report writing.

History Taking

You can use a microcomputer to take all or part of a case history. The client or an informant (e.g., a parent or spouse) answers questions that are displayed on the monitor screen by manipulating a keyboard or other input device (e.g., a touch screen).

The questions may be of the multiple-choice or true-false type or they may require keyboarding short answers. All persons may be asked the same questions or their answers may, at least partially, determine what questions are asked. A short computer tutorial may be used for teaching them how to do the task. The program may print answers in list form and/or generate (write) paragraphs summarizing the information obtained. These paragraphs can be "exported" to a word-processing program for inclusion in an evaluation report. The program is likely to require a password to access history information; this is done to satisfy legal and ethical requirements for confidentiality.

While computers have not been used extensively by speech-language pathologists or audiologists for gathering case history data, practitioners in other health-related fields have used them. The findings of a number of studies suggest that clients are more likely to give accurate information to a computer than they are to an interviewer. They don't try to impress a computer and they regard it as being non-judgmental. Some clients, in fact, tend to regard computers as being intelligent and having the capacity to evaluate and react to information like a human being. According to Murray (1983, p. 98):

> In the 1960s Joseph Weizenbaum [Professor of Computer Science at MIT] developed a notorious program known as ELIZA, which was able to conduct an initial therapeutic interview. As far as Weizenbaum was concerned, ELIZA was something of a joke to prove a point. But other people didn't take her so lightly. Some became convinced that ELIZA really understood them. Weizenbaum was horrified and labeled "delusional" such interactions with ELIZA. And when some psychiatrists hailed ELIZA as a helpmate to close the gap between the demand for therapy and the supply of trained practitioners in clinics, Weizenbaum was appalled.

While reactions to being interviewed by a computer generally tend to be positive, there do appear to be things that can irritate interviewees and, consequently, should be controlled for. One is insufficient choices for responding to questions when a multiple-choice format is used. Another is ambiguities in the questions. A third is having the computer commit breaches of etiquette by not saying "please" and "thank you." Apparently, a machine that engages in human dialogue is expected to evince a polite demeanor.

Case history forms created with a database program that can be filled in by a computer (see Chapter 9) can be used for this purpose. Responses to questions could be printed and/or exported (in whole or part) to a word-processing program where they could be incorporated into an evaluation report. In fact, certain responses from a client's database file could be inserted (merged) automatically into the paragraphs of his or her evaluation report through the use of the word-processing program's mail-merge (print merge) command(s). Almost all database programs can facilitate confidentiality by requiring a password to access files created by them.

Test Selection, Administration, and Scoring

Three main ways that speech-language pathologists and audiologists have used microcomputers clinically is for test selection, administration, and scoring, particularly the latter (e.g., Delgado, Ozdamar, & Miskiel, 1987, 1988; Durnford, Frey, Hazan, & Hoffman, 1994; Marchbanks & Martin, 1985; Mason & Adams, 1984; Rushakoff & Schwartz, 1986; Sheeley, 1984; Stach & Jerger, 1986). They also have used them for analyzing interactions between persons—for example, parents and children (Long & Clezy, 1994; Oratio, 1979) and attributes of speech/language samples (e.g., Baker-van den Goorbergh, 1990; Bakker, Arkebauer, & Boutsen, 1993; Boyd, Rolland, Lyngass, Zutter-Brose, Daggett, et al., 1990; Brinton, Fujiki, Ranck, & Ranck, 1985; Dale & Cole, 1988; Dale & Marriner, 1985; Driscoll & Driscoll, 1984; Elbert, Young, & Bruce, 1981; Gavin, 1987; Hodson & Oller, 1992; Long & Dale, 1994; Long & Fey, 1988, 1990a, 1990b, 1993a, 1993b; Long & Masterson, 1993; Major, 1994; Masterson, Channell, Fey, Hughes, Pollock, & Matesich, 1991; Masterson & Long, 1990; Masterson & Pagan, 1990; Masterson, Spiser-Albert, Laurent, & Waryas, 1994; Miller & Chapman, 1983; Miller & Nockerts, 1993; Oller, 1991; Oller & Delgado, 1991; Oller, Hodson, & Delgado, 1992; Pye, 1988; Riski & Delong, 1982; Rushakoff & Schwartz, 1986; Shriberg & Kwiatkowski, 1985; Somers, 1979; Telage, 1980). These applications are discussed in this section.

Test Selection. There are many tests that could be administered to a client who has a communicative disorder. If those that are required to adequately describe a client's disorder are not administered, management recommendations may not be appropriate. On the other hand, if tests are administered that are unnecessary, the cost of the evaluation will increase unnecessarily. This is particularly likely to be frowned upon in a managed care environment (Vekovius, 1995).

Using database software (see Chapter 9), test database can be created that will both facilitate the test selection process and provide documentation for its being conducted in a cost-effective manner. The record (see Chapter 9) for each test in the database would include fields for recording information relevant to the question(s) that the test could be helpful for answering, including fields for recording the types of disorders, ages, and cultural backgrounds of clients for which a test is appropriate and the specific types of information that a test can provide. These fields would contain the selection criteria for identifying appropriate tests for a client. For a description of the software used to set up a database of this type, see Chapter 9.

Test Administration. You can administer almost any test that has (or can be converted into) a multiple-choice format with a computer. Visual test items (text, drawings, photographs, and/or video segments that contain movies or animation) can be displayed on a monitor screen. And those that are auditory (e.g., speech stimuli or pure tones) can be generated by the digital speech/sound synthesizing circuitry built into most contemporary computers or a peripheral device such as a tape recorder or a pure-tone audiometer. Test items can be multimedia, containing both visual and auditory stimuli. Questions, for example, can be both spoken and printed on a monitor screen.

There are a number of ways that clients could be instructed to respond to items on a multiple-choice, microcomputer-administered test. The most cost-effective probably would be by using the numeric keys on a keyboard: Each choice would have a number (Figure 4.1) or a letter (Figure 4.2) or be selectable by an arrow key or mouse (Figure 4.3). Other possibilities would be by using a touch screen (see Chapter 2), a joystick, or some type of single-switch in conjunction with a scanning response mode (see Chapter 5) or simply indicating the answer by pointing at it on a monitor screen (McCullough, Wilson, Birck, & Anderson, 1994).

Test items do not have to be limited to those with a multiple-choice format; they can also include fill-in-the-blanks (Figure 4.4). Clients, of course, have to be more intact motorically to respond to such items.

It should be possible for this type of program to store your clients' responses to test items on a disk and display them on a monitor screen and/or print them. Furthermore, it may be possible to get the program to analyze their responses in ways you would find helpful and even "write" a paragraph describing the results of the

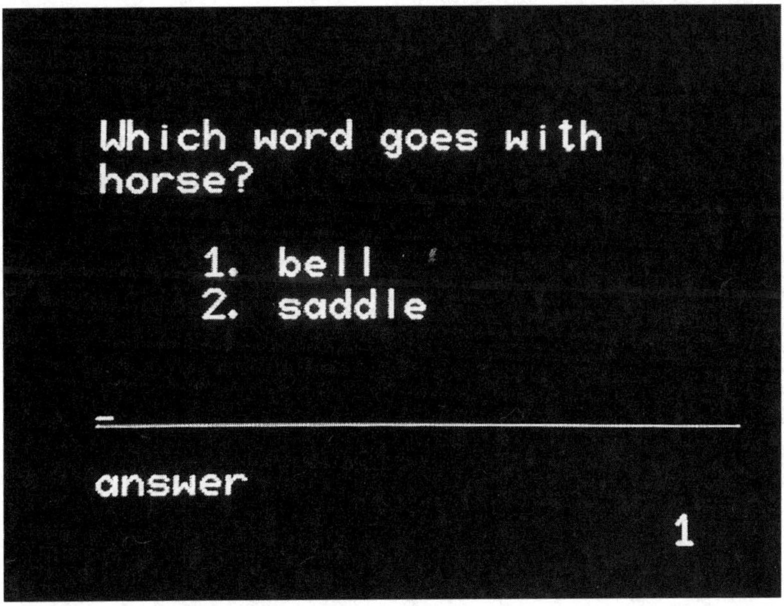

FIGURE 4.1 **A multiple-choice question screen in which each choice has a number (from Smith, 1984).**

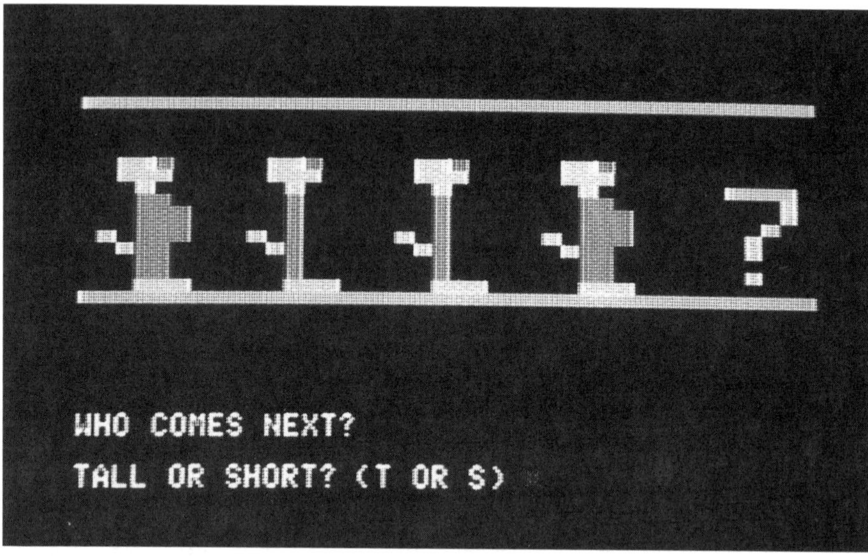

FIGURE 4.2 **A multiple-choice question screen in which each choice has a letter (from Neu, 1985).**

analyses that you can export to your word-processing program for inclusion in the evaluation report. The computer would perform this writing task by filling in the "blanks" in a template (see Chapter 7) that could consist of more than one paragraph.

Test Scoring. Computer test scoring is not limited to data that are generated by having a client interact with a computer. You can also use a computer indirectly to facilitate test scoring: Rather than using it to administer tests, you administer the tests in your usual way and input information about the client's performance on each item (or response to each stimulus) after he or she responds to it (Simpson & Sharpe, 1995). The computer analyzes these data. A computer can be used in this way, for example, to estimate thresholds from audiometric test data (Carterette, 1984). With some such programs (e.g., Sparks, 1972), the computer recommends a stimulus, task, item, or test to administer next. And with others, it makes management recommendations—such as a type of hearing aid (Sims, Knight, & Austin, 1992; Wynne, Culpepper, Mendel, Grote, & Seewald, 1995).

A computer spreadsheet (see Chapter 10) can be used for scoring any test requiring calculations. You would enter the necessary formulas into certain cells of the spreadsheet and the numbers on which calculations are to be based in others. The spreadsheet then would make the calculations automatically. Such a spread-

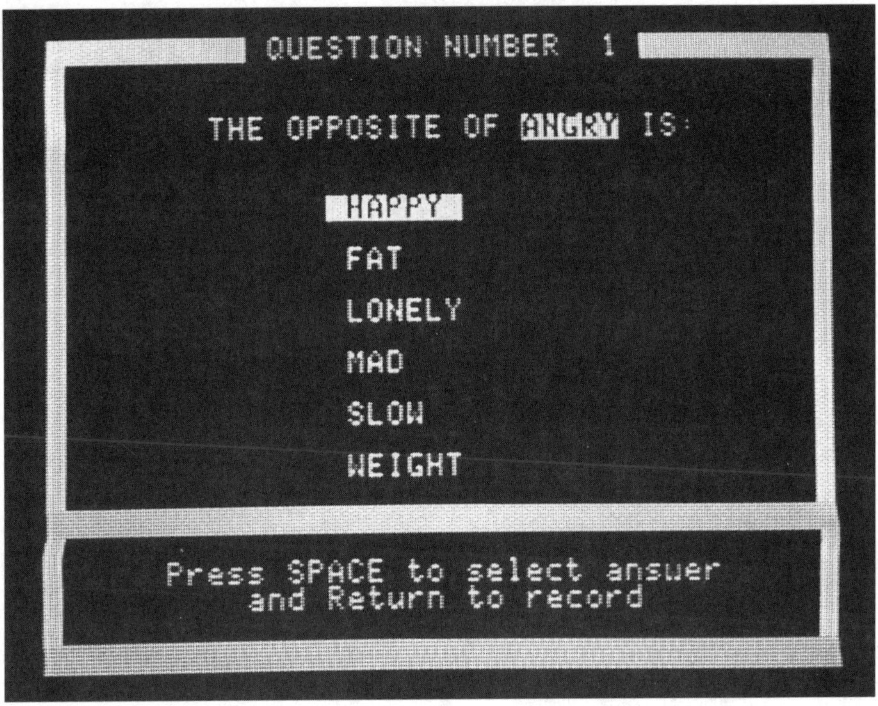

FIGURE 4.3 **A multiple-choice question screen in which choices are made by pressing an arrow key or manipulating a mouse.**

sheet can, incidentally, be saved as a template and reused, so that the next time you had to make the calculations you would merely substitute the client's numbers for those in the spreadsheet cells. The spreadsheet then would redo the calculations. Information needed to develop such a spreadsheet template is presented in Chapter 10.

Speech/Language Sample Analysis

Three types of programs can assist you in performing clinically relevant analyses of speech/language samples: linguistic analysis programs, acoustical speech analysis programs, and physiological speech analysis programs.

Linguistic Analysis Programs. A number of programs do phonological, morphological, syntactic, semantic, and/or other types of *linguistic analyses* (e.g., mean length of response and type/token ratio), including the following: *Articulation Error*

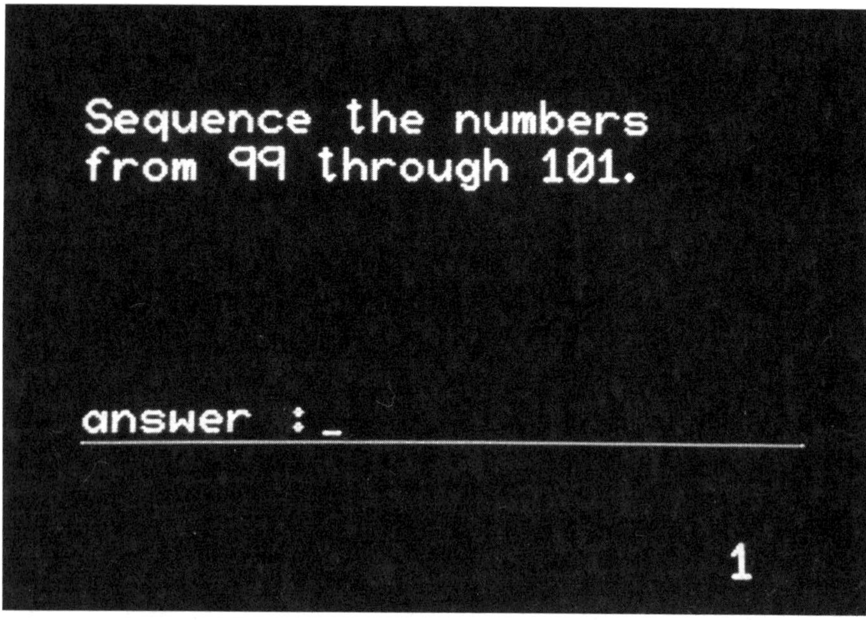

FIGURE 4.4 **A fill-in-the-blank question screen (from Smith, 1984).**

Analysis (Blinn, 1985); *Computer Analysis of Phonological Processes* (Hodson, 1985; Kennedy, 1986; Oller, 1991; Oller & Delgado, 1991; Oller, Hodson, & Delgado, 1992); *Computerized Language Error Analysis Report* (Allen, 1993; Baker-van den Goorbergh, 1990; Baker-van den Goorbergh & Baker, no date; Harn, 1992); *Computerized Language Sample Analysis* (Bowen, 1985; Dale & Cole, 1988); *Computerized Phonological Analysis* (Masterson & Long, 1990; Masterson & Pagan, 1990); *Computerized Profiling* (Long, 1991, 1992; Long & Fey, 1987, 1988, 1990a, 1990b, 1993a, 1993b, 1995; Long & Masterson, 1993; Masterson, Long, Fey, Pye, Oller, Miller, MacWhinney, & Evans, 1995a, 1995b); *Developmental Sentence Scoring* (Channell, Grenfell, & Hilton, 1993; Hughes & Low, 1989, 1990); *Lingquest 1 Language Sample Analysis Program* (Dale & Cole, 1988; Mordecai, Palin, & Palmer, 1985; Wilkinson, Sevcik, Adamson, & Romski, 1989); *Lingquest 2 Phonological Analysis* (Palin & Mordecai, 1982); *Parrot Easy Language Sample Analysis* (Weiner, 1995ii); *PEPPER—Programs to Examine Phonetic and Phonologic Evaluation Records* (Pollock, 1988; Pollock & Dana, 1989; Shriberg, 1985, 1986; Shriberg & Kwiatkowski, 1985; Weston, Schriberg, & Miller, 1989; Wynne, 1987); *Pye Analysis of Language* (Masterson et al., 1995a, 1995b; Pye, 1987, 1988); and *SALT—Systematic Analysis of Language Transcripts* (Dale & Cole, 1988; Long, 1993; Long & Fey, 1990b; Masterson et al., 1995a; Miller & Chapman, 1991; Miller & Nockerts, 1993; Weston et al., 1989; Wilkinson,et al., 1989).

All of the programs described in the preceding paragraph require a word processor file containing a transcription of the sample to be analyzed in which the attributes to be analyzed have been "coded." Consequently, it is desirable that the transcription be made with a word-processing program that creates files that can be "read" by the language analysis program being used. Be aware that the coding of speech/language samples can be time consuming. Some clinicians regard this as being a major drawback to the use of this software.

A computer spreadsheet (see Chapter 10) can be helpful for doing calculations for language analyses when programs of the types discussed in this section are not being used. Both the formulas and numbers needed for doing the calculations are entered into the cells of a spreadsheet, which then computes them automatically. The spreadsheet can be retained as a template and reused by replacing the numbers in it.

Acoustical Speech Analysis Programs. Programs that analyze acoustical attributes of speech samples transform the computer into a *virtual* instrument—one that can mimic such devices as an oscilloscope, a Sonograph, or a Visipitch (McGuire, 1995). Speech samples to be analyzed have to enter the computer through an analog-to-digital converter (see Chapter 12). They can do so either "on line" (i.e., while the client is speaking) or from recordings. A number of attributes of the speech signal can be abstracted and measured in this way, including fundamental frequency (Korabic, Kuo, & Linville, 1986), pitch pertubation (Korabic et al., 1986), and nasalance (McFarlane, 1990a). It is even possible to abstract formant data from speech samples and print spectrograms (Conway & Niederjohn, 1988). Programs that you can use to measure acoustical attributes of a client's speech include public domain, or freeware, programs (e.g., Drumright, Seikel, & Wilcox, 1988; Healey & Tice, 1991) as well as commercial ones such as *LabView* (Espinoza-Varas, 1992; Titze, Wong, Milder, Hensley, & Ramig, 1995), *SoundWave* (Chaney, 1992), *SoundEdit Pro* (Chaney, 1992), *SoundScope* (McCabe & Weinreb, 1995), and *MacSpeech Lab* (Hancock, 1986; Herman, 1989; Rubin, 1987; Scherz, 1993b) for the Macintosh and *Lab Windows* (Espinoza-Varas, 1992), *Dr. Speech Science* (Huang, Minifie, & Lin, 1992), and *IBM SpeechViewer* (Ferrero, Menin, Noventa, & Rosetti, 1993; Friedman, 1989; Kennedy, Radlinski, & Sheridan, 1991; Osredkar & Horii, 1991; Pratt, Heintzelman, & Deming, 1993; Ryalls, 1989; Ryalls, Cloutier, & Cloutier, 1991; Schoenberg, 1995; Zara, 1993) for IBM-compatibles. These programs differ with regard to the acoustical speech analyses they can make and how easily they can make particular ones (Buder & Kent, 1995). They also differ with regard to the reliability with which they can make particular measures (Morris, Brown, & Sapienza, 1995).

A computer spreadsheet (see Chapter 10) can be helpful for doing calculations for acoustical analyses when programs of the types discussed in this section are not being used. Both the formulas and numbers needed for doing the calculations are entered into the cells of a spreadsheet, which then computes them automatically. The spreadsheet could be retained as a template and reused by replacing the numbers in it.

Physiological Speech Analysis Programs. The programs that you would use to analyze (measure) *physiological* concomitants of a client's speech or auditory mechanism functioning pass the electrical signals that contain information about them through an analog-to-digital converter—usually on line. The analysis (measurement) process is essentially the same as the one you would use for analyzing acoustical attributes of a client's speech. Consequently, a single program may be usable for both. One program that can analyze both physiological and acoustical data is *LabVIEW* (Espinoza-Varas, 1992). For an example of such an application, see Bloem (1991) and Barron and Hamill (1991).

Other physiological concomitants of a client's speech that you may seek to analyze with a computer would be abstracted from photographs or other *visual images*. Images can be used from photographs, plotter printouts, x-ray films, slides, motion picture films, or videotapes of parts of the speech mechanism while a client is speaking (Colton, Casper, Brewer, & Conture, 1989; Dengel, Robbins, & Rosenbek, 1990; Logemann, Kahrilas, Begelman, Dodds, & Pauloski, 1989). The images must be digitized before they can be analyzed by a computer. If they were on sheets of paper, a scanner could be used for doing this (see Chapter 2).

A computer spreadsheet (see Chapter 10) can be helpful for doing calculations for physiological analyses, particularly when the measurements on which the analyses are based are not being made by a computer.

Decision Making

Data gathered during an evaluation can be used for making several kinds of decisions, including those pertaining to the etiology of the client's communicative disorder and the prognosis for reducing its severity. Two types of microcomputer programs can provide you with a "second opinion" when making such decisions—pattern recognition and expert system programs.

Opinions from computers should be treated similarly to those from consultants. If the computer agrees with you, you can have more confidence in the validity of your opinion. On the other hand, if the computer disagrees, you should reconsider your opinion. You may, of course, decide to go with it regardless of what the computer says.

In order to know how much weight to give an opinion from a consultant, you need to know on what it was based. Similarly, in order to know how much weight to give an opinion from a computer you need to know how the software programmed it to make decisions.

Pattern recognition programs can help you assign a particular object or event to a category. The category will be determined by data on a number of the object's or event's attributes. It may be possible, for example, to use data on certain acoustic attributes of a client's voice to form an opinion about whether he or she has glottic cancer or some type of noncancerous pathology (see Cox & Morrison, 1983). Or it may be possible to use aphasia test performance data to identify the diagnostic category in which the client best fits (see Beyer, 1988). Furthermore, it may be possible to use data on a client's hearing to make a preliminary hearing aid selection—his or her requirements would be matched with characteristics (attributes) of available instruments (see Craig & Siegenthaler, 1981, and Donnelly, 1982). Classifications of this type may be based, at least in part, on a discriminant function analysis (see Silverman, 1993a, pp. 217-219).

There are several types of diagnostic decisions for which *expert system* software can provide a second opinion. One is whether a client has a communicative disorder—such as whether a preschool-age child is beginning to stutter (*Childhood Stuttering—A Second Opinion*, no date; Silverman, 1985b). A second concerns the etiology of a client's disorder—for example, why a child is slow in developing language or why an adult is having difficulty understanding speech.

Expert system software can also be helpful when formulating statements of prognosis, such as the likelihood that an aphasic will benefit from further therapy (see Figure 4.5 for a screen from such a program by Barsella & Silverman, 1986). As our knowledge base concerning the impacts of specific intervention strategies increases, the accuracy of our statements about the amount that particular clients are likely to benefit from them will improve.

Expert system software can assist you clinically in another way—interpreting a client's test data during an evaluation and making decisions about what additional

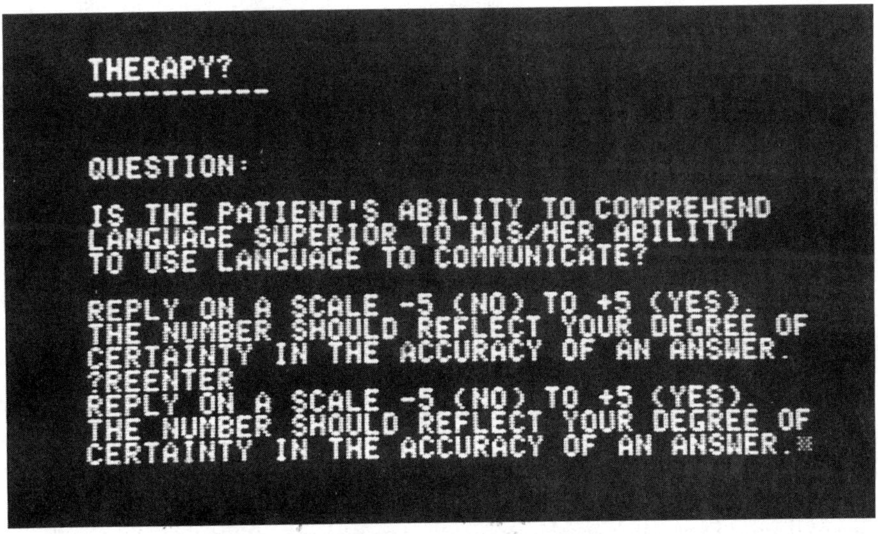

FIGURE 4.5 **A question screen from an expert system program for estimating the likelihood that an aphasic will benefit from further therapy (from Barsella & Silverman, 1986).**

tests should be administered. Expert system software has been used, for example, to help interpret responses to audiometric tests and to make recommendations for further testing based on them (Coupland, 1988; Delgado & Miskiel, 1991; McMillan, Gardiner, & McMillan, 1990; Thornton, Han, Halpin, & Hou, 1992).

The potential of expert system software for facilitating clinical decision making in our field is largely unexplored. Few expert system programs were being marketed to speech-language pathologists and audiologists when this chapter was written. It is likely that such programs could be quite helpful to practitioners in our field judging by the impact that they have had on decision making in other fields (Bull, 1989). They do not require much programming expertise to author because *shell programs* —ones to which you only need to add "content" information—are available for all microcomputers. There is, incidentally, a listing for a BASIC language shell program for the Apple II microcomputer (Naylor, 1983, Chapter 10) that is adequate for creating two-choice (e.g., normal-abnormal) expert system programs (Barsella & Silverman, 1986; Silverman, 1985b). Programs created with a shell such as this one could help you to make the following decisions:

- Whether a client is likely to benefit from a particular management approach
- Whether a client is likely to benefit sufficiently from further therapy to justify recommending it
- Whether a mentally retarded child is sufficiently likely to be capable of learning manual communication to justify a trial program
- Which of two hearing aids would best meet a client's needs
- Whether a client is sufficiently motivated at this time to benefit from therapy
- Whether a client who is severely communicatively impaired is likely to be able to learn to use a particular augmentative communication aid
- Which of two hypotheses is most viable for explaining a client's communicative disorder

There are, incidentally, shell programs for all microcomputers that you can use to create software that will help you to make decisions in which there are more than two choices.

While expert system software doesn't require programming expertise to author because of the availability of shell programs, it does require input from experienced clinicians. The persons whose opinions such programs are intended to simulate are experienced clinicians, not researchers or computer programmers.

Report Writing

One of the main ways that speech-language pathologists and audiologists use microcomputers in the diagnostic (assessment) process is for writing reports. This application is dealt with in Chapter 7.

THERAPY (INTERVENTION) SOFTWARE

Microcomputers have tremendous potential for facilitating the management of communicative disorders. They can generate almost any kind of stimulus and record almost any kind of response. They can provide the reinforcement needed for learning and they can stimulate cognitive processes. They can assist in the setting of goals and provide documentation of their achievement. They can augment a client's ability to communicate. They can help clients learn to modify behaviors that contribute to their disorders by providing appropriate feedback for their attempts to modify them. And perhaps most importantly at present, they can enhance the ability of clinicians to provide high quality services to clients that are cost-effective and consequently, compatible with the managed care model (Vekovius, 1995).

Although the potential of computers to facilitate the management of communicative disorders is enormous, we have a long way to go for this potential to be realized. While ASHA surveys suggest that the majority of speech-language pathologists and audiologists are using computers for report writing, this does not appear to be true for intervention-related tasks (see Chapter 1). The reason may be partially that clinicians are not aware of some of the ways that computers can facilitate their clinical activities and partially that some of the potential intervention applications of computers for clients who have communicative disorders have not been explored. Consequently, we will examine here both what has been done clinically with computers and what it might be possible to do clinically with them.

The programs available to facilitate intervention are of two types. With those of the first type, the clinician uses a computer and the client doesn't. And with those of the second type, the client uses a computer either by himself or herself or together with a clinician or someone else—a paraprofessional or a caregiver. Some of the programs that you can use to facilitate managing your clients' communicative disorders—for example, word-processing, database, drawing, authoring, and education programs—are rarely marketed for this application (Allen, 1990).

Applications Where Clinicians—Not Clients—Use Computers

Five activities for which clinicians use computers to facilitate the intervention process are goal setting, preparing therapy materials, reinforcing and tracking client responses, report writing, and evaluating therapy outcome (auditing). With these, the clinician interacts with the computer.

Goal Setting. Microcomputers have been used by speech-language pathologists and audiologists to facilitate the selection of long- and short-term goals for their clients—particularly school-age children—and to prepare reports (e.g., IEPs) in which goals are specified (see Block, 1991; Iverson, 1990; Iverson & Iverson, 1991;

Jenkins, 1987; Kelly, Richmond, Wesolowski, & Heuer, 1987; Nelson, 1991; Schetz, Miller, & Bernier, 1991; Schuldt & Harding, 1985; Scudder, 1990; Stoker, 1983; Sun, 1990; Swanson & Griffin, 1984; Zemmol, 1985). Some of these papers describe clinician-compiled databases and others describe databases that have been marketed with sets of goals built in (e.g., IEP programs).

You can use almost any database management system software for compiling a database of goals (and possibly subgoals) for persons who have a particular communicative disorder (see Chapter 9). There are several factors that determine the usefulness of such a database. One is the comprehensiveness of the set of goals it can generate. To assess a set's comprehensiveness, check it against the goals you have recommended for clients with this disorder and/or those that are recommended in the clinical literature for such clients.

A second factor that affects such a database's value is the ability of a user to access it with meaningful selection criteria. The criteria should be those that you would ordinarily use to select goals for clients. Such criteria would include information about the client—for example, his or her age, sex, motivation level, and cultural background. It also would include information about the disorder—for example, its severity, the length of time the client has had it, the client's attitude toward it and toward therapy, and its symptomatology and etiology—and previous therapy that the client has received.

A third factor that affects the usefulness of a database is whether goals can be incorporated into reports without having to be rekeyboarded. It is desirable for the program to be capable of saving the goals it recommends in a file that can be "read" by your word-processing program. By using your word-processing program's mail-merge function (see Chapter 7), it would be possible for you to insert goals in reports automatically.

The goals yielded by such a database should merely be regarded as *suggestions*. If they agree with the ones you would have selected without the computer, this would support yours being appropriate. If they disagree, this does not necessarily indicate that yours are inappropriate. What it does mean is that you should carefully think through the probable outcome of adhering to each set of goals and then select the set that seems most likely to be both achievable by and helpful to the client.

Preparing Therapy Materials. Communicative disorders specialists have used computers to prepare items needed for therapy tasks. Such items include printed materials (e.g., exercise sheets) for readers and nonreaders (Blache & Friend, 1985; Montgomery, Walden, & Prosek, 1986; Pentz, 1991). They also include computer software (Bless et al., 1992; Bluestone, 1991, 1992a; Dressler, 1992; Fischer, 1991a, 1992a, 1992b, 1993; Leeper, 1992a; Lieberth, 1992; Lieberth & Martin, 1992).

There are several types of computer software that you can use, alone or in combination, to prepare such items. One of the most useful is word-processing software (see Chapter 7). It can be used for preparing any type of printed material that contains text or a combination of text and drawings. Drawings can be "imported" by word-processing software and combined with text on pages. Most word-processing programs can print pages of almost any size—from those that are small enough to fit in a client's pocket to ones that are poster size; pages that are larger than letter size are usually printed in sections and taped or glued together. A text font and character size combination sometimes can be identified (usually by trial and error) that will at least partially compensate for a client's visual impairments. Text and graphics can be printed in color by most word-processing programs; doing so sometimes can enhance an item's usefulness. Individual text and graphic elements can be stored in "scrapbook" and similar computer files, from which they can be "copied" and "pasted" on practice sheets for individual clients. This approach enables clinicians to tailor practice materials to the needs of individual clients in a way that is likely to be regarded by administrators and third-party payers as being cost-effective.

Another type of computer software that can be used for preparing printed items for therapy tasks is that intended for desktop publishing (see Chapter 7). It can be used for creating the same types of items as word-processing software. However, it offers more options than word-processing software for organizing text and graphics on a page. It can be particularly useful for creating therapy materials that combine text with photographs in black-and-white or color.

A third type of program that can be useful for preparing both printed materials and software for doing therapy tasks is graphic software. This category includes programs for creating drawings and for preparing photographs to be printed (see Chapter 6). It also includes disks containing *clip art*, diskettes and CD-ROM disks that contain large numbers of drawings, sometimes thousands of them. Each contains one or more categories of drawings—for example, animals or common objects found in the home. You can insert copies of these drawings in clinical materials that you create without having to obtain the publisher's permission because the drawings either are not copyrighted or they are copyrighted but the publisher gives you a license (permission) to use them.

A fourth type of program that can facilitate the preparation of software for doing therapy tasks is multimedia authoring software, such as HyperCard (see Chapter 13). Such software enables you to prepare multimedia (containing print, drawings, photographs, video clips, and sound) clinical materials with little or no knowledge of computer programming. Your clients may be instructed to respond to the stimuli displayed on the monitor screen by either verbalizing (or otherwise communicating) their responses to you or by inputing them (with a keyboard, touch screen, or other device) into the computer.

Another type of program that can facilitate the preparation of software for doing therapy tasks in which clients respond to stimuli on the monitor screen by verbalizing (or otherwise communicating) their responses to the clinician is desktop presentation software (see Chapter 8). While such software was never intended to be used for creating therapy stimulus materials, it has a capability that makes it useful for this purpose—it can be used to create and present slide shows. Screens containing text, graphics, or combinations of the two are viewed metaphorically as slides that are being "projected" on a monitor screen. Such slides can be projected in any sequence and can be created *without any knowledge* of computer programming. You can create the graphics for such slides with the desktop presentations program you are using or you can "import" ones that you created with a drawing program or those from a clip art disk.

These are not the only types of programs that can facilitate the preparation of therapy materials, some specialized ones can also facilitate doing so—for example, software for creating animation and virtual reality simulations (see Chapter 15). The types of software that were discussed in this section are general purpose ones to which clinicians are likely to have access.

Reinforcing and/or Tracking Client Responses. While some software of this type only performs one of these functions, most perform both of them. Programs that can do both enable you to reinforce a client's responses to drill stimuli as well as store the data needed to determine the percentage of his or her correct responses. Some of them can compute this percentage for you and/or plot a client's percentage of correct responses over time.

To use such a program to reinforce a client, you could press a preassigned key on the keyboard each time that he or she responded to a stimulus (Pentz, 1987b). If the response was correct, you would press the "positive reinforcement" key, which could result, for example, in a "smiling face" being displayed on the monitor. And if the response was incorrect, you would press the "error" key, which could result in a "sad face" being displayed. The number of correct and incorrect responses—that is, the number of times that each key was pressed—could be tallied by the computer and the percentage of the total number of responses that were correct (i.e., the percentage that were activations of the "positive" reinforcement key) could be computed and, if desired, saved on a disk. You could create the software needed to do these tasks with HyperCard or a similar authoring program (see Chapter 13).

Report Writing. Of course, you can use word processing software to write progress notes and other types of clinical reports. Report writing software is being marketed to speech-language pathologists and audiologists for doing specific types of reports, such as IEPs (see Chapter 7), however, its use is not widespread. The main reason probably is that such reports can be written about as easily with standard word-processing programs using templates (see Chapter 7).

Auditing. All clinicians are now required to document for their employers and for governmental and insurance agencies the impacts of interventions on their clients. The importance of such documentation is likely to increase as the managed care model (Vekovius, 1995) becomes increasingly implemented. Several types of software that can facilitate the preparation of such documentation are discussed in this section.

One type of software that can be particularly useful for preparing auditing documentation is database software (see Chapter 9). You use it to create a database to store the data that you will need. This database would contain a record for each client. The fields in these records would contain the information you need for documentation; you, of course, could also include fields in the records that contain information you use for other purposes. Most database programs permit you to define certain fields as numerical ones and automatically perform calculations on the numbers in them. This feature could allow you to calculate, for example, the number of client sessions of a particular type during a particular time period. While almost any database software can be used for reporting outcome measures, some was developed specifically for doing so (Merson, Rolnick, & Weiner, 1995a, 1995b).

Another type of software that can be useful for preparing auditing documentation is spreadsheet software (see Chapter 10). You could use database software (see Chapter 9) to store the data and spreadsheet software to analyze it. Actually, you probably could use a spreadsheet program for both storing and analyzing data; most spreadsheet programs have database capabilities that should be adequate for this purpose (see Chapter 10).

A third type of software that can be useful for preparing documentation is that for drawing graphs (see Chapter 6). To create a graph with such software, you just have to enter the numbers to be plotted and specify the type of graph (e.g., line, bar, or pie). Graphs created with this software and printed with an ink jet or laser printer are comparable in quality to those drawn by a graphic artist. (In fact, graphic artists now use this software.) Such graphs can be included in year-end reports. They also can be used to document progress for individual clients. For example, a line graph could be used to document changes in the percentage correct of a particular behavior (e.g., the /r/ phoneme) over time. Such documentation could be regarded as more credible (objective and/or scientific) by third-party payers than the same information presented in paragraph form.

A fourth type of software that would be used almost universally for preparing auditing documentation is word-processing software (see Chapter 7). Few clinicians now would prepare any type of report that will be read by persons other than themselves without it.

Applications Used by Clients or Clinicians and Clients Together

Thus far, we have dealt with ways that clinicians can use microcomputers to facilitate the intervention process without having clients interact with them. In this section, we will consider ways that clinicians can facilitate this process by having their clients interact with microcomputers. These include having them use microcomputers for drill practice, simulation, and counseling, and as a "tool" for augmentative communication and writing. The software that they use for doing so may be on a disk in the computer they are using or on one in a computer that they access on-line with telecommunication software (see Chapter 11 and Burk & Bryant, 1993).

Drill-Practice Software. The discussion in this section overlaps some with the preparation of therapy materials described elsewhere in this chapter. The focus here is different—it is on the use of drill-practice software that is not created by the clinician.

Most of the programs that have been marketed to speech-language pathologists and audiologists for "teaching" clients are of this type. The microcomputer is used to facilitate learning by providing opportunities for practice. Its function may be solely to present stimuli—for example, animated pictures of ongoing activities (see Harn, 1986). Clinicians working with persons who are hard-of-hearing or deaf, for example, have used drill-practice programs to provide practice in communicating, speaking, auditory training, and speechreading (Benguerel & Pichora-Fuller, 1988, 1989; Boothroyd, 1987; Boothroyd, Archambault, Adams, & Storm, 1975; Boothroyd, Hanin, & Waltzman, 1987; Boothroyd & Hnath-Chisolm, 1988; Brady & Dickson, 1983; Brooks, Fallside, Gulian, & Hinds, 1981; Dinon & Parsons, 1989; Fujiu, 1989; Gagné, Dinon, & Parsons, 1989, 1991; Grossman, Siders, & Garraway, 1983; Hanin, Boothroyd, & Hnath-Chisolm, 1988; Hight, 1981; Kihneman & Salathiel, 1981; Nickerson, Kalikow, & Stevens, 1976; Nickerson, Stevens, Rollins, & Zue, 1983; Nicolaou, 1988; Pichora-Fuller & Benguerel, 1990, 1991; Pichora-Fuller & Cicchelli, 1986; Quigley & Sanborn, 1992; Sims, 1988; Sims & Clymer, 1986; Sims & Cronic, 1979; Sims, VonFeldt, Dowaliby, Hutchinson, & Meyers, 1979; Tye-Murray & Tyler, 1988; Tye-Murray, Tyler, Bong, & Nares, 1988). And speech-language pathologists have used drill-practice programs for managing their neurologically impaired clients' cognitive, language, and motor impairments (Beck, 1987a; Bloise & Tompkins, 1989; Bluestone & Lefkowitz, 1993; Bracy, 1983; Brown, 1987a; Brubaker & Rolnick, 1985; Craig & Hickey, 1992; Cranley, 1985; Dikeman & Kerman-Lerner, 1989; Dillon & Weiner, 1995a-1995n; Dressler, 1992; Glisky, Schacter, & Tulving, 1986; Hanson & Hooper, 1988; Hinckley, Packard, & Bardach, 1995; Johnson & Kasica, 1984; Katz, 1984, 1986; Katz & Nagy, 1982; Katz, Wertz, Davidoff, Shubitowski, & Devitt, 1988; Katz, Wertz, Lewis, Esparza, & Goldojarb, 1989; King & Hux, 1995; Krogulski, 1988; Loverso & Prescott, 1986; Loverso, Prescott, Selinger, & Riley, 1989; Major & Wilson, 1985; Mills, 1986b, 1986d; Mills, Schatz, & Langmore, 1986; Mills & Thomas, 1981; Mitchell & Owens, 1985; Montgomery & Dean, 1988; Netsell, 1994; Petheram, 1991; Pitts, 1991; Prescott & Loverso, 1985; Raade & Reaburn, 1993; Robertson, 1990; Ruff, Mahaffey, Engel, Farrow, Cox, & Karzmark, 1994; Seron, Deloche, Moulard, & Rousselle, 1980; Vogel, 1988; Weiner, 1995a-1995z, 1995bb-1995hh, 1995jj-1995ww; Wertz, Katz, & Loverso, 1991; Whiteside & Whiteside, 1986).

There are drills for attaining most of the goals for which these programs are intended that can be administered without a computer. Why, then, would you want to use drills that require a computer? There could be several possible reasons. One is that doing so enables you to hold a client's attention for a longer time than you would have been able to otherwise (Ferguson, 1993). Drills tend to be boring because they are repetitious. Consequently, they may not hold a client's attention for a sufficiently long time. If, however, they can be presented in a way that a client finds interesting, they are likely to hold his or her attention longer. Some clients—particularly school-age children—enjoy playing videogames and regard computerized drills as being a type of videogame (see Figure 4.6 for two screens from a language stimulation program that has a videogame format).

A second reason for using a microcomputer to administer drills is that a client experiences less anxiety (is more comfortable) when drills are administered in this way (Colby, 1973). A client, rightly or wrongly, may expect you to be less patient and more judgmental (less tolerant of errors) than a computer, and/or he or she may be less embarrassed about making mistakes when drills are administered by a computer than when they are administered by you.

A third reason why you might want to use a microcomputer to administer drills is that it is a *cost-efficient* way to give the client more practice and stimulation than you could provide otherwise. You would use such drills to *supplement* the practice and stimulation that you provide during therapy sessions (see Figure 4.7 for a screen from a relatively inexpensive alphabet program that could be used for this purpose). Clients could use the drills at your facility or at their own homes. At your facility, they could be assisted by a paraprofessional or volunteer. To enable clients to use the drills at home, you would either provide software that is compatible with a computer that they own or arrange to have them borrow, purchase, rent, or lease a compatible computer. You would probably also have to arrange to have the client performing the drills supervised by someone in the family. A drill administered in this way can be just as effective as one administered by a clinician (Harrison & Engelman, 1992).

Three types of drill-practice software can help clients who have communicative disorders to achieve their goals. The first is drill-practice software that is intended specifically for helping them do so. Most drill-practice software intended for this purpose is currently being marketed for Macintosh and IBM-compatible computers, including those using Windows. Be aware, however, that there is still a great deal of such drill-practice software available for Apple II microcomputers. These computers now can often be purchased (from classified advertisements in newspapers) for a few hundred dollars. Many drill-practice programs of this type for IBM-compatible, Macintosh, and Apple II computers are included in the References and Bibliography

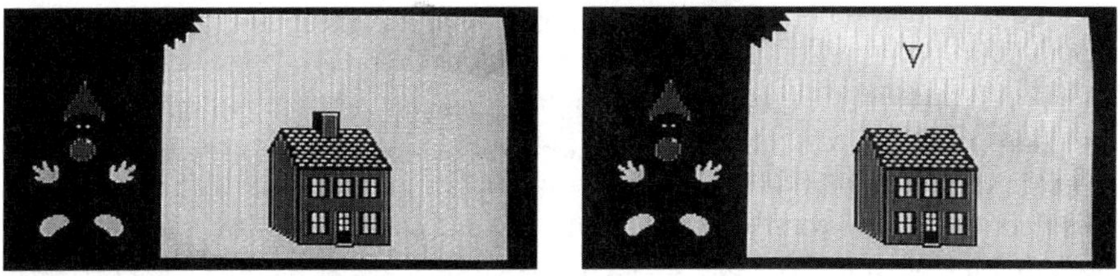

A B

FIGURE 4.6 **A language stimulation program with a videogame format. (A) A pre-response screen. (B) A post-response screen. (From Wilson & Fox, 1991d)**

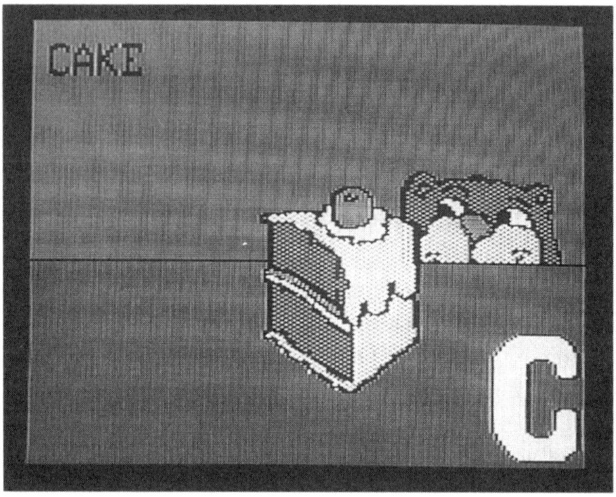

FIGURE 4.7 **A screen from an alphabet program that a client could use at home to supplement therapy. (From Optimum Resources, 1986)**

at the end of the book. Computer program listings are labelled. Many reviews of such programs also are included in the References and Bibliography; these are also labelled. Furthermore, there is a directory of publishers of clinical software in Appendix C that includes those who market drill-practice programs.

The second type of drill-practice software that can help clients with communicative disorders to achieve their goals is software intended for educational purposes. Educational software that a clinician can use for this purpose as is or with minor modification is available for all microcomputers (see Boyd & Denenberg, 1992; Burns, 1985; Orwig & Hodges, 1982; Schetz & Sheese, 1989; Williams & Watt, 1993). You may find software in the public domain—not copyrighted—particularly useful. These are referred to as freeware (see Chapter 3) and can be downloaded from computers that can be accessed through the Internet and another telecomputer network (see Chapter 11). Included in this group are "shell" programs for creating drills having a multiple-choice format. Some of these shells provide videogame-type reinforcers such a "hang man." There also are freeware shell programs for creating drills that require fill-in-the-blank and other types of responses.

The third type of drill-practice software that can help clients with communicative disorders to achieve their goals is software that clinicians create with an authoring program, such as HyperCard (see Bless et al., 1992; Bluestone, 1991, 1992a; Dressler, 1992; Fischer, 1991a, 1992a, 1992b, 1993; Leeper, 1992a; Lieberth, 1992; Lieberth & Martin, 1992). This option is discussed in the section of this chapter on preparing therapy materials and in Chapter 13.

Some drill-practice programs teach concepts as well as provide practice for learning them. Programs of this type—which sometimes are referred to as CAI (computer-assisted instruction) or tutorial programs—have been helpful to both clients and clinicians (see Bull, Cochran, & Snell, 1988; Hadjian, Drumm, & Haynes-Drumm, 1994; Hughes, Fey, Kertoy, & Nelson, 1994). For information about creating them, see Chapter 13.

Simulation. These programs tend to be more sophisticated than drill-practice ones (Bermejo, 1985). Their goal is to promote understanding or insight by *simulating events*. According to Ma (1985, p. 10): "Here learning is less a commodity than a process. It is characterized by an intellectual thrill (the great 'aha!')—an experience all to rare. . . . And because the burst of realization feels good, it's habit-forming."

Speech-language pathologists and audiologists have used simulation programs in several ways. Audiologists have used them to train clinicians to do hearing testing (Domico, 1986; Durham, Thelin, & Muenchen, 1993; Finley, 1984; Glascoe, 1984a; Hood & Zimmerman, 1980, 1981; Mitchell, 1986; O'Rouke-Jackson, 1985; Pawluk, 1986; Robins, 1996; Smith, 1990; Townsend, 1989b; Yanz & Siegel, 1985). Certain of the keys on a computer keyboard are used to simulate audiometer controls and the computer is programmed to respond like a person who has a particular kind of hearing loss. Audiologists have also used simulation programs to train clinicians to take case histories (Lotterman & Barry, 1985).

Speech-language pathologists have used simulation programs to train students to do therapy with stutterers (Meyers & Strang, 1988). They have also used them to train clients to use various types of augmentative communication devices (Mizuko, 1991). The computer is programmed to simulate a particular type of dedicated communication device (see Chapter 5).

Speech-language pathologists and audiologists to date have used simulation programs primarily for training clinicians. There are several ways they probably could use them with clients other than for simulating dedicated augmentative communication devices (Mizuko, 1991). One would be for training clients to react appropriately under such circumstances as being patronized or teased. The computer would be programmed to respond to the client's responses (made using a multiple-choice format) as the person he or she is confronting would be likely to do. Another would be to increase young children's comprehension of semantic/pragmatic "rules" by using computer simulations of object manipulation tasks (Duncan, Skarakis-Doyle, & Haaf, 1993). A third would be to simulate a context that would facilitate client-clinician interaction during therapy. For example, the monitor screen could simulate a window of a car that is touring a zoo. The client would view the various animals that the clinician wanted him or her to learn to name through this "window". The HyperCard program (see Chapter 13) could be used to create the necessary software.

Another clinical activity for which simulation software may be helpful is parent/caregiver training. Situations could be simulated to which we want parents/caregivers to learn to respond appropriately. For example, situations could be simulated in which a preschool child is being disfluent and/or reacting to being disfluent in a particular way. The parent/caregiver could either respond to questions about the child's speech or the child's reactions to being disfluent using the computer or discuss the situation being depicted with the clinician. The software needed for this type of simulation could be created with HyperCard (see Chapter 13).

The behaviors that a clinician attempts to modify with a simulation program can be involuntary ones—such as, reacting to particular stimuli with anxiety. For example, a clinician could use systematic desensitization incorporating a microcomputer simulation of a telephone to reduce the extent to which a stutterer reacts to one with anxiety. The use of virtual reality instrumentation could make the simulation more realistic (see Chapter 15).

Tools. With programs of this type, clients use microcomputers as tools for doing something, one of the main tasks for which they use them in this manner is augmenting their ability to communicate. Some severely communicatively impaired children and adults rely on microcomputer-based augmentative communication devices for partially or totally meeting their communication needs (see Chapter 5).

Some persons use microcomputers (with modems) to communicate by telephone. Incidentally, the devices that most hearing-impaired persons use for this purpose (i.e., telecommunication devices for the deaf or TDDs) are actually *dedicated* microcomputers—ones that have been programmed to do a single task (see Chapter 15).

Microcomputers can also be used as tools by clients who are not severely communicatively impaired. Word processing programs with spell-check commands, for example, can be used by aphasics who have limited ability to spell (Clarke & Aagaard, 1990).

Parent (Spouse) Counseling. You can use a microcomputer to provide members of a client's family with essential information on his or her communicative disorder (e.g., Lieberth, 1992; Silverman, 1985c; Wynne, Martin, & Matt, 1995). Interactive CAI (Computer Assisted Instruction) tutorials for this purpose can be created with HyperCard and similar authoring programs (see Chapter 13). An interactive CAI tutorial is one in which the user responds to questions displayed on the monitor screen using a keyboard, touch screen, or other input device (see Chapter 2). Figure 4.8 illustrates a screen from such a tutorial.

The content of a tutorial intended to provide family members with information about a client's communicative disorder(s) is apt to be quite similar to that of a pamphlet that could be used for the purpose. Why, then, use a computer? A computer tutorial is likely to hold their attention longer than a pamphlet because of its novelty and the fact that it is interactive—they are required to respond in some way to what they see on the screen and/or hear. Perhaps the best strategy would be to use both. That is, after a family member completes the tutorial he or she would be given a handout (possibly a pamphlet) that restates the main points in the tutorial.

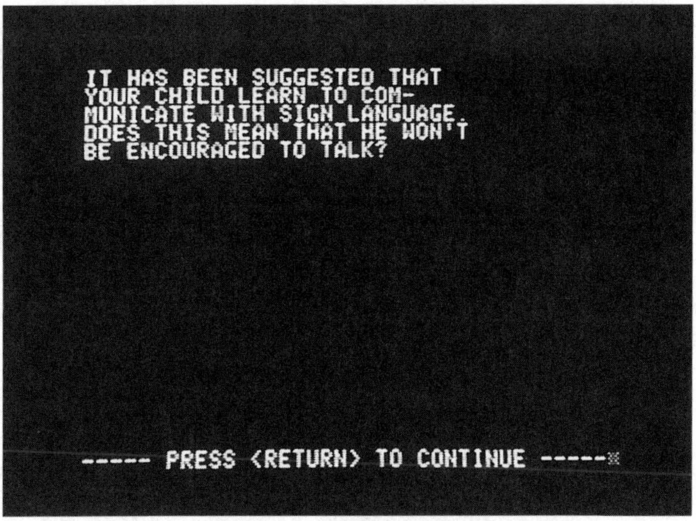

FIGURE 4.8 **The opening screen from an interactive CAI tutorial (from Silverman, 1985c).**

CONSIDERATIONS FOR EVALUATING AND DESIGNING SOFTWARE TO BE USED BY CLIENTS

Some clinical software that has been marketed for use with children and adults who have communicative disorders appears to have been designed by persons who were more knowledgeable about computer programming than about clients who have these disorders. Attributes that influenced this conclusion included the following:

- Displaying printing on the screen that is relatively small. This is particularly inappropriate for drill/practice software intended for aphasics who often have visual problems as well as language ones.
- Displaying instructions on the screen that are too complex to be easily understood by clients who will be using the software. This, like the previous item, is particularly inappropriate for drill/practice software intended for aphasics because their language deficits often include cognitive and reading ones.
- Displaying extraneous text and/or graphics on screens. Many children and adults with whom we work tend to be distractible. Consequently, the only stimulus material displayed should be that to which we want the client to attend.
- Using drawings that are too abstract. Many of the children and adults with whom we work have cortical damage and consequently, are likely to evince

abstract/concrete imbalance (Silverman, 1995). They may not be able to associate, for example, a simple line drawing of a cup with the three-dimensional object that it is intended to depict.

- Using the same reinforcer repeatedly. In some drill/practice software, a single reinforcer is displayed over and over again following a correct response. This reinforcer may be a phrase (e.g., "Correct!") or a graphic (e.g., a "smiling" face). Frequent use of a reinforcer can result in its becoming meaningless.
- The motor requirements for doing a task exceed the abilities of many clients for whom the software is intended. They may have to respond too quickly or they may have to manipulate an input device in a way that exceeds their ability to do so. Clients who are too motor impaired to use a keyboard, for example, may be expected to select items displayed on the screen by moving the cursor to them (i.e., pointing to them) using a mouse.
- The items displayed cannot be modified. For example, in a drill/practice program intended for aphasics in which the items are words and/or phrases, the vocabulary used cannot be modified to meet a client's functional needs.
- The program is unlikely to hold a client's interest for the length of time that it is intended to be used. This can happen for a number of reasons, including the task(s) in it ceasing to be challenging.

The bottom line here is that clinical programs that contain highly sophisticated programming are not necessarily more effective—or even as effective—for accomplishing clinical goals as those containing relatively unsophisticated programming, such as ones you could create with an authoring program such as HyperCard (see Chapter 13).

▶ 5

Augmentative Communication

One aspect of management for which the use of microcomputers is widely accepted is augmenting the communication of persons who are severely communicatively impaired. Such persons—particularly those who have a severe motor impairment—are using microcomputers to enhance their ability to communicate as well as learn, control their environments, and play (Beukelman, Traynor, Poblete, & Warren, 1984; Brandenburg & Vanderheiden, 1987; Bruno, 1994; Clark, 1993; Cohen & DeRuyter, 1982; Colby, Christinaz, Parkinson, Graham, & Karpf, 1981; Costello & Sauer, 1990; Fishman, 1987; Franzwa, 1991a; Fried-Oken, 1989; Gibbs, 1988; Harlan, 1988; Higgins, Baker, Nyberg, & Kushler, 1989; Hillinger, Fox, & Wilson, 1981; Kimmerly, Fox, & Wilson, 1982; Klatt, Tetschner, Tiao, & Pisoni, 1984; Korabic & Silverman, 1983; Korabic, Silverman, & Rosera, 1987; Lawler, 1990; Layton, 1991; Lee & Thomas, 1990; Meyers, 1984; Mills & Thomas, 1983a; Mizuko, 1992, 1993; Mizuko & Hornstadt, 1992a, 1992b; Mizuko, Hornstadt, & Erickson, 1993; Morris & Ray, 1991; Ross, Butt, & Williams, 1991; Rushakoff, 1984d; Rushakoff & Lombardino, 1983, 1984; Salciccia, 1986; Schwartz, Koller, & Koczot, 1984; Shane, 1985, 1990a, 1990b, 1990c; Shannon, Staewen, Miller, & Cohen, 1981; Silverman, 1995; Venkatagiri, 1992, 1994; Wertz, 1983).

A microcomputer can enhance a severely communicatively impaired person's ability to communicate by augmenting his or her ability to acquire and provide information and express feelings by printed and/or spoken messages. Printed messages can be in a natural language, such as English, or in a language consisting of drawings, such as Blissymbolics (Blissymbolics Communication International, 1992a, 1992b; Silverman, 1995). They can be displayed on a monitor screen and/or printed by a computer printer. Messages can be just spoken or they can be both printed and spoken.

Microcomputers can be helpful to persons who are severely communicatively impaired in ways other than augmenting their ability to communicate. They can help them with their *education*. Programs are available for almost all primary, intermediate, and high school subjects. A computer is patient and doesn't make a person feel bad about himself or herself for taking longer than usual to understand a concept. Furthermore, computers can enable some persons who are too motor impaired to write to do written assignments.

Another way that microcomputers can assist some persons who are severely communicatively impaired is by enabling them to control some aspects of their *environment*. They can use a microcomputer to turn electrical devices on and off and manipulate other controls. They can use a microcomputer, for example, to turn a television set on, adjust the volume, and change channels. Other devices that they can control in this manner include telephones, wheelchairs, book page turners, thermostats, and room lights.

A microcomputer can also increase the options for *recreation*. Game programs are available for all microcomputers. Some can be controlled by a special switching mechanism if a person's motor ability isn't adequate to manipulate the switching mechanism that is supposed to be used (e.g., a joystick or keyboard). There are also recreational programs other than games (e.g., drawing programs) that can be controlled in this way.

Finally, microcomputers can enhance the ability to communicate by mail and telephone as well as face-to-face, thereby increasing options for employment and personal relationships for persons who are severely communicatively impaired.

WHAT ARE MICROCOMPUTER-BASED AUGMENTATIVE COMMUNICATION DEVICES?

There are two general types of microcomputer-based augmentative communication devices. The first are *dedicated* to (used exclusively for) communication (Figure 5.1 is a photograph of one such device). Some generate speech, others generate printed messages, and still others generate both. All of the ones that are being marketed now are portable and can be battery operated. Their software is usually on PROM or EPROM chips (see Chapter 2). These devices tend to be relatively expensive because the market is not large enough for them to be mass produced. For further information about dedicated communication devices, see Chapter 5 in Silverman (1995).

Most of the components of the second type of communication device can be purchased at a local computer store. They include a microcomputer (now usually a laptop) and peripherals such as a printer and a speech synthesizer (if the computer doesn't have speech synthesizer circuitry). The same special switching mechanisms that are used to control dedicated communication devices can also be used to control them. These communication devices tend to be less expensive than dedicated ones because most of their components are mass produced.

One advantage of microcomputer-based communication devices over dedicated ones is that they can be used for applications other than communication, including

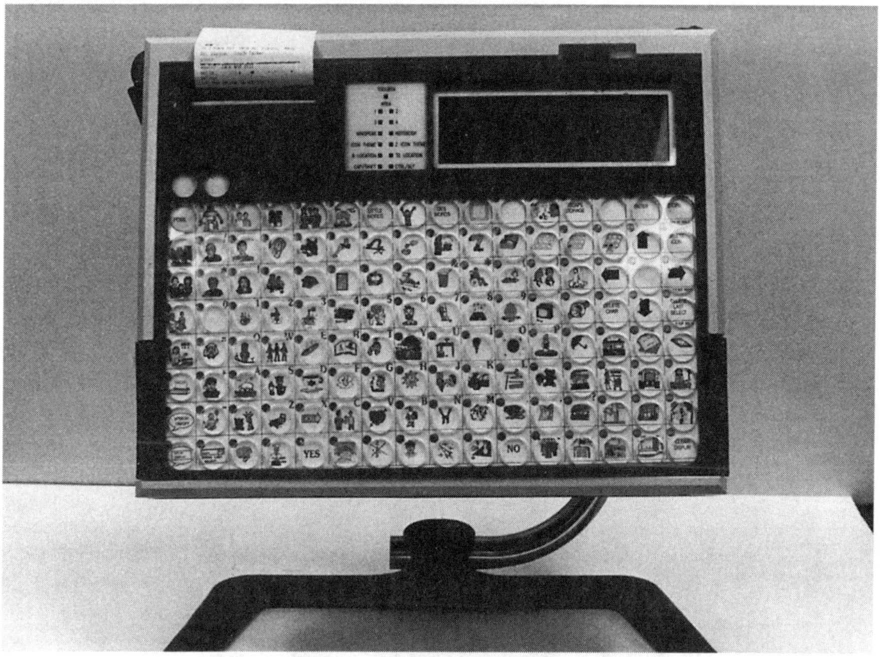

FIGURE 5.1 **A dedicated microcomputer-based augmentative communication device.**

learning, environmental control, and recreation. They can, in fact, be used for doing any task for which the necessary software and peripherals are available.

You can have a client use either a desktop or a laptop (portable) microcomputer for augmentative communication. A desktop computer, however, is likely to be too large to mount on a wheelchair. Laptop computers can be mounted on wheelchairs with the same types of devices that are used for mounting dedicated communication aids on them (Figure 5.2).

Hardware and software components of microcomputer-based augmentative communication aids are described in the next two sections. While the focus is on microcomputer-based communication aids rather than dedicated ones, much of the information presented applies to both types.

HARDWARE COMPONENTS

Most of the hardware components of a microcomputer-based augmentative communication aid can be purchased locally. They include a microcomputer with sufficient RAM to run the software; a disk drive for loading the software into the computer; a

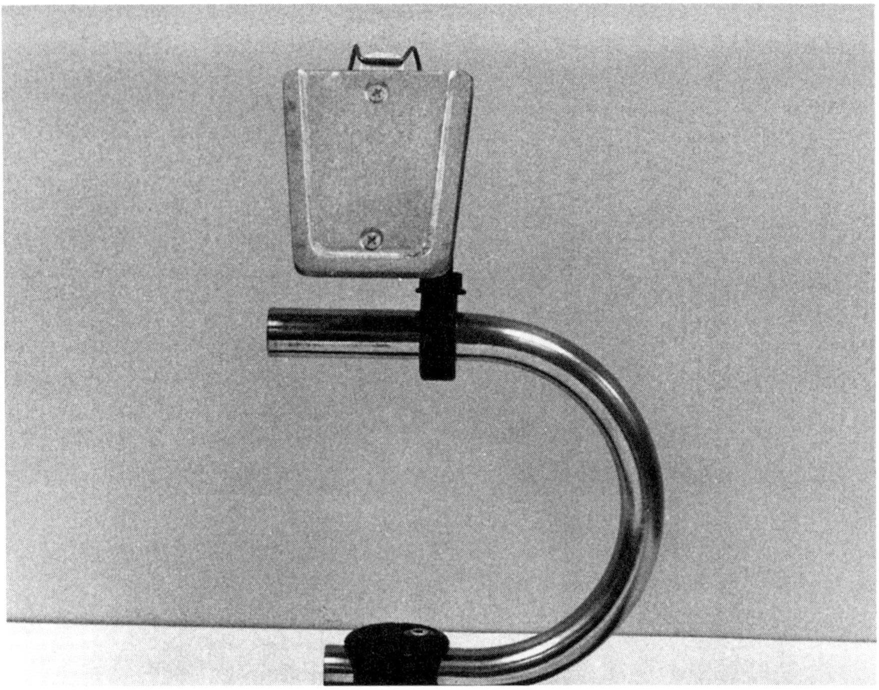

FIGURE 5.2 **A device that can be used for mounting a laptop computer on a wheelchair.**

switching mechanism that enables the person to do what is necessary to generate messages; a monitor, printer, and speech synthesizer for "displaying" the messages that are generated; and a power supply. The requirements for each of these are described below.

The Microcomputer

Almost any microcomputer can be adapted for augmentative communication. Even obsolete inexpensive ones intended for hobbyists—such as the Radio Shack Color Computer, the Commodore 64, and the Timex-Sinclair 1000—can be used for this purpose (Hugghins, 1987; Korabic & Silverman, 1983; Korabic, Silverman, & Rosera, 1987). The most frequently used microcomputers for augmentative communication when this chapter was written were the Apple II, the Apple Macintosh, and IBM compatibles.

One problem you may encounter if you recommend that a client purchase a microcomputer (e.g., a Macintosh or an IBM compatible) for augmentative communication is that he or she cannot afford to do so and third-party funding isn't available. One solution is to recommend the purchase of a used microcomputer. I probably would recommend the Apple II, particularly the IIc model, which has a built-in disk drive. These microcomputers—which can often be purchased used for less than $300—are the ones that were used most often for augmentative communication during the 1980s. A great deal of software and hardware is available to adapt them for this use (see Brightman, 1988). Their main limitation is that they relatively large and do not have a built-in hard drive or monitor. They can, however, be powered by a 12-volt automobile, motorcycle, or electric wheelchair battery.

Storage Devices

Augmentative communication software can be stored on and loaded into the CPU from a diskette, a hard disk, or an EPROM chip (see Chapter 2). Diskettes and hard disks are used more often than EPROM chips. The latter are used mainly—but not exclusively (see Korabic, Silverman, & Rosera, 1987)—for doing so with *dedicated* communication aids (see Chapter 5 in Silverman, 1995).

Output Devices

All microcomputer-based augmentative communication aids either generate or indicate message components. *Generated* message components may be spoken, printed, or signaled by a code (e.g., a buzzer may may be used to communicate "I need help!").

Message components can be *indicated* rather than generated. The alphabet, for example, could be displayed in rows and columns on a monitor screen (Figure 5.3). The cursor would move from letter to letter, remaining with each a predetermined amount of time (e.g., two seconds). When the cursor was with the next letter in the user's message, he or she would activate a switch thereby causing the letter to be added to a word at the bottom of the screen (Figure 5.3). This process is referred to as *linear scanning*.

The output devices that have been used for augmentative communication include: monitors, printers, speech synthesizers, noise and light generators, modems, and environmental control modules. Some of the ways that they have been used for communication and environmental control are described here. The devices themselves are described in Chapter 2.

Computer Monitors. Both desktop computer monitors and those that are built into laptop computers can be used for augmentative communication.

Printers. Many microcomputer setups for augmentative communication include a dot-matrix or inkjet printer (see Chapter 2). For microcomputers mounted on wheelchairs, a small battery-powered printer intended for laptop computers is most practical.

A	B	C	D	E	F
G	H	I	J	K	L
M	N	O	P	Q	R
S	T	U	V	W	X
Y	Z	1	2	3	4
5	6	7	8	9	0

MY NAME IS FRANK

FIGURE 5.3 **The alphabet arranged in rows and columns on a monitor screen for linear or row-column scanning. Messages are printed letter-by-letter at the bottom of the screen.**

Speech Generators. Almost all microcomputers can generate speech. The ability to do so can facilitate both face-to-face and telephone communication. Some microcomputers (e.g., the Macintosh) have the necessary circuitry built into them. While computer-generated speech is almost always intelligible, it may not sound entirely "natural." Processes that generate words from digitized speech samples rather than synthesize the phonemes in them from formant and other acoustical data tend to produce speech that is more natural sounding.

Modems. Modems make it possible for persons who are severely communicatively impaired to communicate (and consequently, interact) with persons outside of their homes. It is *not necessary* that the persons with whom they want to communicate have a microcomputer. It is only necessary that they have a telephone; they can use a telecommunication relay service to connect them (See Chapter 11 and Silverman, 1993b, 1995).

The simplest form of computer communication via telephone—the transmission of computer-generated speech—does not require a modem. It is only necessary that you place the telephone headset close enough to the computer that it can transmit the speech generated by it.

Environmental Control Modules. These are used to turn electrical devices on and off and otherwise control them. They can be helpful to some clients who are severely communicatively impaired because the condition that causes them to be severely dysarthric may also impair the functioning of their upper extremities.

You can link devices that you want a client to be able to control in this manner to a computer, either directly or indirectly. If they are *directly linked* to a computer, they are connected to it by a cable. This type of linkage is usually not desirable if the person is seated in a wheelchair and the device being controlled is not on the wheelchair.

Devices that are *indirectly linked* to a computer are "connected" to it by sound, light, or radio waves rather than a cable. The technology is similar to that used for television set and VCR remote controls. A sound, light, or radio wave *transmitter* is attached to the computer, and an appropriate *receiver* is attached to the device. The use of this type of linkage is particularly advantageous for persons in wheelchairs who want to control devices that are not mounted on their chairs.

Switching Mechanisms (Input Devices)

There are a number of special switching mechanisms and modifications to standard ones that can enable clients who have a neuromuscular disorder to use a microcomputer. Some are described in this section. There is additional information about these and others in Chapter 5 of Silverman (1995).

Keyboards. It may be possible for some of your motor-impaired clients to use a standard keyboard "as is." That is, they may be able to press the keys—each of which is a switch—with a finger (or another part of the hand), a toe (or another part of the foot), or a head or mouth stick. While the speed at which they can type in this manner is likely to be relatively slow, it may be adequate for doing some tasks (e.g., short-answer homework assignments).

If a client isn't sufficiently intact motorically to use a standard keyboard, it may be possible for him or her to do so if it is modified. One of the most common modifications is installing a keyguard (Figure 5.4). This is a sheet of plastic or metal the size of the keyboard that is mounted a fraction of an inch above it. There is a hole in the keyguard above each key. To press a key, a finger or other object (e.g., a headstick) is inserted into the appropriate hole in the keyguard. This device makes it less likely that keys will be pressed accidentally. Keyguards can be purchased for some computer keyboards. They can also be fabricated fairly easily from a keyboard-size sheet of plastic: All that is required is to have someone (perhaps a family member) drill a lot of holes.

There are special keyboards available for persons who are not sufficiently intact motorically or visually to use a standard keyboard with a keyguard. Four of them are described below.

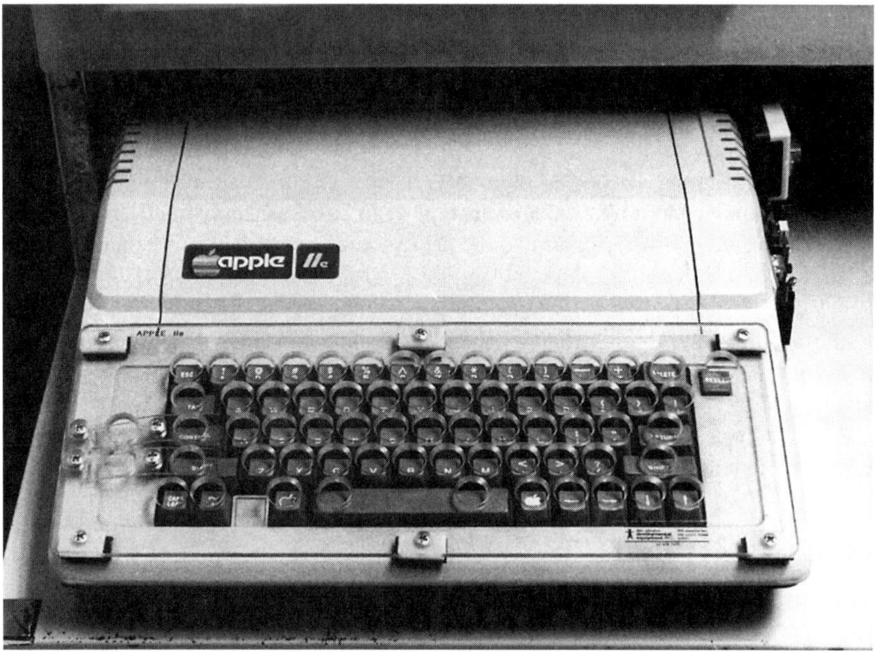

FIGURE 5.4 **A computer keyboard with a keyguard installed.**

Large-key keyboards (Figure 5.5) can compensate for some visual and motor disturbances. Because the keys are larger than those on a standard keyboard, they are both easier to see and activate.

Keyboards with small keys (Figure 5.6) can compensate for some visual field disturbances and limitations in hand or head movement. A client with a visual field disturbance may be unable to see enough of a standard-size keyboard at a time to use it reliably. And a client's range of hand or head movement (if he or she is using a headstick) may be too limited to do so.

Keyboards with photoelectric switches can enable some quadriplegics to use microcomputers. They usually have the same numbers of switches as standard keyboards. Keys are activated by directing a beam of light at them from a device that is attached (usually by a strap) to the user's forehead (Figure 2.5). For further information about photoelectric switches, see Chapter 5 in Silverman (1995).

Keyboard emulation software makes it possible for quadriplegics to run programs requiring the use of a keyboard (e.g., word processing software) by activating a single switch. Most such software displays a keyboard on the monitor screen and causes the cursor to move from key to key every few seconds (Figure 2.5). Activating any kind of a switch (e.g., those described in the next section) when the cursor is on the key the user wants to activate causes it to be activated. Consequently, a quadri-

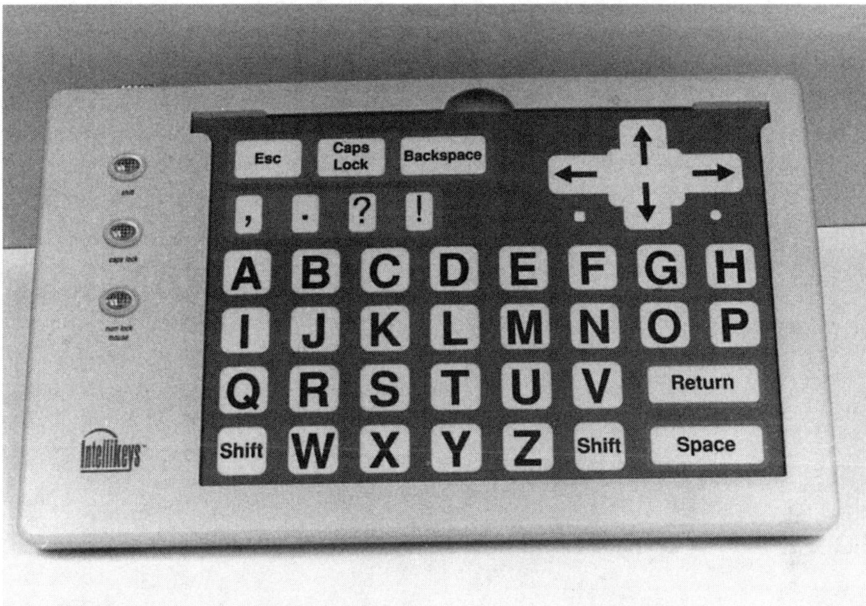

FIGURE 5.5 **A large-key keyboard.**

plegic can do anything with a keyboard emulator that an able-bodied person can do with a keyboard—although more slowly.

Special switching mechanisms. There are a number of types of switches that a client can use alone or in combination with keyboard emulation software to control a microcomputer. Since some programs do not require the use of a keyboard, keyboard emulation software isn't always necessary. A cable usually is used to connect the switch to the computer. The cable may be plugged into the computer's joystick port. Some of these switches are described in this section, and there is additional information about them in Chapter 5 of Silverman (1995).

Push switches have been used most often for augmentative communication because they are the least sophisticated mechanically and, consequently, the least expensive and most reliable. They are activated by applying pressure to (i.e., pushing) a surface. Many types of surfaces have been used including plates (Figure 5.7), hand paddles (Figure 5.8), and vertical shafts (Figure 5.9).

Position switches (also known as *tip-tilt* switches) are activated by a particular movement of a body part, for example, an arm (Figure 5.10). They usually consist of a small globule of mercury and two wire ends in a glass envelope (Figure 5.11). The switch is "on" when its position is such that the globule of mercury touches both wire ends.

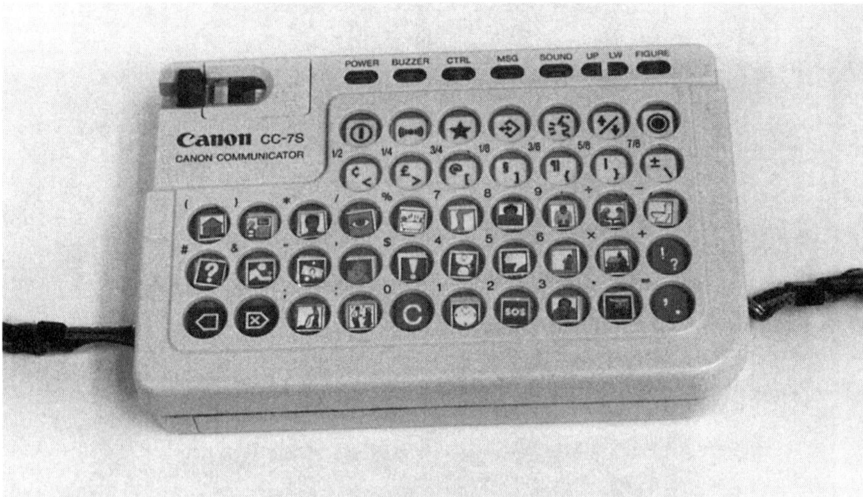

FIGURE 5.6 **A keyboard with smaller than standard size keys.**

Pneumatic switches (also referred to as *suck-blow* switches) are activated by blowing into or sucking on the end of a tube (Figure 5.12).

Sound controlled switches are activated by a noise. The noises that activate them can be generated by a device (e.g., a whistle) or by the vocal tract (e.g., a cough, hum, or prolonged vowel).

Light-controlled switches are activated by directing a beam of light at a photoelectric cell or by interrupting a light beam that is directed at such a device. Photoelectric cells that are activated in the first of these ways can be arranged in rows and columns to simulate keyboards. The client would activate ("press") a key by directing a beam of light on it from a device that is attached by a strap to his or her head (Figure 2.5).

Myoswitches are activated by muscle action potentials. Electrodes are attached to the client's skin over the muscle fibers that he or she contracts to activate the switch. Myoswitches would only be used with clients who are so severely impaired motorically that they are unable to easily activate other types of switches. For further information about myoswitches, see Chapter 6 in Silverman (1995).

EEG-switches are activated by changes in brain waves (Zarrella, 1995). A pair of electrodes are attached to a client's skin over a particular location on his or her skull. The client is trained to activate a switch by changing a brain wave pattern in a particular way that the computer can recognize (Zarrella, 1995). These, like myoswitches, would only be used with clients who are so severely impaired motorically that they cannot easily activate other types.

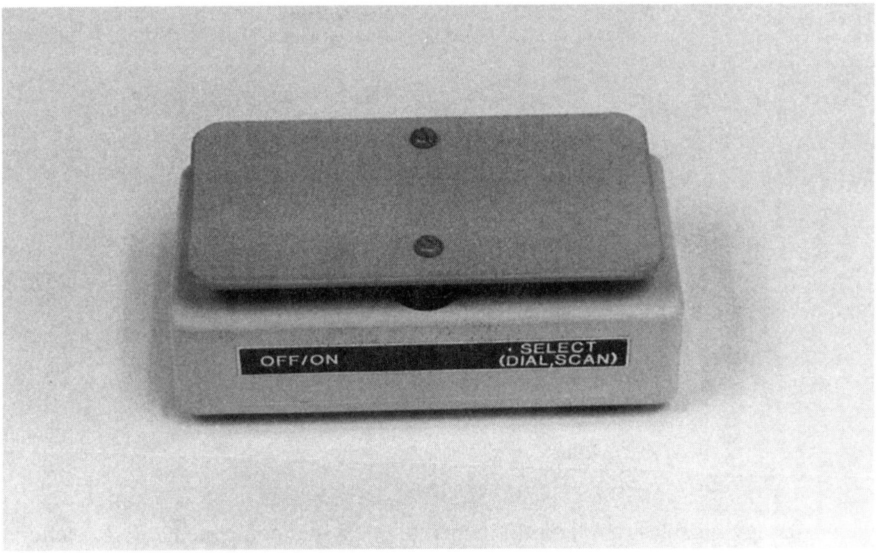

FIGURE 5.7 **Push-plate switching mechanisms.**

Power Supply

Standard house current (110 volts in the United States) is used to power augmentative communication aids that utilize desktop microcomputers. Both batteries and house current are used to power those that utilize laptops. A client probably would use house current to power a laptop when it is practical to do so because the charge in its batteries is likely to be adequate for only a few hours of use.

SOFTWARE

A number of programs are available for microcomputer-based augmentative communication (Benjamin, 1991; Beukelman, Garrett, Lange, & Tice, 1988; Birch & Birch, 1990; Blissymbolics Communication International, 1992a, 1992b; Brightman, 1988; Cohen, 1987; Don Johnson Developmental Equipment, 1990; Fletcher, 1986; Franzwa, 1991a; House & House, 1994; Huer, 1991; King, 1990; Layton, 1991; Mayer-Johnson Company, 1990; Meyers, 1990; Odom, 1991b; Russel, 1990; Shane, 1990a, 1990b, 1990c; Simmons, 1987; *Talk:About*, 1994; Venkatagiri, 1989a, 1992). Each is compatible with one or more of the following strategies for selecting (generating) message component: direct selection, scanning, and encoding. These three strategies are described below.

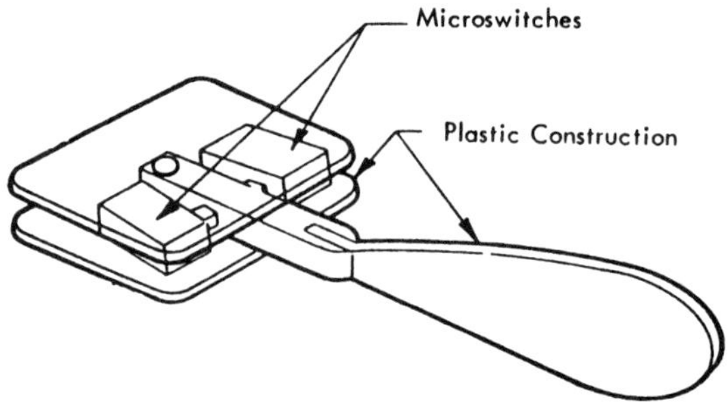

FIGURE 5.8 **A hand paddle switching mechanism.**

Direct Selection

This strategy enables a client to generate message components (e.g., letters) directly—usually with a keyboard that is manipulated by a hand, a foot, or a head-stick (see Bruno & Stoughton, 1984). It is the most efficient (most rapid and least fatiguing) of these strategies. Several types of software that can be used with it to generate message components are described below.

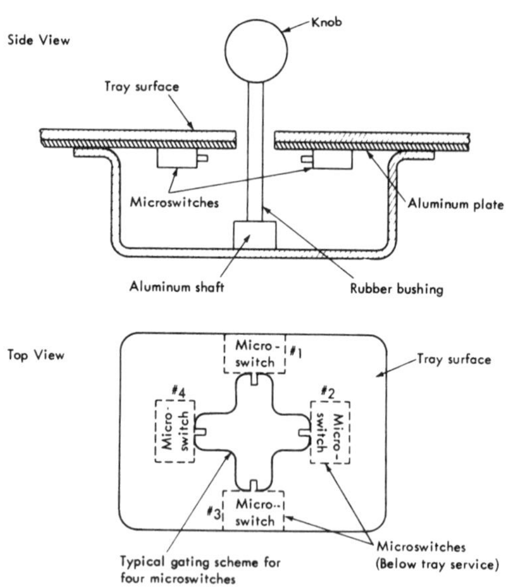

FIGURE 5.9 **A joystick.**

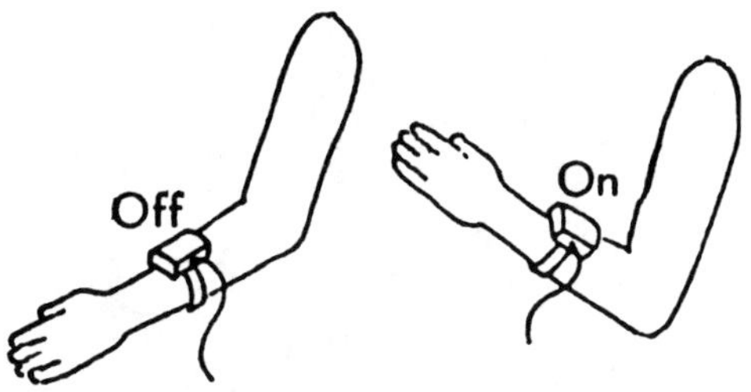

FIGURE 5.10 **A tip-tilt switch strapped to the arm.**

Word-Processing Programs. These programs enable a client to type messages with a standard keyboard or with one that has large, small, or other special kinds of keys. They can be used for generating messages on a monitor screen for face-to-face communication as well as letters and other documents.

Keyboard-Based Speech Generating Programs. These programs reconfigure a keyboard so that spoken messages can be generated with it. Phonemes, letters, words, and phrases needed for synthesizing a message are generated by pressing (or otherwise activating) keys and combinations of keys. Some of these programs will generate printed messages as well as spoken ones.

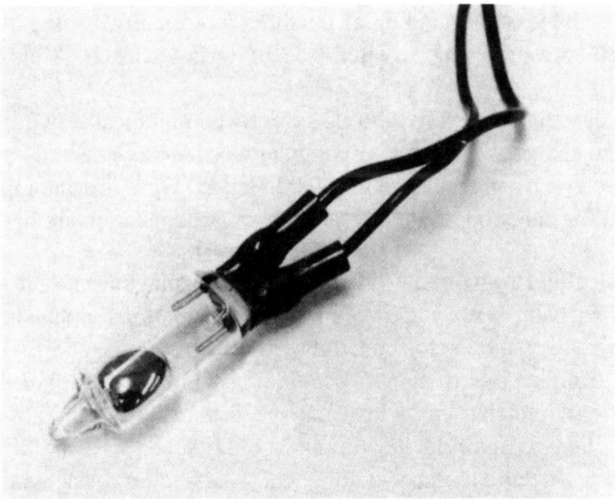

FIGURE 5.11 **A tip-tilt switch mechanism in the "off" position.**

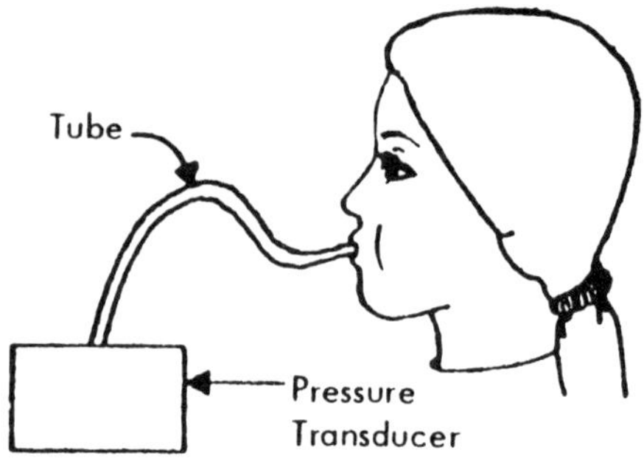

FIGURE 5.12 **A suck-blow switch.**

Pictographic Symbol Programs. These programs enable a client to communicate with pictograms, such as Blissymbols or Picsyms (see Blissymbolics Communication International, 1992a, 1992b). Such message components (pictograms) can be generated by direct selection in two ways. One is to reconfigure a keyboard to draw the components on a monitor screen—there would be a specific key or key combination for each symbol. The other is to indicate which of a group of symbols displayed on a screen (usually in rows and columns) communicates a message (wholly or partially) by moving the cursor to them with a keyboard or other input device—such as a trackball or mouse (see Chapter 2 and Silverman, 1995).

Scanning

This strategy is the least demanding of the three motorically. All the client has to be able to do is to activate a single switch (see Butterfield, 1991). Almost any type of switch can be used.

Scanning can enable persons who are severely communicatively impaired to communicate. It can also enable them to use regular word processing and other productivity software because it can emulate a keyboard. Several types of scanning software that can be utilized for either communication or keyboard emulation are described below.

Alphabet Scanning Programs. These programs display on a monitor screen (usually on the upper half) in rows and columns the letters of the alphabet, digits, punctuation marks, and symbols for functions such as spacing (see Figure 5.3). The cursor moves from symbol to symbol (beginning with the symbol at the left end of the top row). The clinician can adjust the speed that the cursor moves: The more impaired the client is motorically, the slower the speed that the clinician would select. The client selects a message component (e.g., a letter) by activating the switch when the cursor is adjacent to it. The message component selected is printed on the screen—usually the lower half. This process is repeated until the entire message or document is displayed. Some screen displays that are generated by these programs contain a "print" symbol. When the cursor is stopped on it, the content of the screen (minus the scanning display) is printed. Some of these programs (with a speech synthesizer) can cause the computer to "voice" characters as they are being scanned, or printed on the screen, or both.

Clients use one of two scanning strategies for selecting message components with these programs: linear or row-column (Figure 5.13). With *linear* scanning, the cursor moves from symbol to symbol in the first row, beginning at the left end. From the right end of the first row it goes to the left end of the second row. This process continues until it gets to the right end of the last row. The cursor moves from here to the left end of the first row and continues moving in this manner. The client activates the switch when the cursor is adjacent to the symbol that he or she wants to communicate (print). Formulating a message in this way can, of course, be very time consuming.

Row-column scanning is less time consuming than linear scanning. With this strategy, the continual movement of the cursor from symbol to symbol is limited to the first row. When the cursor is in the column containing the symbol the client wants to communicate, he or she activates the switch. The cursor then moves downward in that column. When it reaches the symbol the client wants to communicate, he or she activates the switch a second time. This prints the symbol on the screen and returns the cursor to the left end of the top row. The process is repeated until the entire message has been printed. With some of these programs, the continual movement of the cursor occurs in the first column rather than in the top row: Activating the switch causes the cursor to move from symbol to symbol in the row it was in when the activation occurred. Row-column scanning is more efficient than linear scanning because the cursor can reach target symbols by a more direct route (Figure 5.13).

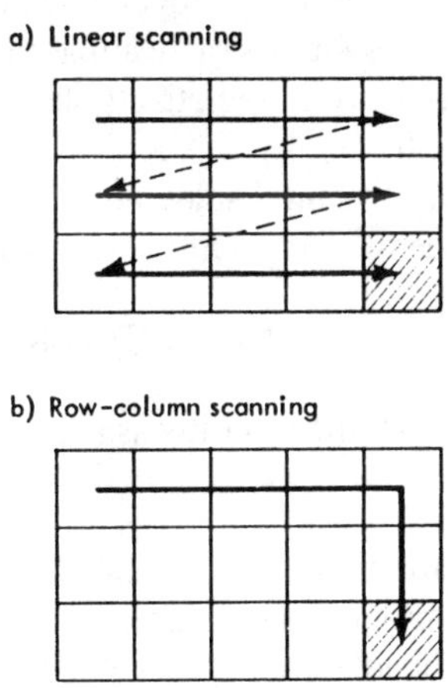

FIGURE 5.13 **Two scanning strategies—linear and row-column.**

Matrix Scanning Programs. These programs divide a monitor screen into cells (rectangles) that are arranged in rows and columns. In each cell there is a message component (e.g., a word/phrase or a pictogram). The message components in the cells may be generated by the program or printed on a transparent sheet (e.g., that used for overhead transparencies) that covers the monitor screen. The client activates the switch when the cursor is in the cell that contains the next component of his or her message. Either a linear or row-column scanning strategy can be used.

Some programs of this type can generate more that one screen ("page") of message components. They utilize a two-step scanning process. The process begins with a screen displaying one or more rows of page numbers. The client stops the cursor when it is adjacent to the number of the page containing the next component of his or her message. That page then appears on the screen and the user repeats the scanning process to select the message component.

Encoding

A code is used here for selecting or generating message components. The client either memorizes the code or refers to it on a chart. Two codes that have been used for this purpose are described below.

Morse Code. The client inputs messages as patterns of dots and dashes (Figure 5.14). The patterns are translated by the computer into alphanumeric characters (letters and numbers) and displayed on the monitor screen (see Beukelman, Traynor, Poblete, & Warren, 1984; King, 1990; King, Noel, Rounds, & Bergo, 1991; Shannon, Staewen, Miller, & Cohen, 1981).

A client can use either a direct-selection or a linear scanning strategy to enter Morse code. He or she can enter it by direct selection with either one or two switches. If it is done with two switches, activating one would input a dot and the other a dash. If a single switch is used, a relatively short activation would input a dot and a relatively long one a dash.

A client could use a four-element display on the monitor screen, similar to the following, to enter Morse code by using a linear scanning strategy:

DOT DASH NEW LETTER NEW WORD

The client would stop the cursor whenever it was adjacent to the next element of the code for his or her message.

Numerical Codes. These are number codes. Each letter, phoneme, word, phrase, and punctuation mark that a program can generate is assigned a two- or three-digit code. A two-digit code can handle 100 message components (00-99) and a three-digit code, a thousand (000-999). A client can generate a message by entering the codes (digits) for its components, in the appropriate order, directly with a keyboard or indirectly by using a single-switch linear scanning strategy.

Symbol	Code	Symbol	Code
A	.-	V	...-
B	-...	W	.--
C	-.-.	X	-..-
D	-..	Y	-.--
E	.	Z	--..
F	..-.	1	.----
G	--.	2	..---
H	....	3	...--
I	..	4	....-
J	.---	5	.....
K	-.-	6	-....
L	.-..	7	--...
M	--	8	---..
N	-.	9	----.
O	---	0	-----
P	.--.	Period	.-.-.-
Q	--.-	Comma	--..--
R	.-.	?	..--..
S	...	Error	....
T	-	Wait	.-...
U	..-	End	.-.-.

FIGURE 5.14 **The International Morse Code.**

PERSONS WHO ARE SEVERELY COMMUNICATIVELY IMPAIRED BECAUSE OF DEAFNESS

The focus in this chapter has been on augmenting the communication of persons who are severely communicatively impaired for reasons other than deafness. The reason for this focus is that AAC specialists historically have not been the ones responsible for augmenting the communication of the deaf. Microcomputers have been used a great deal to augment their communication abilities. For example, computers have been used to augment the classroom notetaking abilities of mainstreamed hearing-impaired students (Kozma-Spytek, Bakke, & Chute, 1995).

6

Creating Drawings, Graphs, and Other Types of Figures

The programs that we have discussed thus far—those for evaluation, therapy, clinical decision making, and augmentative communication—are intended specifically for the management of communicative disorders. Other types of software not specifically intended for clinical activities can facilitate your performing some clinical tasks. Clinical applications of one of them—programs for creating drawings, graphs, and other types of figures—are described in this chapter.

How can the ability to create drawings, graphs, and other types of figures facilitate your clinical activities? There are a number of way that it may be able to do so, including the following:

- Generating pictographic symbols and other graphics for clinical materials, including communication boards (Ashbaugh, 1988; Chial & Kelly, 1987; Lieberth & Martin, 1992; Nye & Pentz, 1987; Phonological Project, Waisman Center on Mental Retardation and Human Development, University of Wisconsin-Madison, 1987; Quinoa, 1988; Shriberg, no date).
- Laying out and printing communication boards (Birch & Birch, 1990; Huer, 1991; Mayer-Johnson Company, 1990; Mizuko & Hornstadt, 1992b; Mizuko, Hornstadt, & Erickson, 1993).
- Preparing printed and computer-administered therapy materials, particularly for nonreaders (Blache & Friend, 1985; Bull & Cochran, 1992; Dressler, 1991, 1992; Harn & Ruder, 1987; Pentz, 1991; Scherz & Koch, 1991; Weiner, 1983).
- Preparing graphs and other figures for reports (Wynne, Friedman, Friedman, & Renshaw, 1993).

- Producing printed forms—for example, those for recording hearing test results (Chial & Kelly, 1987; Walence, 1985).
- Preparing computer-administered tutorials and producing overhead transparencies, slides, videotapes, and handouts for inservice presentations, including multimedia ones (Allen, 1993; Bull & Cochran, 1992; Charpied, 1993; Clarke & Kneil, 1990; Fischer, 1991a, 1991b, 1992b; Larrick, 1992; Lieberth, 1992; Tatchell, Letson, Zlotolow, & DeLauro, 1993).

This list is limited to applications that have been the topic of reports in the speech-language-hearing literature. Undoubtedly, there are others that either have been made but not reported or could be made.

My main objective in this chapter is to acquaint you with the graphic software that you would use for doing clinical tasks such as those mentioned above. This software is available for both Macintosh and IBM-compatible (MS-DOS and Microsoft Windows) platforms.

PAINTING AND DRAWING SOFTWARE

While both painting and drawing programs can be used to create drawings or modify ones that have been scanned into a computer (in either black-and-white or color), they do it differently. Several practical implications of the differences in how they "draw" are discussed in this section.

Paint Programs

Paint programs create drawings (on a screen simulation of a desktop—see Figure 6.1) that consist of rows and columns of tiny dots known as *pixels*. There can be fewer than 100 or more than 300 pixels to the inch. The shape of the dots can be either round or square. The more pixels there are to the inch in a drawing, the less obvious it will be that the drawing is composed of dots.

Illustrations created with paint programs are sometimes referred to as being *bit mapped graphics*. A bit map is the machine language code (see Chapter 3) that generates the pixels in a drawing created with a paint program. For black-and-white drawings that aren't "gray scale," the status of each pixel is designated by one bit in the bit map. More than one bit is needed to designate each pixel in a gray scale drawing; the pixels in these drawings can be shades of gray in addition to black and white. More than one bit also is needed to designate each pixel in a multicolor drawing.

As I have previously indicated, pixels in a non-gray-scale black-and-white illustration are either black or white. Lines in drawings that have a white background consist of black pixels. If all of the pixels that form a line are black, the line will

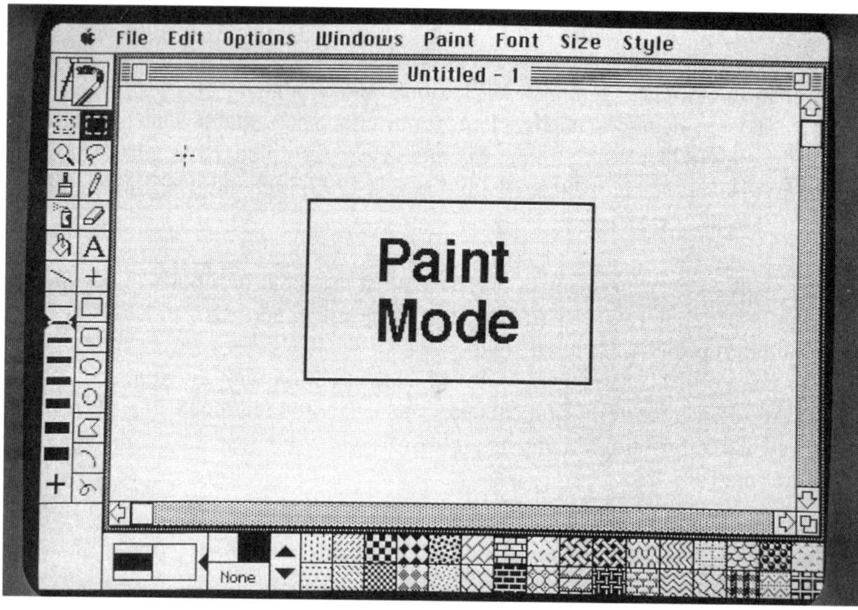

FIGURE 6.1 **The monitor screen "desktop" for a typical paint program.**

appear to be black. However, if only some of the pixels forming the line are black (e.g., every other pixel), the line will appear to be gray. The smaller the percentage of black pixels in a line, the lighter the gray (Figure 6.2). Erasing consists of changing black pixels to white ones if the background is white. If the background is black, it consists of changing white pixels to black ones.

You "paint" by manipulating "tools" with a mouse or other input device. The tools usually are designated by icons. Figure 6.1 is a photograph of the monitor screen "desktop" for a typical paint program. The tool icons are on the left side of the screen. Selecting the "pencil" icon enables you to draw lines; the "A" (alphabet) icon to print words (e.g., "paint mode"); and the "rectangle" icon to draw rectangles. When you manipulate a tool, the program changes the color of some of the pixels in the bit map.

Collections of clip art are a source of graphics for drill-practice materials (see Chapter 4), communication boards (see Chapter 5), and other clinical applications. Clip art is graphics distributed on diskettes and CD-ROM disks (in collections of hundreds or thousands), usually not copyrighted (i.e., they are in the public domain).

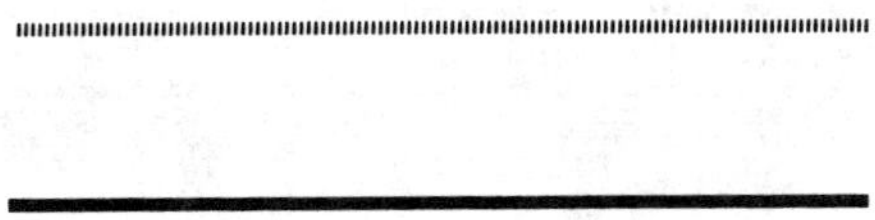

FIGURE 6.2 **Two lines that vary in "darkness" because the number of black pixels in them differ.**

Some are in a file format that a paint program can import. Clip art graphics can be used as is or modified with a paint program.

Draw Programs

Draw programs differ from paint ones in the way that they manipulate pixels. Draw programs do it by issuing *commands*. The computer file for a graphic created with a draw program contains a listing of the commands required to draw it. The computer file for a graphic created with a paint program, on the other hand, contains a bit map that designates the color of each pixel in it. All of the commands that are issued by draw programs manipulate more than one pixel.

There are several languages in which draw programs may issue commands, two of the most common being *QuickDraw* and *Postscript*. The former is used by the Macintosh and the latter by both the Macintosh and by IBM-compatibles. Each time a "tool" is used to change a drawing, instructions are added to or deleted from the file for that drawing.

One advantage that draw programs have over paint ones is that a component of a graphic (e.g., a line or a word) can be manipulated without affecting the others—it can be added to, deleted, moved, and made larger or smaller. A component of a graphic made with a paint program can only be manipulated without affecting the others if the background is white.

A second advantage that draw programs have over paint programs is that drawings can be enlarged without making their dot structure more obvious. The number of dots to the inch printed by an inkjet or laser printer is the same regardless of the size of the drawing. Since drawings created with a paint program have a fixed dot structure, enlarging them is equivalent to viewing them through a magnifying glass—dots appear to be larger and further apart.

The main disadvantage that draw programs have when compared to paint ones is that it is not as easy with them to manipulate individual pixels. This is particularly likely to be a limitation when you are creating graphics with a great deal of fine detail and/or irregular shapes.

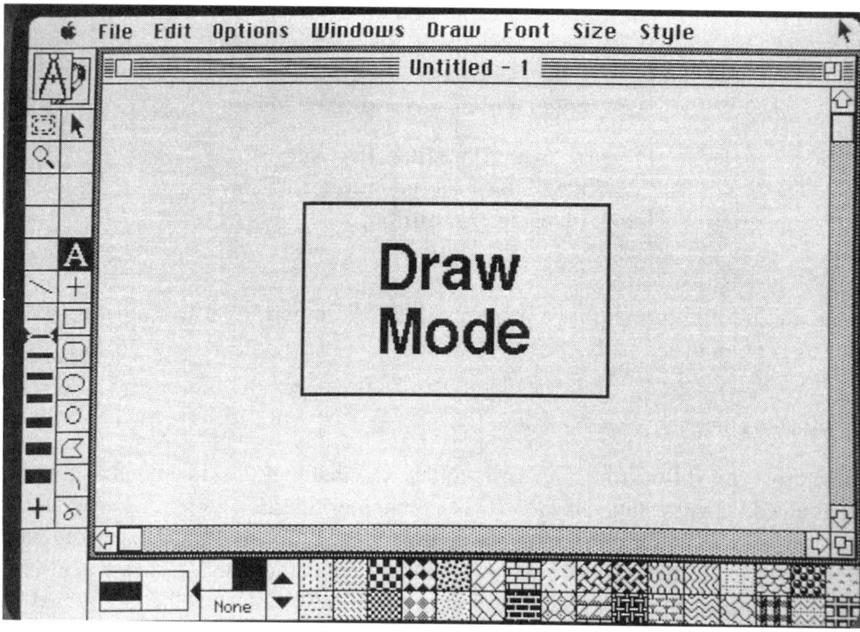

FIGURE 6.3 **The monitor screen "desktop" for a typical draw program.**

Draw programs, like paint ones, use tools that you manipulate with a mouse or other input device (Figure 6.3). These tools, however, are not identical to those for paint programs (compare the tools on the left side of the screen in Figure 6.1 with those on the left side of it in Figure 6.3).

Collections of clip art, as I indicated in the section on paint programs, are a source of graphics for drill-practice materials (see Chapter 4), communication boards (see Chapter 5), and other clinical applications. Some are in a file format that a draw program can import. These can be used as is or modified.

Combination Paint and Draw Programs

These programs contain both paint and draw "layers" that can be used by themselves or combined. When used by themselves, they create graphics identical to those created by other paint and draw programs. When the layers are combined, they create graphics that contain both paint- and draw-type components. The program used for Figures 6.1 and 6.3 is of this type. Note the paint brush icon in the upper left corner of the screen in Figure 6.1 and the compass icon in the upper left corner of the screen in Figure 6.3. Placing the cursor on the desired icon and pressing the button on the mouse changes the layer from a paint to a draw one and vice versa.

PHOTOGRAPH REPRODUCTION AND ENHANCEMENT SOFTWARE

There are programs with which you can both modify and prepare black-and-white and color photographs for printing with an inkjet or laser printer or a printing press. Almost all of the photographs that are reproduced now in books, magazines, newspapers, catalogues, newsletters, journals, and other types of documents are processed in this way.

Photographs have to be "translated" into a *halftone* format, which consists of small dots, before they can be printed with a printing press or computer printer. There is software available for doing this. The dots in halftone renderings of photographs vary in size and spacing. Those that are fairly large and/or close together in black-and-white photographs give the impression of a relatively dark gray and those that are fairly small and/or widely separated, a relatively light one. (To learn more about the halftone process, examine some photographs in a newspaper or magazine with a magnifying glass.)

Photographs must be *digitized* before you can modify and print them with a computer. You can do this in three ways. The first is to take them with a special camera that records images on a hard disk rather than on film. The second is to have them reproduced digitally on a CD-ROM disk (see Chapter 2) from transparencies or negatives. (The Eastman Kodak Company offered this service when this chapter was written.) And the third is to digitize them using a scanner (see Chapter 2).

Photographs can be modified in a number of ways after they are digitized. Their size can be changed—either reduced or increased. Parts of them can be deleted—they can be *cropped*. Their contrast can be increased or reduced. They can be retouched—a plain background can be substituted for a distracting one. Labels can be added. If they are black and white, they can be colorized. And two or more can be combined—e.g., one person's head can be "grafted" on another person's body. (This, incidentally, is how they produce the photographs of beings that are part alien and part human in supermarket tabloids.)

GRAPH-GENERATING SOFTWARE

If you are like most speech-language pathologists and audiologists (particularly if you are one who has administrative responsibilities), you occasionally have to draw graphs. There is software that can draw them. Some are programs that are intended for other purposes. If, for example, you have access to a sophisticated spreadsheet program, such as *Microsoft Excel* or *Lotus 1-2-3* (see Chapter 10), you already have the necessary software.

These programs do not require you to have any artistic ability. You enter numbers and labels (Figure 6.4) and the computer does the rest. You can generate almost

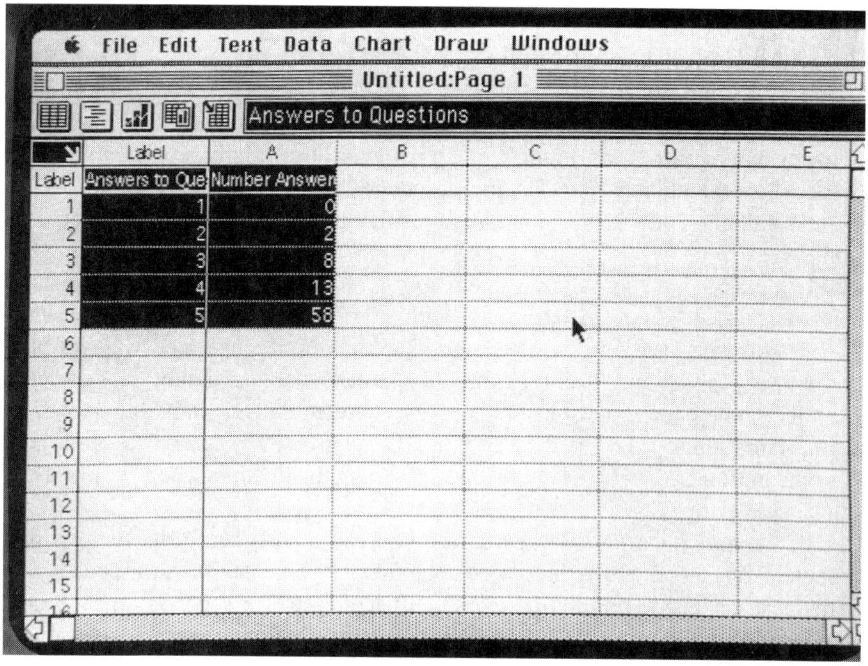

FIGURE 6.4 **The data screen for a graphing program.**

any type of graph with them—including pie (Figure 6.5), two-dimensional bar (Figure 6.6), and three-dimensional bar ones (Figure 6.7)—in black-and-white or color. They can be printed with an inkjet or a laser printer. Graphs produced in this way can be as high a quality as those drawn by a graphic artist; in fact, this is how most graphic artists now produce them.

DESKTOP PRESENTATION SOFTWARE

Many persons who give in-service and/or other types of presentations use overhead transparencies or slides to both highlight main points and supplement what they have to say. In Chapter 8, software is described that you can use to both facilitate the planning of a presentation and prepare overhead transparencies or slides (as well as speaker notes and handouts) for it.

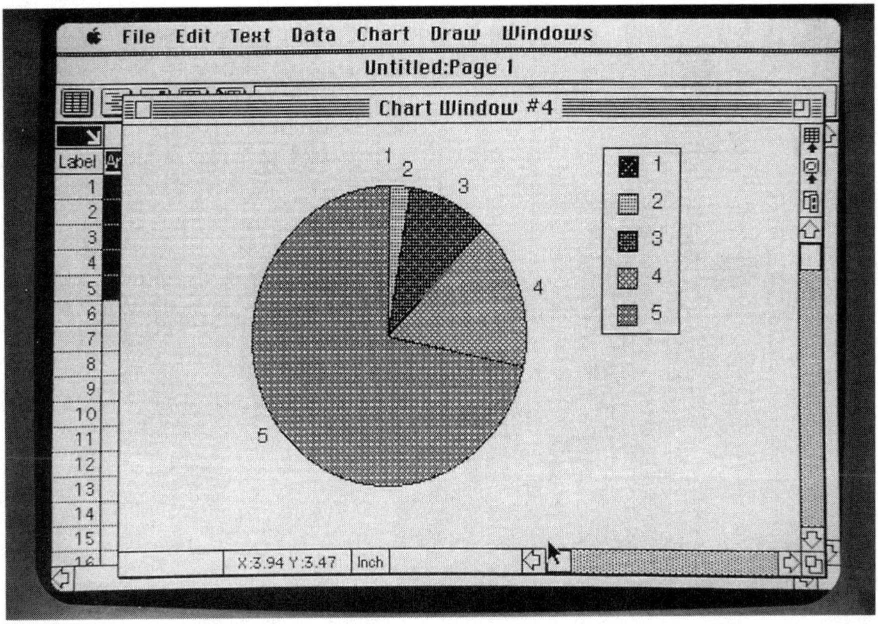

FIGURE 6.5 **A pie graph screen generated from the data in Figure 6.4.**

FORM-GENERATION SOFTWARE

All speech-language pathologists and audiologists use forms. Software is available for laying out and printing them. The forms generated can contain drawings (e.g., graphs on which to plot hearing test results) as well as text. Copies can either be printed as needed with an inkjet or laser printer or in quantities with a photocopy machine.

Most programs of this type have the necessary word-processing capability to fill in the forms they generate. Consequently, they can either print forms before or after they have been completed. Some of these programs store information used to fill in blanks in a database file (see Chapter 9).

While it is relatively simple to lay out and print forms with form generating software, they can also be laid out and printed with word-processing (see Chapter 7), painting, and drawing software (the latter are described elsewhere in this chapter). You can use a computer to fill in and print a form created with these types of software by using a blank copy of the form as a template (i.e., a copy that you saved as a "read only" file).

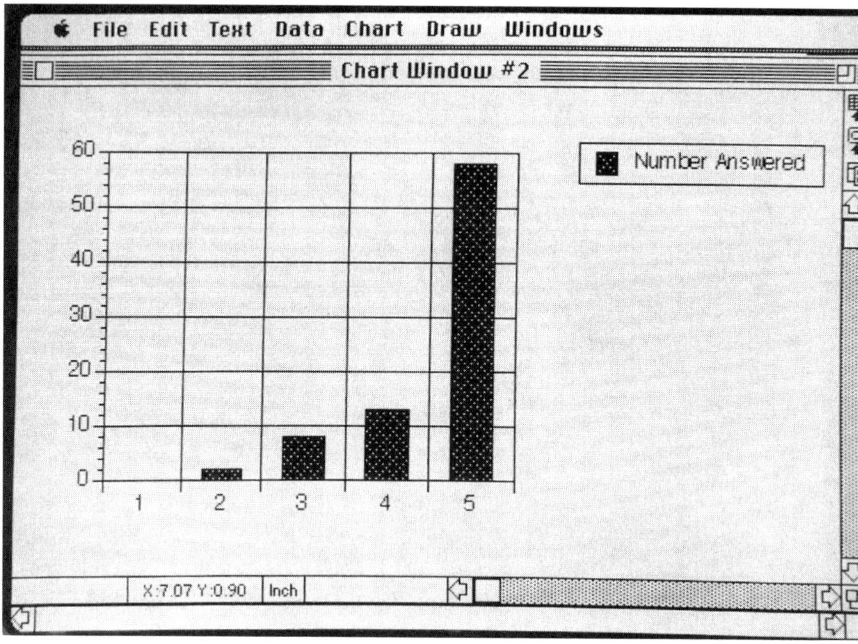

FIGURE 6.6 **A two-dimensional bar graph screen generated from the data in Figure 6.4.**

SIGN- AND POSTER-MAKING SOFTWARE

You probably have to make signs or posters occasionally (e.g., to announce in-service presentations or meetings). Signs up to billboard size can be laid out and printed with a computer in black-and-white or color. Signs and posters that are larger than a sheet of legal size paper would be printed in segments and taped together. They could then be copied with one of the wide paper roll machines (intended for blueprints and other large plans) that are available at many copy shops. These machines can print posters up to 36 inches wide and almost any length. One of the most popular programs for making small signs when this chapter was written was *The Print Shop*, available for Apple II, Macintosh, and IBM-compatibles.

SOFTWARE FOR CREATING GRAPHICS FOR MULTIMEDIA PRESENTATIONS

This software creates photographs, drawings, and moving pictures for interactive tutorials (e.g., for teaching clients Ameslan or speechreading) and other types of

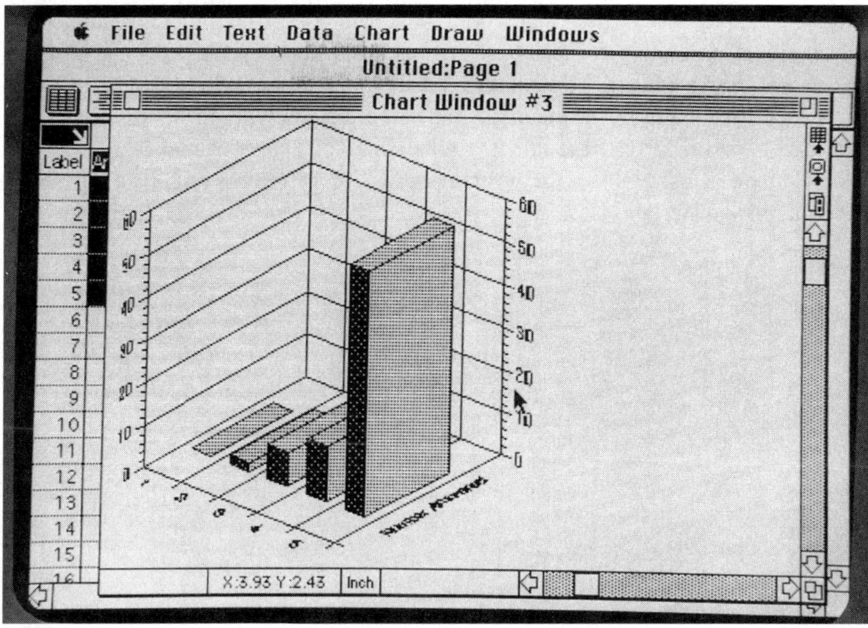

FIGURE 6.7 **A three-dimensional bar graph screen generated from the data in Figure 6.4.**

multimedia presentations. The presentations are stored on a CD-ROM disk or a hard drive (see Chapter 2) and can be viewed on a monitor screen in either black-and-white or color. For further information about multimedia presentations, see Chapter 8.

LEGAL CONSIDERATIONS WHEN USING GRAPHIC SOFTWARE

All drawings, photographs, videotapes, moving pictures, and *parts thereof* that are less than fifty years old (with the exception of clip art that is designated as being in the public domain—see Chapter 3) should be regarded as being copyrighted regardless of whether they have been published and regardless of whether there is a copyright notice on them. If you use one created by someone else—even if you modify it considerably—without the written permission of the copyright owner (the person who created it if there is no notice to the contrary), you can be sued for copyright infringement. If there is a copyright notice on it, the amount can be $25,000 (statutory damages) or more plus attorney fees. A bill was being considered by Congress when this chapter was written that would make works on which there was no copyright notice also eligible for statutory damages and attorney fees. Even if this bill isn't passed, you could still be sued for a substantial amount. While the likelihood of being sued for copyright infringement for using a work without permission is not very great—particularly if the use is a noncommercial one—it makes no sense to place yourself at risk. Obtain the written permission of the copyright owner before using graphics materials.

7

Word Processing and Desktop Publishing

Most speech-language pathologists and audiologists are now using microcomputers with word-processing software for writing clinical reports (Bacon & Shearer, 1989; Fein, 1983, 1984; Fersting, 1984; Fitch, 1993; Hughes, Lehman, Soukanec, & Tatchell, 1993; Silbar & Konarska, 1984; Simmons & Condon, 1993). These include evaluation and progress reports (Allen, 1993; Baker-van den Goorbergh & Baker, no date; Bryant, Tonkovich, Horowitz, & Tan, 1992; Cassidy, Koller, & Schwartz, 1984; Dalston, 1983; Friedrich, LaRue, & Smyke, 1981; Han, Hou, & Thornton, 1993; Harn, 1992; Katz & Porch, 1987; Krueger, 1985; Krueger & Barker, 1983; Kurtis, 1990; Lotterman, 1984b, 1985; Oshrin & Terrio, 1991; Schuldt, no date; Schwartz, 1988c; Schwartz, Koller, & Cassidy, 1984; Sonies & Larkins, 1982; Weiner, 1995aa) and IEPs (Block, 1991; *Goalquest: IEP Writer*, no date; Iverson, 1990; Jenkins, 1987; Kelly et al., 1987; Nelson, 1991; Schetz et al., 1991; Schuldt, no date; Schuldt & Harding, 1985; Scudder, 1990; Sun, 1990; Swanson & Griffin, 1984; Weiner, Polackoff, & Provenzano, 1995; Zemmol, 1985). They also are using them for administrative reports (e.g., year-end summaries, budgets, and grant applications), research reports, and professional correspondence. Furthermore, some speech-language pathologists and audiologists are using them alone or in combination with desktop publishing software for preparing various types of publications, including brochures describing their clinical programs and booklets for client/family counseling.

Why did clinicians switch from typewriters to microcomputers for preparing reports? There appear to have been several reasons. One is that it was the "in thing" to do. Writing with a typewriter was (and still is) regarded as being old fashioned. Some clinicians undoubtedly initially switched for this reason.

Clinicians switched from typewriters to microcomputers for writing reports mainly because doing so enabled them to reduce the amount of time they had to spend. There are several reasons. First, using computers enabled them to edit and revise reports without having to retype them. Keyboarding errors can be corrected invisibly, and words, sentences, and even paragraphs can be added, deleted, and/or moved to different locations. This latter feature makes it possible to write sentences and paragraphs in a sequence different from that in which they will appear in the report. You could, for example, begin to draft the recommendation section of an evaluation report either during the evaluation while recommendations are being made (using a laptop computer) or immediately following it—while the recommendations are still fresh in your mind. And you could write sentences describing a client's performance on various diagnostic tests immediately after they are administered and/or scored. If you did either of the above with a computer different than the one you use for writing reports, you could transfer the material to the other computer and incorporate it into the report. This could be done even if the word-processing programs being used were different and the computers were of different types—if one was a Macintosh and the other was an IBM-compatible—by utilizing a file translator program (see Chapter 3).

A second way that word-processing software reduces the amount of time it is necessary to spend on report writing is by making it possible to use of *templates*. These are standard sentences and paragraphs that can be incorporated into reports (for examples, see Cassidy, Koller, & Schwartz, 1984; Newman, Jacobson, & Weinstein, 1993; and Appendix A in Silverman, 1992b). Some of them contain blanks that you fill in: For example, in a paragraph describing a client's performance on an aphasia test, blanks would be used for reporting the client's overall and subtest scores. And in a paragraph describing the results of a pure-tone audiometric test, they would be used for reporting his or her hearing thresholds at the frequencies tested. Sentences and paragraphs that do not contain blanks could pertain to aspects of speech, language, or hearing that are screened and found to be within normal limits—for example, they could present the results of the routine pure-tone hearing screening of a client with a speech or language impairment whose hearing is within normal limits.

A third way that using word-processing with a computer can reduce the amount of time it is necessary to devote to report writing is by making "writer's block" less likely to occur. You can temporarily skip paragraphs on which you feel "blocked" and later rearrange them.

A fourth reason why the use of word-processing software is likely to reduce the amount of time spent on report writing is that you don't have to type final drafts. After the computer file for a report has been edited, one or more copies (hopefully, error-free) can be printed.

My overall objective in this chapter is to introduce you to word-processing and desktop publishing, particularly as they relate to report writing and other aspects of your clinical functioning. Features of word-processing and desktop publishing software are described that can make the preparation of reports and other clinically relevant documents more efficient.

WORD-PROCESSING SOFTWARE

The application for which speech-language pathologists and audiologists have been using using computers the longest is report writing (Bacon & Shearer, 1989; Fein, 1983, 1984; Fersting, 1984; Silbar & Konarska, 1984). Consequently, I decided to use report writing to illustrate how word-processing software can enable you to do certain clinical tasks more efficiently. The comments made about using it for report writing, of course, also apply to using it for other purposes.

There are several steps in writing reports with a word processor. The first is producing a rough draft. While this is usually done on a computer, it can also be done in whole or part on a legal pad and later keyboarded. You may find that combining the two works best for you—for example, you may draft recommendations in the therapy room by hand immediately after making them.

Paragraphs should be saved on a diskette or a hard disk after they are drafted rather than waiting until the report is completed. A power failure or a computer malfunction can result in your having to redraft a lot of material if you don't save often. Actually, authors of word-processing texts agree that documents being drafted should be saved at least every fifteen minutes. I do so about every five minutes. These authors also recommend that at least one back-up copy of files (documents) be made on a different disk (or disks). This provides insurance against material being lost if a disk is damaged or accidentally erased.

After a report has been drafted, it is edited and formatted for printing. All of the editing can be done on a computer, or a draft can be printed and at least partially edited on paper before doing so on a computer. The editing process may include using the computer to identify and correct grammatical and spelling errors and to access a thesaurus to find words that are more appropriate than some that were used. Almost all word-processing programs have these capabilities.

After a report has been edited, it is formatted for printing. Instructions are added that tell the computer how to print it. These instructions specify, for example, the font, size, and style of type (e.g., plain or boldfaced) for each word; the spacing between letters, lines of text, and paragraphs; and the widths of margins.

The final step in the process is printing the report. A *near-letter-quality* dot-matrix printer, a laser printer, or an inkjet printer is used for this purpose. A near-letter-quality dot-matrix printer is one that prints characters that do not have an obvious dot structure—they are formed by relatively small dots. Extra copies of reports can be printed by the computer or the original can be photocopied. Photocopying, incidentally, makes the characters produced by dot-matrix printers appear more solid (i.e., they tend to have a less obvious dot structure).

The process described above for drafting, editing, and printing documents is appropriate when all three will be done using the same software (e.g., Microsoft Word or WordPerfect) and on computers with the same operating system (e.g., MS-DOS, Microsoft Windows, or Macintosh—see Chapter 3). If all three are not being done with a single word-processing program on computers having the same operating system, it will be necessary before a switch is made to save the document in a format that is compatible with the program and computer on which it will be worked on next. Some word-processing programs for IBM-compatible and Macintosh computers have the capability to save files in the other formats. There are also utility programs that translate file formats from that for one computer operating system to another (see Chapter 3) and from that for one word-processing program to another.

There are a number programs that can facilitate the writing of reports. Some were created specifically for doing this task and others for general word-processing. Both types are described below.

Special Word-Processing Software

There are word-processing programs that can facilitate the writing of clinical reports. Several types are described below.

Test Performance Summarizers. These programs print a summary of a client's performance on a particular diagnostic test. **Computer Managed Articulation Diagnosis** (Fitch, 1985b), for example, prints a four-page analysis of error patterns by distinctive features. **Computerized Assessment of Intelligibility of Dysarthric Speech** (Beukelman, Yorkston, & Traynor, 1984) prints a sheet listing several measures of single-word and sentence intelligibility. And **Systematic Hearing Aid Prescription** (Moomaw, no date) prints a hearing aid prescription.

Session or Task Performance Summarizers. These programs print a summary of a client's performance on specific intervention-related tasks. **Computer Managed Language Treatment** (Fitch, 1985c), for example, prints the total number of responses, the percent that were correct, and the highest level achieved during particular sessions. And **First Categories** (Wilson & Fox, 1991a) prints for particular lessons what level was worked on, what interface was used, the nouns and categories presented, and the accuracy of the client's response to each.

Individual Education Program (IEP) Generators. These programs are intended for public school speech clinicians. They generate therapy goals (objectives) in IEP format for children who have speech, language, and/or hearing disorders. Some can be used for any type of disorder and others for only a single type. Examples of the former are **Goalquest: IEP Writer** (no date) and **Planning Individualized Speech and Language Intervention Programs** (Berryman, Johnson, & Toman, 1984). An example of the latter is **Automated IEP System—Hypernasality Goal Bank** (Schuldt, no date).

Word-Processing Programs for Writing Reports. These are word-processing programs that have been optimized for writing particular types of reports. **CDTS-Initial/Final Report** (Schuldt, no date), for example, contains an initial and final report format that may be modified so that each client receives a personalized report. And **Parent Reporting** (no date) is intended for periodically informing parents about their children's progress. Programs of these types can be simulated by using a template with standard word-processing software. A template is a word-processor file that contains a report with blanks to be filled in. To use it, a copy is made of the template and the blanks are filled in.

Standard Word-Processing Software

Word-processing programs are available as separate packages or packaged with other applications. Such packages are referred to as *integrated programs*. Examples are Microsoft Works and Claris Works. The applications in them usually include ones for word-processing, managing databases (see Chapter 9), creating spreadsheets (see Chapter 10), drawing (see Chapter 6), and telecommunication (see Chapter 11). While word-processing programs that are separate packages—such as Microsoft Word and WordPerfect—offer more features than those that are components of an integrated program, the latter are likely to be sufficiently flexible to meet most, if not all, of your needs. Integrated programs, incidentally, cost no more than separate word-processing ones. Consequently, if the word-processing component of such a package is sufficiently flexible to meet your needs, by purchasing it rather than a separate word-processing program, you would be getting "for free" the software needed for the other applications in the package.

Word-processing programs enable you to process (manipulate) words in a number of ways. Each of these manipulations is initiated by issuing a command. Some of the commands (e.g., the one for word-wrap) are issued by the computer rather than the user.

The commands that can be issued by word-processing programs facilitate one of two aspects of document creation: writing/editing or screen/printer formatting. Some of the commands that you would use routinely when doing clinical reports are described in this section.

Writing/Editing. These commands enable you to type reports and edit them. They include the following:

- CURSOR CONTROL COMMANDS. The cursor is a line or patch of light that "tells" the computer the location of the next letter or larger alphanumeric unit you want to manipulate. For example, it could indicate where the next letter you type should be inserted or the location of a word that you want to delete. The position of the cursor can be changed with a keyboard or a device such as a mouse or trackball (see Chapter 2). The arrow keys on most, if not all, keyboards allow you to move the cursor one or more units (characters, spaces, or lines) in four directions—up, down, right, and left. Furthermore, almost all word-processing programs have keyboard commands that enable you to change the position of the cursor by a word, a line, a sentence, a paragraph, a screenful (or "page"), and move it to the beginning or end of a document.

- WORD WRAP AND HYPHENATION. *Word wrap* is a command that the computer executes automatically unless otherwise instructed—a *default* command. Word-processing programs, unlike typewriters, do not require a key to be pressed at the end of a line. They will automatically begin a new line when the number of characters and spaces in one exceed the line length specified when the right and left margins were set. If the line length is exceeded part way through a word, the command automatically moves the word to the beginning of the next line.

  An alternative to word wrap is *automatic hyphenation*. Hyphenation can also be done manually: The computer indicates the locations in a word where it is appropriate to insert a hyphen and does so at the one selected by the user. A hyphen that is inserted in a word by a computer is removed by it if sufficient characters are added to or deleted from a line to result in the word no longer requiring hyphenation.
- SCROLLING. This command allows you to read and edit a document (e.g., a report) that is too long to be displayed on the screen in its entirety. Its called scrolling because metaphorically the document is regarded as being printed on a scroll with the screen being a "window" located between the two rolls through which portions of it can be viewed. Manipulating a keyboard, mouse, or trackball causes the "scroll" to be wound forward or backward, thereby changing the portion of it that can be seen through the window—that is, displayed on the screen.
- DELETION. All word-processing programs have commands that delete letters, words, lines, and larger blocks of text. You can issue these commands with a keyboard and/or a device such as a mouse or trackball. Most word-processing programs retain the last block of text that was deleted in memory and have an undo command that enables you to retrieve it.
- INSERTION. This command enables you to add text to a document simply by indicating where it should be inserted (with the cursor) and either typing it or "moving" it from elsewhere in that document or another document. A space is created to accommodate it, regardless of its length.
- BLOCK MOVEMENT. This enables you to move a block of text from one location to another. The block can be as small as a single letter or as large as several hundred pages. Two commands are needed to move a block of text: The first "cuts" it from one location and the second "pastes" it in another. A clinician would use these commands to rearrange the sections of an evaluation report before printing if he or she had found it advantageous to write them in a sequence other than the appropriate one.
- SEARCH AND REPLACE. All word-processing programs have a command that enables you *find* each occurrence of a sequence of characters (e.g., a particular word) in a document. You can use this command to locate information quickly by searching for one of the words in the paragraph containing the information. You

can also use it to mark sentences and paragraphs that you want to be able to locate quickly and display on the screen (e.g., ones that need further editing). You would type a group of characters near them that do not appear in the document (e.g., xxx). To display the material, you would search for these characters. They, of course, would have to be deleted before the document was printed.

These program also have a command that enables you to substitute other characters (for example, words) for ones that have been searched for and found—that is, to *replace* them. You can have the computer make the substitution for all occurrences of the characters in a document or you can have the computer display each occurrence on the screen and decide on a case-by-case basis whether to make it. This routine is particularly useful for locating and correcting words that you have misspelled the same way a number of times in a report—such as a client's name.

Search and replace commands are not restricted to locating and changing groups of characters. They can also be used to locate and change particular types of formatting. They could be used, for example, to locate all of the words in a document that are underlined and then change them to italics.

- SAVE. This command enables you to save what you have written on a diskette and/or a hard disk. It's good practice to get into the habit of doing so every ten or fifteen minutes while you are drafting or editing a document. If this isn't done a power outage or command error (e.g., one that deletes material you don't want to be deleted) can result in your having to redraft or re-edit a considerable amount of material.

Screen/Printer Formatting. All word-processing programs have *default settings*. These specify how documents will be formatted on the monitor screen and printed. There are many such settings, including ones that specify the type font, size, and style (e.g., plain or italics) to be used; the top, bottom, left, and right margin widths; and the spacing between lines and paragraphs. When a default setting is not appropriate, you can change it by issuing a command. The settings you can change include the following:

- TYPE FONT. Font-related commands enable you to select a font in which to display characters (and other symbols) on your monitor screen and print them. There are thousands of fonts available. See Figure 7.1 for several examples of ones that are appropriate for use in clinical reports. A particular font can be used for any amount of text, including a single character (e.g., an arrow, Greek letter, or other symbol that is not in the text font being used).

  Fonts differ from each other in several ways. One of the most significant is whether they have *serifs*. These are horizontal lines that are added to the tops and/or bottoms of some letters. The *Bookman* and *Times* fonts in Figure 7.1 have serifs and the *Avant Garde* and *Helvetica* ones do not. The latter are referred to as *sans-serif* fonts because they lack them. The difference that serifs make can easily

English text (Avant Garde)
English text [Bookman]
English text [Helvetica]
English text [Times]

FIGURE 7.1 **Four representative type fonts. The name of the font is in brackets.**

be seen by comparing the letter "l" in the word "English" in the *Bookman* and *Times* fonts in Figure 7.1 to those in the *Avant Garde* and *Helvetica* ones in this figure. Note that there are horizontal lines at both the top and bottom of "l" in the former but not in the latter. Serif fonts tend to be easier to read than san-serif ones. Both serif and san-serif fonts may be combined in a document: When this is done, the serif font usually is used for the text and the san-serif one for the headings. (Times and Helvetica, incidentally, go well together for clinical reports.)

A second way that fonts differ is whether characters in them are *monospaced* or *proportional*. Characters that are monospaced, like those on a typewriter, all take up the same amount of space—the letter *i* takes up the same amount of space as the letter *m* (Figure 7.2). For characters that are proportional, the amount of space allotted is determined by its width—the letter *i* would take up about one-fifth the space of the letter *m* (Figure 7.2). Proportional fonts are used for typesetting books and journals and should be used when documents are printed with a laser or inkjet printer, unless a typewritten appearance is desired. Because there is less space between characters when proportional fonts are used, words take up less space (Figure 7.2). Also, when proportional fonts are used, only a *single space* is needed between sentences (Williams, 1990). Consequently, more words can be printed on a page of a report with a proportional font than with a monospaced one.

```
A second way that fonts differ is whether
characters in them are monospaced or
proportional.
[Monospaced font]
```

A second way that fonts differ is whether characters in them are *monospaced or proportional.*
[Proportional font]

FIGURE 7.2 **A sentence printed with a monospaced and a proportional font.**

Text [Bitmapped Font]

Text [Truetype Font]

FIGURE 7.3 **Words printed with a bitmapped font and a TrueType font.**

A third way that fonts differ is *how characters are generated* by the computer. The way that it generates them determines both how "solid" characters appear to be (the smaller the dots used to form them the more solid their appearance) and the types of printers on which they are likely to be used. The three main types of fonts based on how characters are generated are bit-mapped, PostScript, and TrueType. *Bit-mapped* characters usually don't appear to be solid because they are formed from relatively large dots (Figure 7.3). They are used mainly with dot-matrix printers. Characters in PostScript and TrueType fonts, on the other hand, almost always appear to be solid (Figure 7.3) because they are formed from relatively small dots (300 or more to the inch). They are used mainly with laser and inkjet printers (see Chapter 2 for information about the printers mentioned in this paragraph).

A fourth way that fonts differ is the *size* of the characters that they generate on the screen and print. Their size is determined by their height, which is specified in *points* (in Figure 7.4 there are 12-point, 24-point, 36-point, 48-point, and 60-point versions of the *Times* font). A point is 1/72nd of an inch. The font size that is usually used for clinical reports is either 10-point or 12-point.

Text [12-Point]

Text [24-Point]

Text [36-Point]

Text [48-Point]

Text [60-Point]

FIGURE 7.4 **A word printed in 12-point, 24-point, 36-point, 48-point, and 60-point versions of the *Times* font.**

A fifth way fonts differ is the *style* of the characters that they generate. The four styles that you probably will find most useful for clinical applications are plain, bold, italic, bold italic (Figure 7.5). Incidentally, the combination of *Times* plain for text and *Helvetica* bold for headings works well for clinical reports.

A sixth way that fonts differ concerns the characters they can generate. Almost all can generate the characters that appear on the keyboard. The two main types that can't generate keyboard characters are symbol fonts (e.g., those that generate mathematical or international phonetic symbols or many types of bullets for lists) and fonts for languages that don't use our alphabet (e.g., Hebrew, Russian, Arabic, Japanese, Chinese, Greek, and Hindi). While almost all fonts generate characters that do not appear on the keyboard, they differ with regard to which ones and how many. Some fonts can generate more than 200 characters. Both Macintosh and Windows operating systems have *keyfinder* utilities that indicate the key or key combination that will generate a particular character in a particular font.

- SPACING. All word-processing programs have commands for adjusting the spacing between lines and paragraphs and most have them for changing (increasing or reducing) the spacing between some characters when they occur together in words. Adjusting the spacing between lines of type is referred to as *leading*. The amount can be specified as it is on a typewriter (i.e., single space, space-and-a-half, or double space) or in points. The amount of leading between paragraphs can be set to be a little greater than that between lines of type. Changing the spacing between some characters in words is referred to as *kerning*. This is done frequently, for example, when *f* is followed by *i* or *l*: the space between the characters is eliminated (Figure 7.6).

Text [Plain]

Text [Bold]

Text [Italic]

Text [Bold-Italic]

FIGURE 7.5 **A word printed in plain, bold, italic, and bold-italic versions of the *Times* font.**

find [Not kerned] find [Kerned]

flat [Not kerned] flat [Kerned]

FIGURE 7.6 **The effect of kerning when when *f* is followed by *i* or *l*.**

- PARAGRAPH ALIGNMENT. All word-processing programs can align paragraphs in the following four ways: flush left, flush right, centered, and justified (Figure 7.7). A paragraph is any word, line, or group of lines that was terminated by pressing the return key.
- MARGINS AND INDENTATIONS. All word-processing programs have commands for setting right, left, top, and bottom margins. The margins on each page of a multi-page document can be different. Furthermore, the right and left margins of the paragraphs on a page do not have to be the same width. This makes it possible for paragraphs containing direct quotations to be set off from the others by increasing their right and left margins by about one-half inch.

  There are two types of indentations. One results in the first line of a paragraph being indented. The other, which is known as a *hanging indent*, results in

All word-processing programs have commands for
aligning paragraphs in four ways: flush left, flush
right, centered, and justified. **[Flush left]**

All word-processing programs have commands for
aligning paragraphs in four ways: flush left, flush
right, centered, and justified. **[Flush right]**

All word-processing programs have commands for
aligning paragraphs in four ways: flush left, flush
right, centered, and justified. **[Centered]**

All word-processing programs have commands for aligning paragraphs in four ways: flush left, flush right, centered, and justified. **[Justified]**

FIGURE 7.7 **Alignment of paragraphs flush left, flush right, centered, and justified.**

all of the lines in a paragraph other than the first being indented. This type of indentation is used mainly for paragraphs that are items in lists, including *bulleted* ones as shown in Figure 7.8. The black dots that are used in this list to set off items are a type of bullet.

- HEADERS AND FOOTERS. These are lines of text that are printed at the tops or bottoms of the pages in a multi-page document. Those printed at the top of a page are called *headers* and those printed at the bottom are called *footers*. A different header or footer can be printed on right and left *facing pages* of documents that are bound like a book. *Page numbers* can be included in headers or footers, either alone or with text. The pages in this book have headers that include text and page numbers.
- TAB SETTINGS. These commands enable you to do everything that you can with a tabulator key on a typewriter and more. You can, for example, set tabs that will automatically line up the decimal points in columns of figures.
- PAGE BREAKS. These programs automatically divide documents into pages and indicate on the screen where page breaks will occur when a document is printed. Most have commands that enable you to eliminate "widows" and "ophans" if you want to do so. A *widow* is the last line of a paragraph that appears alone at the top of the next page and an *orphan* is the first line of a paragraph that appears alone at the bottom of a page. They eliminate widows by inserting page breaks that result in the first paragraphs of pages having at least two lines. Furthermore, these programs have commands that enable you to remove and insert page breaks manually if any of the ones that the program inserts are unacceptable.
- PAGE SETUP AND PRINT. These commands control the printer; *Page setup* commands set it to print on a sheet of a particular size. For clinical reports the setting usually would be *US letter*. They also set the orientation of the paper: vertical ("portrait") or horizontal ("landscape"). The *print* commands include ones for setting the number of copies and selecting the pages to be printed (all or certain ones) and the quality of the printing (e.g., "draft" or "best").

There are two kinds of indentations:

- The first line of a paragraph is indented and all other lines begin at the left margin.
- The first line of a paragraph begins at the left margin and all other lines are indented.

FIGURE 7.8 **Two paragraphs in a bulleted list that were formatted by the hanging indent command.**

Other Software Routines. Most of the commands that we have discussed thus far are essential for report writing. There are others that are not essential but make doing so more efficient. You may be able to issue them with your word-processing program or you may have to use other programs that are compatible with it. The following are several examples:

- SPELL CHECKING. Spell checking identifies the words in a document that are not identical to those in the program's dictionary. For each, you are given the option of letting the word remain as is or correcting it. If the computer is "told" to correct a word, it will suggest alternative spellings. The computer will replace the one in the document with the one that you select. Because the dictionary is unlikely to contain all of the technical terms and names that you include in reports, some words that you spell correctly are likely to be flagged by the program. Such words can be added to the program's dictionary. Because spelling errors in a document can reduce its author's credibility, it is desirable to spell-check all clinical reports and related correspondence.
- GRAMMAR CHECKERS. Grammar checkers flag *possible* grammatical errors, punctuation errors, and awkward wordings and generate suggestions for correcting or modifying them. They search for punctuations and wordings that are in their "error" dictionary. For each one they find, they give you the option of leaving it as is or changing it. While I usually find such checking to be aggravating because many of the wordings that are flagged are acceptable to me, I nevertheless feel that doing it improves my writing sufficiently to compensate for the aggravation it produces. The use of one of these checkers can be made less aggravating and more efficient by removing wordings from the program's "error" dictionary that you find acceptable.
- THESAURUS. The thesaurus suggests synonyms for a word that you mark with the cursor (e.g., by highlighting it) and they enable you to replace the word (if you decide to do so) with the synonym you select.
- WORD COUNT. This command can be particularly useful when you are writing something that has a specified word limit, such as an abstract or letter to the editor. Be aware, however, that things may be counted as words that really aren't—for example, quotation marks.
- INDEX. This command creates an index for books, manuals, relatively long reports, proposals, and other documents. You mark the words that you want to include in the index with a code that is invisible to the printer when the document is printed. If a document will be printed from pages other than those generated by your word-processing program (e.g., if it is the manuscript for a book or manual that will be typeset), you will have to use the "Insert Page Break" command to make pages begin and end where they do in the document. Otherwise, the page numbers in your index are unlikely to be accurate.

- MACROS. Macros program your keyboard so that frequently used multi-step word-processing functions are performed or frequently used words, phrases, sentences, and paragraphs are keyboarded by simultaneously pressing two or three keys. The computer "records" a series of keypresses when commanded to do so, assigns a two- or three-key combination to them (e.g., the "shift" key, the "option" key, and the "S" key), and "plays them back" when these keys are pressed. Mouse movements can be included in macros. Macros can be programmed to automatically repeat themselves a specific number of times or until they reach the end of a document. Macros can be saved in a file and more than one set of them can be created.

  Macros could be used in several ways to facilitate writing clinical report. You could, for example, create a macro that would automatically keyboard all of the headings (at their appropriate locations) that you routinely use in them. You could also create macros that would automatically keyboard sentences and paragraphs that you use frequently; there would be a macro for each such sentence and paragraph.
- MAIL MERGE. Mail merge enables you to print "personalized" form letters—ones that contain "blanks" (names, addresses, salutations, etc.) that are filled in by the computer. Each appears to the recipient to have been individually typed. School clinicians, for example, could use it for reports that they send to parents periodically about their children's performance and progress.

  The process involved in getting set up to use mail merge is a three-step one. First, you create a database file that contains the specific words and phrases you want inserted in each person's letter. You may do so with the word-processing program or a compatible database one (see Chapter 9). Second, you write the letter and insert a "code" where each word or phrase is to be placed. The code for a particular entry will include the name of the *field* in the database (see Chapter 9) that contains the information to be inserted. And third, both the form letter file and the database file are loaded into the computer and the letters are printed. Whenever the computer encounters an entry code while printing a letter, it retrieves the appropriate word or phrase from the recipient's record in the database and prints it.
- TABLES. Most word-processing programs have commands that facilitate the aligning of words and numbers in the rows and columns of tables. They also have commands that enable you to draw vertical and horizontal lines to set off headings from items and items from each other.
- TELECOMMUNICATIONS. These commands enable you to transmit documents (e.g., faxes) over telephone lines (see Chapter 11).
- OUTLINING AND ORGANIZING. With these commands you can organize a document prior to drafting it. They may generate an outline or a series of boxes containing "ideas" (each of which is an electronic file card) that you connect (Simpson, 1995). You can expand the text in an outline file into a document with your word processor.

DESKTOP PUBLISHING SOFTWARE

Desktop publishing software enables you to produce high-quality *camera ready* printed pages in black-and-white or color. The plates used for printing pages are made by photographing them. Pages set up with such software are not restricted to text. There can also contain photographs and drawings. The pages for almost all professional books, manuals, and journals are now prepared in this way.

What types of publications might you be able to produce using desktop publishing software? There are many, including questionnaires and other clinical forms, stationery, year-end reports, research reports, flyers, invitations, books, booklets, brochures, newsletters, employee manuals, grant applications, and posters.

For some publications (e.g., questionnaires and other clinical forms), pages printed on a 300-dot-per-inch laser or inkjet printer are adequate for camera-ready copy. Others—particularly those containing photographs and color illustrations—require higher quality. To produce the latter, you could give the printer the pages on disk rather than as camera-ready copy. He or she would produce camera-ready copy by printing the pages with a high-quality printer—one that can generate 1200 or more dots per inch—in black-and-white or color. This, incidentally, is how the pages of most of your recent books (including this one) were produced.

A key feature of desktop publishing software is that it enables you to combine text and graphics into pages that appear on the monitor screen as they will when printed. You can import material (text and graphics) that you produced with other programs. Once imported, they can be manipulated in various ways. Drawings and photographs can be enlarged or reduced, cropped, and "pasted" on a page wherever desired. Text can be altered with regard to font, point size, leading, and kerning and made to "flow" around the graphics. Text can also be made to flow from column to column and from page to page.

Most contemporary word-processing programs (such as Microsoft Word and WordPerfect) have some desktop publishing (page layout) capabilities. They can import graphics produced with other programs, size and crop them, and place them on a page. They can also manipulate text in various ways, including causing it to flow around graphics. The files they generate can be printed by high resolution printers to produce camera-ready copy. Consequently, a desktop publishing program is not always needed to lay out pages for some types of publications, including questionnaires and other clinical forms.

While it is relatively easy to generate camera-ready copy, it is not easy to do it well. To do so, you have to understand the basic elements of graphic design, such as what fonts to use and how to lay out pages in an artistic manner. There are a number of books available that describe these in the context of page layout for desktop publishing. These book assume no previous experience with or knowledge of graphic design. Three that I have found particularly helpful are *Design for Desktop Publishing* (Miles, 1987), *Looking Good in Print* (Parker, 1990), and *The Non-designer's Design Book* (Williams, 1994).

THE COMPUTER IS NOT A TYPEWRITER

Many of us were taught to write with a typewriter rather than with a computer. Some of the typing rules we learned were necessitated by several limitations of typewriters that are not so for computers. One such limitation is characters being monospaced rather than proportionally spaced. A second is an incomplete character set (e.g., no true quotation marks). A third is the inability to conveniently change fonts and point sizes. And the fourth is an inability to produce characters in italics and/or boldface. Williams (1990) suggests that when writing with a computer we should ignore a number of typing rules. Those that are applicable to clinical reports include the following:

- *Having two spaces after periods.* Because proportionally spaced characters are closer together than monospaced ones, not as much space is needed to separate sentences visually. Consequently, use only one space after periods, colons, exclamation points, question marks, and quotation marks. Note that only one space is used to separate sentences in books that are typeset with proportionally spaced fonts.
- *Using inch marks (") and foot marks (') for quotation marks.* The character sets for all fonts that would be used for word-processing or desktop publishing contain opening double quotes (“), closing double quotes (”), opening single quotes (‘) and closing single quotes (’). Use real quotation marks.
- *Using foot marks (') for apostrophes.* The closing single quote (’) should be used for apostrophes rather than the generic foot mark.
- *Using two hyphens instead of a dash.* Computer font character sets contain a dash (—) as well as a hyphen (-). Consequently, there is no need to simulate one with two hyphens.
- *Underlining.* If it is being done to indicate italics, use *italic characters*. If it is being done to emphasize words, use *italic characters*, **boldface characters**, larger characters, or those in a different font instead.
- *Creating headings in capital letters.* Headings in all caps are hard to read. To make headings stand out visually, use boldface characters, larger characters, or those in a different font.
- *Using the space bar to line up columns of words and numbers.* This method does not work with proportionally spaced fonts. Use tabs instead.

8

Desktop Presentation and Multimedia

Regardless of whether you are employed in an educational or medical setting, it is quite likely that you will occasionally be expected to give oral presentations to professional and/or consumer groups—including the general public. Professional groups are likely to include staff meetings and multidisciplinary team staffings of clients. Presentations that you would be expected to give to the general public are likely to be a component of your employer's marketing strategy.

You will also be called upon to provide information—give presentations—to clients and their families. If you are an audiologist, you will probably advise clients about the use and maintenance of hearing aids. And if you are a speech-language pathologist, you may give presentations to the parents of young children who are "at risk" for beginning to stutter about appropriate ways to react to their disfluency.

You can make presentations—even to clients and their families—more effective by augmenting what you say with audio- and videotapes, charts, graphs, or other audiovisual aids. According to Meng (1988, p. 143):

> A 1986 study by the University of Minnesota showed that use of graphics increased a presenter's persuasiveness by 43 percent. Speakers using visual aids were perceived as being better prepared, more professional, clearer, more interesting, and more concise when compared with speakers who didn't use visuals.

Software is available for IBM-compatible and Macintosh computers (e.g., PowerPoint) that can facilitate both the preparation and delivery of audiovisual aids (Allen, 1993; Kouri & Savage, 1993; Lieberth, 1992; Tatchell, Letson, Zlotolow, & DeLauro, 1993). Some of this software generates text and graphics for presentations that utilize flipcharts, overhead transparencies, on-screen video, and/or slides. Other programs of this type generate presentations that integrate sound (including speech) and movies with text and graphics. The latter are referred to as *multimedia* presentations.

Some of the "products" you can create with presentation software that should enable you to communicate more effectively with fellow professionals, clients, their families, and others are described in this chapter. There are also some suggestions here for planning and giving presentations in which audiovisual aids are used.

PLANNING THE PRESENTATION

The planning process begins with the creation of an outline containing the text and other material (e.g., graphs and drawings) for the overhead transparencies, flipcharts, slides, or on-screen video that the speaker intends to use. The outline can be created with either word-processing or presentation software. It specifies both the topics that will be discussed and their order. Topics can be added, deleted, or modified, and their locations and levels of subordination can be changed.

The outline for a presentation, in addition to indicating its content, functions as a visual-auditory-verbal *storyboard.* It indicates the underlying layout structure of the presentation in *frame* sequences. Each frame—which is a main heading in the outline—contains the text and graphics for creating the visual (if it is not a tape segment) and notes for comments you should make while it is being shown. There is a frame for each visual (e.g., overhead transparency) or tape segment. If a frame is for a tape segment, it should contain the script for that segment and notes for comments you should made before or after it is played. Tape segments may be recorded on audio- or videotape, a videodisk, or a computer disk.

Decisions made during the development of the storyboard for a presentation—the information to present and how to present it—are perhaps the most crucial in determining its effectiveness. The following recommendations by Rabb (1990, p. 40) can be helpful when making these decisions:

> As you generate ideas for your presentation, keep your objectives in mind and evaluate each idea accordingly. Work from your content outline, visualizing different ways to present each point. There's no single "right" way to approach your subject. Experiment; develop several alternative solutions. Evaluation and selection will come later. Don't try to get from start to finish in one step. Just let the ideas flow and see where they take you.

SELECTING A VISUAL MEDIUM AND CREATING VISUALS

After the storyboard for a presentation has been developed and the decision has been made to use visuals that aren't "movies," the next decision is the *medium* to use. There are six possibilities: posters, flipcharts, flip books, overhead transparencies, 35-millimeter slides, and on-screen video.

Flip Books, Flipcharts, and Posters

Flipcharts are poster-size pages of presentation material (charts) that are bound together into a large book (usually with rings) and attached to a floor easel. You turn pages when it is appropriate to do so. *Posters* are similar to flipcharts except the pages are not bound together. They are mounted on stiff backing boards; foamcore is best when they are to be placed on an easel because it is lightweight and doesn't sag or buckle. *Flip books* are similar to flip charts except that the pages are smaller and the easel is placed on a table or desk. You—the presenter—would be seated during the presentation. These presentation forms are most effective when used with relatively small audiences: under twenty people for flipcharts and posters and fewer than five for flip books. These forms are the only media that do not require electrical equipment.

Pages for flip books can be laid out from the storyboard outline and printed with desktop presentation software. Figures 8.1, 8.2, and 8.3 illustrate the process. The screen in Figure 8.1, from a desktop presentation program, contains a segment of such an outline. The outline could have been created with the program or "imported." Note that the icon for an outline in the row at the bottom of the screen is highlighted (darkened). The *bullet chart* in Figure 8.2 was created by selecting the icon to the right of the outline one (with a mouse). And the *tree chart* in Figure

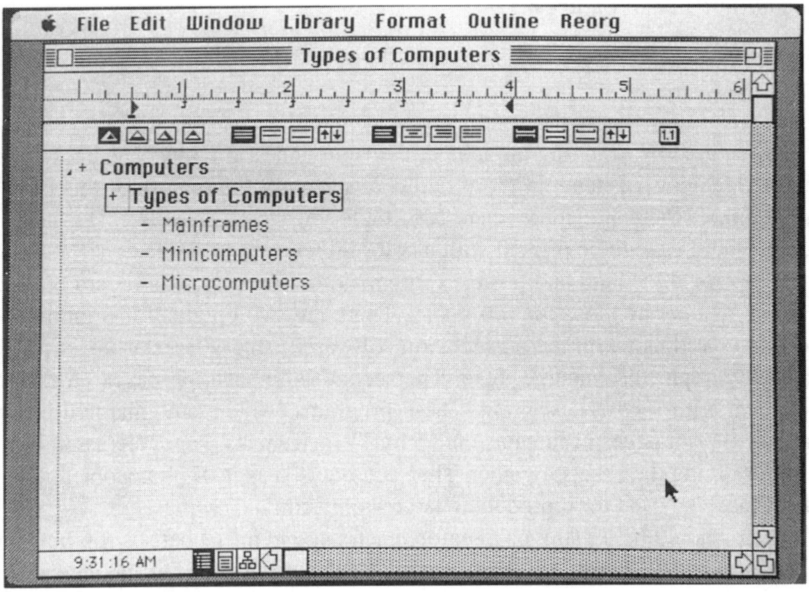

FIGURE 8.1 **A screen from a desktop presentation program containing a segment of an outline.**

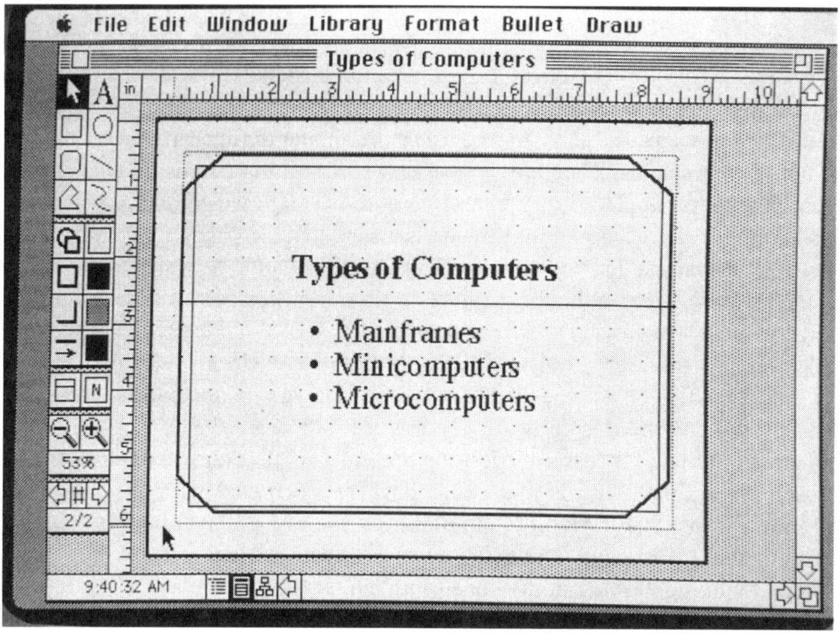

FIGURE 8.2 **A bullet chart created by selecting the icon to the right of the outline one in Figure 8.1.**

8.3 was created by selecting the icon at the right end of the row. The backgrounds and arrangements of items in these two charts are not the only ones this program can generate; there are more than 100, including some in color. The latter, of course, would have to be printed with a color inkjet or laser printer.

Pages for flip charts and posters can be laid out from the storyboard outline in the same manner as those for flip books. There are two options for printing them. The first is to do so with the presentation software (using a laser or inkjet printer), then photographically enlarge them. The second is to save the pages on disk and print them with a *poster program*. These programs (which can enlarge up to billboard size) print pages in sections on 8.5 by 11 inch sheets. Pages are assembled by taping or gluing the sheets together. They can be used as is or photocopied with the type of machine used for reproducing large architectural drawings.

There should be a blank page before each page in a flipchart or flip book. You display these when there is no relevant visual for your remarks. Displaying visuals at times other than while they are being discussed is likely to distract and possibly confuse your audience.

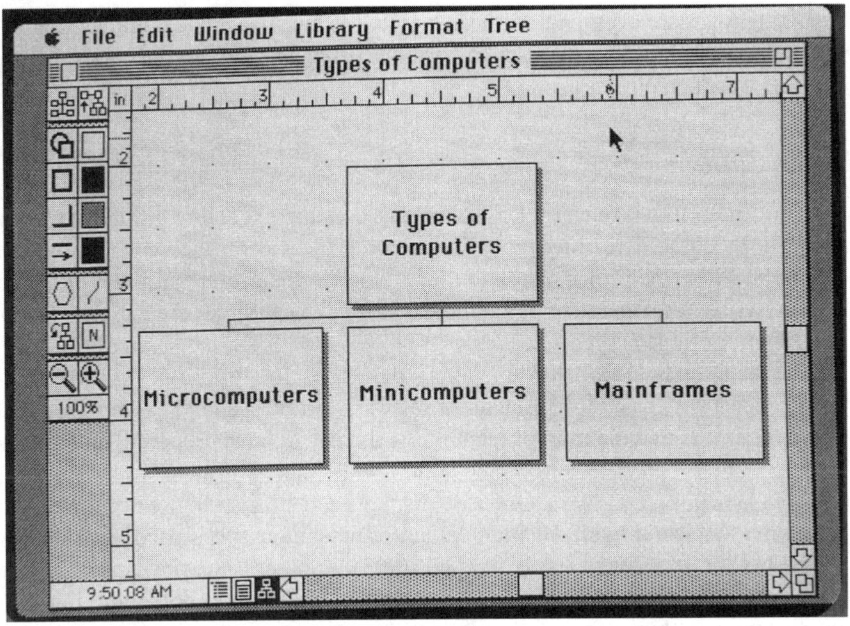

FIGURE 8.3 **A tree chart created by selecting the icon at the right end of the row in Figure 8.1.**

Overhead Transparencies

Overhead transparencies (overheads) are sheets of transparent film—usually 8.5 by 11 inches—on which are reproduced text and/or graphics in black-and-white or color. The lights in the room usually do not have to be turned off for them to be legible when projected on a screen. You can usually insert and change them yourself without disrupting your presentation because the projector is almost always close to where you are standing. Overhead transparencies are most effective for audiences of fewer than 100 people.

The techniques described in the preceding section to lay out pages for flip books can be used (with desktop presentation software) to lay out them for overhead transparencies. They can be printed with a laser or inkjet printer directly on sheets of overhead transparency film or on sheets of paper and photocopied on this film. You can mount your overheads in cardboard or plastic frames with openings of approximately 7.5 by 9.5 inches. Doing so really isn't necessary, however, if you handle them carefully.

Overhead transparencies, incidentally, can also be created with word-processing (see Chapter 7) and drawing (see Chapter 6) software. However, it is more time consuming to create overheads with such software because the text and graphics in them must be laid out by the user rather than being laid out automatically by the computer (from an outline).

35mm Slides

Slides on 35mm film (1 inch by 1.5 inches) can contain text and/or graphics in back-and-white or color. They ordinarily cannot be projected on the screen in normal room light. Since the projector usually isn't close to the presenter, he or she either needs an assistant to operate it or a remote control device. Slides are the most practical medium for large audiences.

The same techniques used for laying out pages for flip books and overhead transparencies with desktop presentation software can be used to lay out slides. The only difference is that the ratio of length to width has to be appropriate—that is, the length must be 1.5 times as long as the width. Slides can be made from the resulting computer files in several ways. One is to display each slide on a monitor screen and photograph the screen with a 35mm camera. The shutter speed used, incidentally, must be 1/30 of a second or less (Charpied, 1993). Another is to print each on a sheet of paper (as you would produce a page for a flip book) and photograph it with a 35mm camera. A third way is to send the diskette on which the slide file was saved to a *service bureau*. The service bureau will make 35mm slides from the magnetic image using special photographic equipment.

On-Screen Videos

On-screen videos are actually slides. The graphics/text for each is produced in the same way as for a slide, but it is stored as a magnetic image on a computer disk rather than as a photographically generated image on 35mm film. The presentation software enables the computer to simulate a slide projector. The monitor is the screen. For relatively large audiences, special monitors are available that both function and look like overhead transparency projectors; they have a monitor screen where the lighted "window" is on an overhead projector (Figure 8.4).

The main limitation of on-screen videos is that you need a computer to do a presentation. You either have to carry one with you or arrange to rent one. If a presentation is being given to a very small group (e.g., a client and his or her family), a laptop can be used.

The software "slides" for a presentation can be stored on a diskette, a hard drive, or a CD-ROM disk. A diskette can be used if the presentation is relatively short and the slides do not include scanned photographs. A hard disk can be used for storing almost any size presentation, including those that contain scanned photographs. A CD-ROM disk can also be used to store almost any size presentation, and is particularly advantageous to use for storing those where many of the slides contain color photographs. The images can be stored on a CD-ROM disk either directly using the computer or indirectly from 35mm slides. With regard to the latter, the Eastman Kodak Company has developed a process for transferring images from 35mm slides to CD-ROM disks that is relatively inexpensive. The text slides for a presentation, incidentally, can be copied with a 35mm camera (from a monitor screen or printed sheets) on color transparency (slide) film and sequenced with the photographs for transfer to a Kodak CD-ROM disk.

CREATING AUDIOTAPES AND VIDEOTAPES

If the audiotaped speech/language samples that you plan to include in a presentation are not usable as is, a computer may enable you to modify them. If the samples were not digitally recorded (with a computer), they would have to be converted to digital form with an analog-to-digital converter (see Chapter 12). There is software with which you can increase the signal-to-noise ratios in them by eliminating or attenuating distracting background noise. This software can also enable you to modify the samples themselves through selective filtering—for example, it can enable you to modify speech samples to simulate for an audience what a person with a sensorineural hearing loss hears by filtering high frequency information from them. Furthermore, it enables you to "cut" segments from speech samples and arrange ("paste") them in a desired sequence. This sequence can include drawings, photographs, and/or movies (with or without animation) as well as other segments from speech samples. Presentations that include various types of visual media or combinations of visual and auditory media are referred to as multimedia ones. Special software (e.g., Authorware, ToolBook, and HyperCard—see Chapter 13) is available for

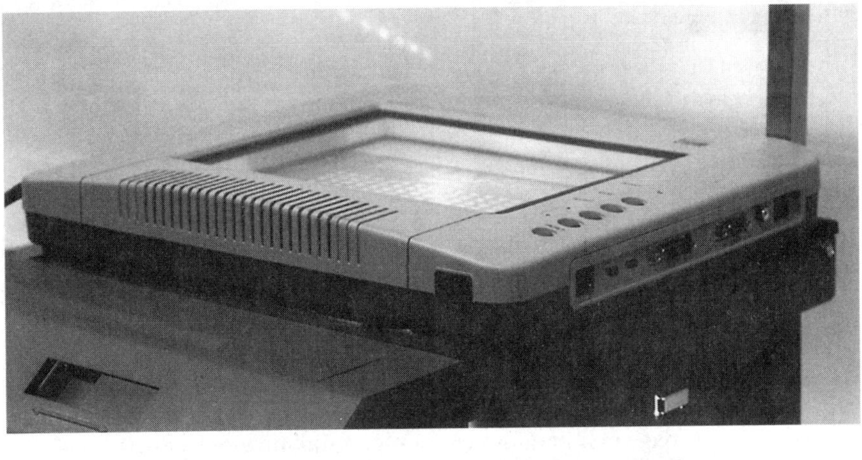

FIGURE 8.4 **An overhead projector-type of computer monitor.**

assembling them. Such presentations can include videotape segments that have been converted from analog to digital form (see Chapter 12) so that they can be displayed on a monitor screen.

Computers can also facilitate the preparation of videotape presentations. They can be used to create titles and subtitles. Almost any "painting" or "drawing" software can be used for this purpose (see Chapter 6). Also, there is software that can facilitate the process of assembling them. After the videotapes, audiotapes, photographs, and drawings (including titles and charts) that contain the material to be included in the presentation are put into the computer, pieces/segments can be "cut" from them and "pasted" into the presentation videotape at appropriate locations. Transitions of various kinds (e.g., fades) between the pieces/segments of the presentation can be generated by the software and added. The "images" to be included in the videotape are sent from the computer (through a cable) to a videotape recorder in the appropriate sequence.

Computers can also enable you to enhance videotape presentations in other ways. They can, for example, enable you to create "windows" through which two or more images can be displayed simultaneously. They can also enable you to animate drawings—for example, to show how data displayed in a graph changed over time.

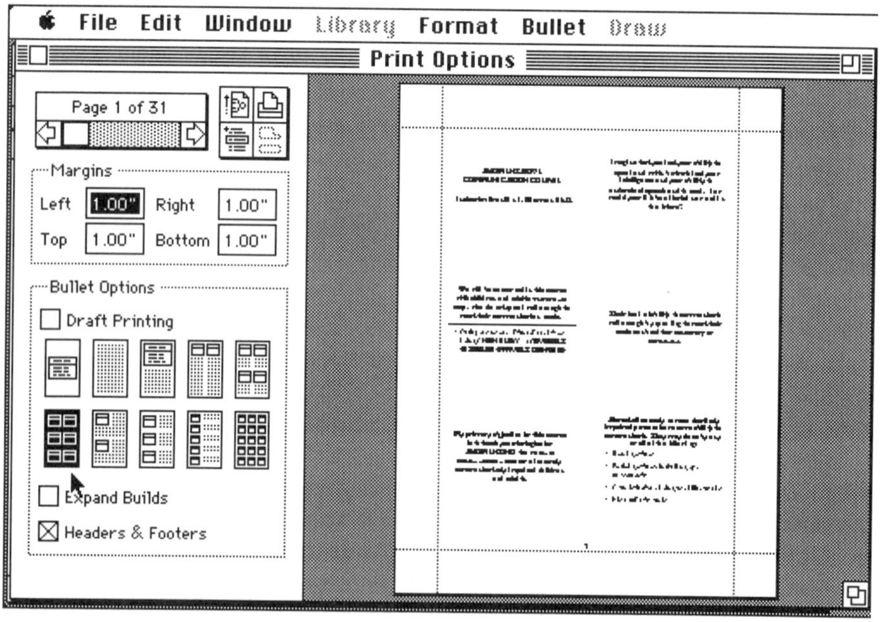

FIGURE 8.5 **A page of a handout containing miniature reproductions of some of the overheads or slides shown during a presentation.**

With some animation software, it is only necessary to create the beginning and end drawings of a sequence: the computer generates the animation for the transition between them.

CREATING SPEAKER NOTES AND HANDOUTS

These programs can generate and print handouts that contain miniature reproductions of your overheads or slides (Figure 8.5). You can print as few as two or as many as twelve on a page. I usually print six on a page. You can, incidentally, do a presentation using just the handouts without projecting the overheads or slides.

These programs can also generate sets of speaker notes. The number of pages in a set is equal to the number of slides or overheads. Each page contains a miniature reproduction of a slide or overhead, usually at the top. You can write or outline the comments that you plan to make on it with the program's word processor.

MAKING THE PRESENTATION

You can use the computer to present as well as create audio-visual material. A computer can be programmed to present the material (e.g., on a monitor screen), control devices that do so (e.g., a laser videodisk player), or both.

You can store the audiovisual material for a presentation on a hard drive, a CD-ROM disk, or both. CD-ROM disks tend to be most practical for storing photographs (including photographs of drawings and charts). You can have them recorded on CD-ROM disks by a photofinisher who does so utilizing the Kodak or a similar process.

You can display visual material on a computer monitor, on a screen using an overhead projector-type computer monitor (Figure 8.4), or on a large-screen television set. The former tends to be most practical for audiences of five or fewer. Audio material can be played through the computer's built-in speaker or an external one. An external speaker is likely to yield higher quality sound than a built-in one.

Overhead projection-type computer monitors and large-screen monitors can be used for audiences larger than five. The largest audience for which this would be practical would be determined by the size of the monitor or projection screen being used and the arrangement of seats around it. It is usually less costly, incidentally, to link a computer to a standard monitor than to purchase an overhead projection-type computer monitor.

The types of presentation devices that can be controlled by a computer include audiotape recorders, videotape recorders, CD-ROM players, slide projectors, and videodisk players. A computer can be programmed to turn them on and off at specified times (or intervals) during a presentation, either singly or in combinations of two or more. A computer can be programmed, for example, to control three slide projectors, each of which projects an image on a different portion of a large screen. By also programming the computer to control an audiotape recorder or a CD-ROM player, you could produce a multimedia presentation that an audience could experience merely by throwing a switch. Some museums and historical sites offer such presentations.

DESIGN CONSIDERATIONS

The effectiveness of visual aids (visuals) is determined by their design as well as their content. A number of guidelines are summarized in this section for designing posters, flipcharts, flip books, overhead transparencies, 35mm slides, and on-screen videos. For further information about designing them, see Holcombe and Stein (1983) and Rabb (1990).

Text Visuals

Perhaps the most common error people make when preparing text visuals is placing too much text on each. Audience members do not tend to carefully read overheads and other visuals that contain a great deal of text. Consequently, such visuals tend to be less effective for communicating. To be effective a visual should:

- Have no more than six lines of text
- Have no more than forty characters per line
- Use phrases rather than sentences

Other design guidelines for maximizing the effectiveness of text visuals include the following:

- Use a plain typeface, such as Helvetica
- Use upper and lower case type, not just upper case
- Use bullets (for example, • or ⇨) or Arabic numerals for listings
- Use color, boldface, or larger-size type for emphasis

Graphic Visuals

The most common error that people make when preparing graphic visuals is the same one they make when preparing text ones—that is presenting too much information. You should limit both the text and graphics on your visuals to what is absolutely necessary!

Specific Considerations

Overhead Transparencies. Guidelines are given in the presentation literature for maximizing the effectiveness of overhead transparencies other than the general ones for text and graphic visuals that have already been mentioned (see Holcombe & Stein, 1983; Rabb, 1990). They include the following:

- Work within a horizontal 7.5 by 9.5 inch space.
- Do not include borders unless they are absolutely necessary. They tend to distract from the image they surround and limit readability. The more elements in an overhead, the less attention each one commands. Use borders and lines for separation and clarity only when blank space alone can't do the job.
- The same basic background and typeface(s) should be used throughout a set of overheads. You don't want the audience's attention diverted from what you are attempting to communicate.
- Have as much contrast as possible between the color of the background and that of the text and/or graphics—if, for example, the background is dark, use light lettering. Blue backgrounds, incidentally, tend to be effective for color overheads.
- Use no more then one overlay on any overhead. An overlay is a second transparency that is mounted in the same frame as the overhead with a single strip of tape (which functions as a hinge). When the overlay is in contact with (on top of) the overhead, both are projected.

Flip Charts and Flip Books. Most of the design considerations for these are the same as for overhead transparencies. Others include the following:

- Choose a size for the pages that is appropriate for the size of the audience. They should be large enough for the visuals they contain to be read/seen easily by all members of the audience.
- Design the visuals so that they look good in a *vertical* format. A layout that is appropriate for overheads may not be appropriate for these because the format used for overheads is *horizontal.*
- Mount the pages so that you can turn them easily while making the presentation. Take your height into consideration if you will be standing while doing so.
- Place a blank page between each page containing a visual.

Slides. The guidelines for preparing slides are generally the same as those for overheads, flipcharts, and flip books. There are, however, some special ones, including the following:

- Design all visuals based on the 2-to-3 ratio for a slide. The absolute size of a visual is not too important because it will be reduced photographically to 1.0 by 1.5 inches either from a sheet of paper or from a monitor screen.
- Slides can be either black and white or color. Audiences tend to pay more attention to color than to black-and-white ones (Rabb, 1990).
- Either a vertical or horizontal format can be used.
- The slides should be numbered on their cardboard mounts. The numbering should be done in pencil so that it can be changed if a slide is to be used in more than one presentation.

On-screen Videos. Design considerations for on-screen videos are essentially the same as for slides. The main difference is that they have to utilize a horizontal format because computer monitors have this format. The length-width ratio used for laying them out should be that of the monitor screen on which they will be viewed.

9

Database Management Systems (DBMSs)

You, like all speech-language pathologists and audiologists, store information and organize it in a way you can retrieve it efficiently. You also utilize information that has been stored and "indexed" for efficient retrieval by others. The "device" that is used to *store, organize, and retrieve* such information is referred to as a *database management system* (DBMS).

All DBMSs have a device for storing and organizing data. The device may be a *book*. The "white pages" of the telephone book is an example of a database that utilizes this device. The data—the names, addresses, and telephone numbers of persons who reside in a particular community—are stored (printed) in the book and are organized ("indexed") for rapid retrieval by their names being ordered alphabetically.

The device used by a DBMS for for storing and organizing data can also be a container. An example is a filing cabinet in which client folders are stored. All of the pertinent information or data concerning a client would be in his or her folder, and the folders would be arranged alphabetically ("indexed") by last name.

Traditionally, as I have indicated, information in DBMSs has been recorded on sheets of paper that are stored in a book or a container. An alternative approach is to store them in a computer. Records are recorded and stored on *disks* (e.g., usually hard disks or CD-ROM disks) and indexed in ways that permit their rapid retrieval. After being retrieved, they can be viewed on a monitor screen and/or printed on sheets of paper, envelopes, or mailing labels. The computer that contains the database can be located in the same building as the one used to retrieve information from it or in a different building—even one thousands of miles away. If the computers were in different buildings, they would either be connected to each other by cables (if they were part of a network) or telephone modems (see Chapters 2 and 11).

There are a number of DBMS programs available for microcomputers. Some—like FileMaker—are intended solely for database management and others—like those in Claris Works and Microsoft Works—are components of integrated programs that also enable you to do other tasks, including word processing (see Chapter 7). They also make it simple for you to integrate database information with other applications—for example, to print form letters with a word processing program in which the information used to fill in blanks comes from a database file (see Chapter 7).

FOR WHAT TASKS CAN YOU USE DATABASE SOFTWARE?

What can you do with microcomputer-based DBMSs that you cannot do—or do as well—with traditional paper-based methods? There are a number of record-keeping (clerical) tasks that database software may enable you to do efficiently (Nelson, 1991). One task is maintaining client records and billing (Alberti & Hyde, 1983; Ball, Anderson, & Schweitzer, 1986; Cassidy & Wynne, 1990; Charpied, 1995; Dale, 1984; Diaz, Hillman, Gress, Bunting, & Doyle, 1993; Domico, 1985; Dustrude, 1990; Elliot, Vegely, & Falvey, 1971; Emanuele, 1994; Harden, Harden, & Norris, 1977; Hood & Miller, 1982; Kamara & Kamara, 1976; Karnell, 1992a, 1992b; Karnell & MacCracken, 1992; Kersting, 1983; Krueger, 1985; Martin, 1991; Mueller & Peters, 1976; Oliveira, 1991; Ostergren & Rodel, 1987; Peterson, 1977; Rushakoff, 1986; Sanders, 1986b; Vogen, 1985). Information can be retrieved more rapidly from client records if they are stored in a computer (using database software) than if they are stored in filing cabinets. The types of information about a caseload that can be retrieved quickly if client records are stored in a computer DBMS include the following:

- Specific information about a client. This is equivalent to searching for it in his or her folder. Doing so by computer is likely to be faster because you can use the software's "find" command to locate information almost instantaneously. If the information is on sheets of paper in the client's folder, the folder would have to be searched, which would almost always take longer.
- The names and numbers of clients in your caseload who have a particular type of communicative disorder (e.g., a conductive hearing loss) or who share some other attribute (e.g., are in the 0-to-3 age range). Such data are needed for year-end and other institutional reports (Krueger, 1985). Getting it by examining client folders would almost always take longer.
- The names of the clients—both past and present—with whom you have used certain intervention approaches. You need this information to assess their effectiveness. Most contemporary database programs, incidentally, have commands that could print form letters (with envelopes or mailing labels) to clients inquiring about the status of their communicative disorder(s) or could dial their telephone numbers if you wanted to followup by phone.
- The names of all of the clients in your caseload who should be scheduled for re-evaluation. You, of course, would have to establish criteria for identifying them

(e.g., having been in therapy for six months). You could also use your database software to identify times when reevaluations could be scheduled and to print form letters informing clients about them.

- Billing and payment information. You could, for example, retrieve the names of all of your clients for whom payments have not been received for more than 60 days after bills were sent. Furthermore, you can probably use your database program to calculate and print bills (with envelopes or address labels).

A second task for which you can use database software is the storage and retrieval of clinically relevant information (Buchanan & Jones, 1987; Diaz et al., 1993; Harden et al., 1977; Miller & Nockerts, 1993; Perez, Alba, Reimer, & Oboudi, 1993; Wiepsuj,et al., 1992). The content of such a database could be therapy goals for IEPs (Block, 1991; *Goalquest: IEP Writer*, no date; Iverson, 1990; Jenkins, 1987; Kelly et al., 1987; Nelson, 1991; Schetz et al., 1991; Schuldt, no date; Schuldt & Harding, 1985; Scudder, 1990; Sun, 1990; Swanson & Griffin, 1984; Zemmol, 1985), directories of devices for augmenting the speech or hearing of persons who are communicatively impaired (Corell, Ludvissen, & Birk-Nielsen, 1983; Vanderheiden, 1990; Vanderheiden, Snyder, & Kelso, 1992), descriptions of community referral resources, or bibliographies of clinically relevant literature (Litke, 1991). A database of this type that you use may have been created by someone other than yourself.

A third task for which you can use database software is laying out and printing forms. Clinicians use forms for a number of purposes, including recording case history and test data. Some database programs—such as FileMaker—have the "tools" needed to lay out complex ones (see Sosinsky, 1991). Forms created in this way can be filled in prior to being printed and used for writing reports, including initial evaluation ones (Bluestone, Lefkowitz, & Boole, 1994; Bluestone, Lefkowitz, Violock-Boole, McLean, & O'Neil-Pirozzi, 1993).

Other tasks for which you can use database software include appointment scheduling (Valentine, 1995a); printing form letters and mailing labels; maintaining bibliographies; creating assessment, tutorial, and other learning tasks; storing and printing therapy stimuli (word lists, sentence lists, etc.); and inventorying items that are despensed, such as hearing aids (Brown, 1982). Incidentally, if you are on the faculty of a speech-language pathology or audiology training program, you can use database software for tracking your students' progress toward meeting ASHA-CCC requirements (Mahaffey, 1973; Sansone & Acker, 1993; Sawyer & Sawyer, 1994). The Macintosh HyperCard and similar programs can be used for some of the applications mentioned in this paragraph (see Chapter 13).

DATABASE TERMINOLOGY

A prerequisite for learning to use database management software is understanding the terminology used to describe both the hierarchical organization of data within a database and the layouts used for data entry and display. This terminology is defined in this section.

Hierarchical Organization of Data within a Database

The levels on which data are organized within a database are depicted in Figure 9.1. The lowest level consists of *characters*—individual letters or numbers. The amount of secondary memory that a computer can access (see Chapter 2) determines the maximum number of characters there can be in a database. Each character consumes approximately one byte of a disk's storage capacity. Consequently, a 120 megabyte hard drive can store databases that contain approximately 120,000,000 characters. And a CD-ROM disk can store databases that contain 550,000,000 characters and possibly more.

The next level in the hierarchy consists of data elements or *entries*. An entry is a word or phrase (i.e., a grouping of characters) that designates a single piece of information. A client's street address would be an entry.

The third level in the hierarchy consists of records and fields.

Records are logical groupings of entries. In a client database, all of the entries pertaining to a particular client could be combined to form a record.

Each entry in a record is assigned to a *field*. A field is a category within a record

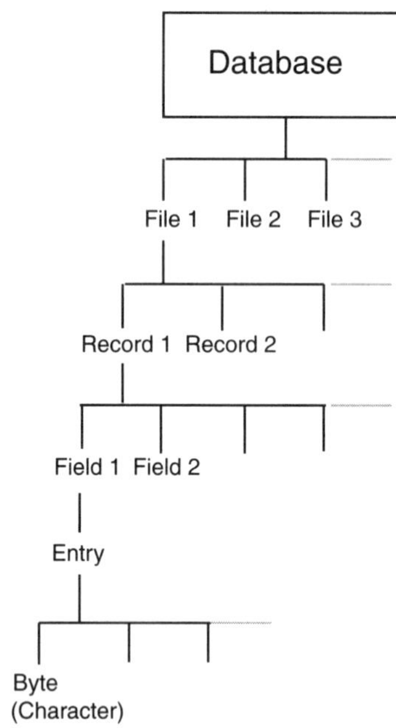

FIGURE 9.1 **Hierarchical organization of data within a database.**

that "holds" a single data entry. For example, in a client database, *last name* would be a field that would be expected to "hold" an entry in every client's record. In some fields, however, there may not be an entry in every record. There wouldn't be an entry, for example, in the field *apartment number* in the records of clients who live in single-family homes.

When creating a field, you must specify the *attributes* of a data entry that would be appropriate to assign to it. The appropriate data entry for a field may not be text. It may be a date, a drawing, or a photograph. It may also be a number that the program calculates. Most database programs can do relatively complex calculations that involve addition, subtraction, multiplication, and/or division as well as other arithmetic operations.

The next to the highest level in the hierarchy consists of *files*. These are logical groupings of records. For example, all of the records in a client database that contain the same fields—in whole or part—can be combined to form a file. The fields do not have to be identical in all of the records in a file.

The highest level in the hierarchy is the *database*. Some databases consist of a single file. Others consist of a group of files that have been logically integrated to minimize redundancy and facilitate the retrieval of entries and records that are stored in more than one file. Redundancy is minimized by reducing the need for particular data entries to be stored in more than one file.

Layouts

You are unlikely to use all of the fields in a database for a particular application. For example, you would use only the "name" and "address" fields from the records in a client database to create address labels. All database programs have commands for specifying what fields are to be displayed (on the monitor screen) and printed and how the entries in them are to be arranged, or laid out. A *layout* is an arrangement of fields, possibly combined with graphic elements (drawings and photographs), that can be displayed and printed. As such, it is a type of *form*. You can create many layouts (forms) and switch between them.

Database output layouts—layouts for printing reports—are referred to as *reporting structures*. The layout (form) for a data-entry screen may not be the same as that for a reporting structure. It could only be the same if you were including all of the fields in a record in a report you were preparing—for example, if you were printing all of the information in a client's record.

TYPES OF DATABASES

There are four basic types of databases: flat-file, hierarchical, relational, and networked. Some database software can create several of them (e.g., both flat-file and relational databases).

Flat-File Databases

This is the type that speech-language pathologists and audiologists appear to use most often. These databases—also referred to as *file managers* and *file handlers*—have a relatively simple structure. They store records in files that are independent of each other. Consequently, changing an entry in a field in one file (e.g., an address) will not change it in the same field in other files that you maintain on your computer. You can search only one file at a time. If the records that contain the information you need are stored in more than one file, you must access more than one file to retrieve them. The software that you would need to create this type of database is usually less expensive than that you would need to create the other types.

Each file in a flat-file database can be conceptualized as a *two-dimensional array of records and fields*. The records would be rows and the fields columns (Figure 9.2). This type of array is similar to that used in spreadsheets (see Chapter 10). In fact, spreadsheet software can be used for relatively small flat-file databases that don't require sophisticated layouts for reporting structures.

Hierarchical Databases

These databases organize data much like a family tree or an organizational chart. They contain three types of records. The record at the highest level in the database—at the top of the "tree"—is called the *root record*. The root record connects the various branches, which are referred to metaphorically as *parent records* and *child records*.

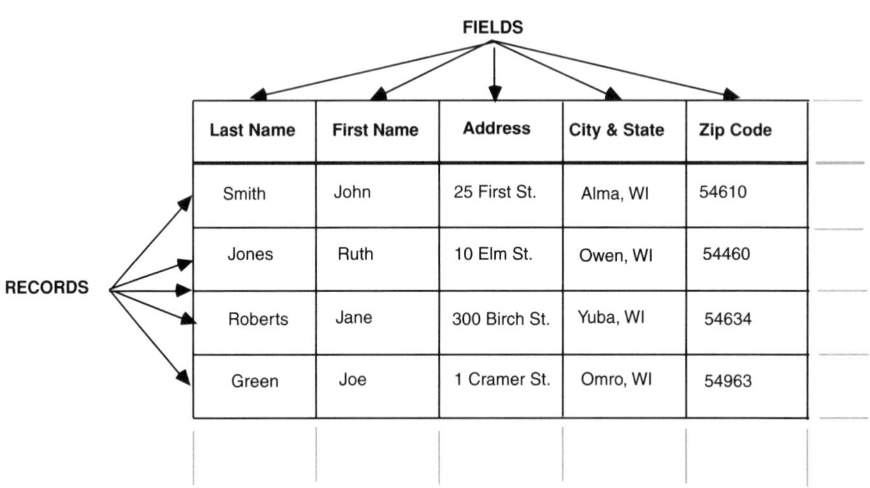

FIGURE 9.2 **A flat-file database conceptualized as a two-dimensional array of records and fields.**

A parent record can have many child records, but each child record can have only one parent record. If your telephone company used a hierarchical database for computing charges, your name, address, and telephone number would be fields in the parent record and your incoming and outgoing calls and charges would be child records.

Hierarchical databases link together groups ("files") of records, but only in certain ways. To retrieve data from a child record, it is necessary to descend the "tree" (the root record) to the "branch" (the parent record) to which it has been assigned. Only certain data entries can be retrieved conveniently from sets of records that are organized in this manner. All data entries are not linked together. The links between them are determined by the database designer when he or she designates some records as *parents* and others *children* and specifies how parent records are to be linked with the *root* record.

While this type of organization rarely is used for microcomputer databases, some large organizations (e.g., hospitals) do use it for the financial records they maintain on minicomputers or mainframe computers.

Relational Databases

These databases can create records with data entries from different sources. These entries do not have to be in the same file or in the same type of record. Because entries can be cross-referenced, they do not have to be "written" in the database more than once. Consequently, files in a relational database can be structured to be less redundant than those in a flat-file one. In a client database, for example, a client's date of birth, address, and telephone number would not have to be "written" in every document for it to be easily retrieved and displayed.

Relational databases can construct files from other files. The user defines a link or relationship between certain fields in one or more files that causes a new file to be formed. The records in this new file contain the entries in these fields. For example, in a client database that has a relational structure, the name and address fields (with entries) could be used to form a new file—one for printing mailing labels.

Software for creating relational databases is available for microcomputers. However, it tends to be more expensive and difficult to learn to use than that for creating flat-file databases. Consequently, you probably would only find it advantageous to use it for databases for which flat-file software is inadequate. It has been estimated, incidentally, that flat-file software is adequate for more than 95 percent of database projects (Sosinsky, 1991). This is particularly true for flat-file programs that are *pseudorelational*. Such programs have commands for looking up information in other files.

Networked Databases

A network is a system of cables (electrical connections) and associated hardware and software that links two or more computers together. Computers so linked are part of a network and can access data on each others hard drives or CD-ROM disks (see Chapter 11 for additional information about computer networks).

Networked database software can synthesize records and files from data entries on computers at various locations in a network. If, for example, the computers containing the "card catalogues" for a number of college and university libraries were linked to form a network, you could determine by accessing the network whether any of them had a book that you needed.

PLANNING A DATABASE

Your first and perhaps most important task when planning a database is deciding what information (data entries) to include and how is to organize, retrieve, and use it. You need to do this before defining fields because how data entries are to be used can determine how they should be defined. If, for example, you are a school clinician and plan to use your client record database for writing form letters, parents' first and last names should be in separate fields because their last names will be needed for salutations.

A good way to ensure that a database will contain all pertinent fields is to create the output reporting structures (forms) you will be using before defining them. While almost all database programs will allow you to add and redefine fields after data entry has begun, doing so can be very time-consuming because the records that have already been entered will have to be modified.

After you have defined and created fields and reporting structures, the next step is to select database software. Choose the "simplest" program that will meet your needs. There are several reasons. The first is cost. Relatively simple programs (e.g., flat-file ones) tend to be less expensive that relatively sophisticated ones (e.g., relational ones). The second is ease of learning. Relatively simple database programs tend to take less time to learn to use than relatively sophisticated ones. The third is amount of memory needed. Relatively simple database programs require less RAM to operate and less disk space to store than relatively sophisticated ones. And the fourth one is speed. Relative simple (flat-file) database programs tend to retrieve information faster than relatively sophisticated (relational) ones. The only possible advantage of using a database program that is more sophisticated than the one your application requires is that you (or your institution) already own it. For most databases that speech-language pathologists and audiologists are likely to create, flat-file programs should be adequate.

Your next task is to create a data entry form and to write instructions for using it. The form should be as simple and intuitive as possible. If a database will have only one reporting form—which means that all of the fields will be used—the data entry form should be laid out the same way. If, for example, a database is to be used solely for printing mailing labels, the layout of fields on the data entry form should be similar to that of information (name, street address, etc.) on a mailing label. You should write instructions for the data entry form even if you are the only one who will be entering data. The instructions should specify unambiguously the information that should be in the data entry for each field. While you may assume that you will never forget what this information should be, this is not a safe assumption to make based on personal experience and that of colleagues.

A consideration in designing databases—particularly ones that contain client records—is maintaining *confidentiality*. To maintain confidentiality, you need a "mechanism" for controlling access. Almost all database programs offer such a mechanism—*password protection*. Password protection gives access only to users who know the password and can limit what a user can access. For example, the password used by your secretary to access a client database could conceal all information but that needed for billing.

Another consideration when designing is database is developing a backup strategy. Disks can fail and data can be deleted by mistake. The loss of information in a database—particularly one containing client records—can be disastrous. Consequently, you should back up your databases periodically on diskettes, a different hard disk, or on a tape intended for backing up hard disks. If the entries in a database will not fit on a single diskette, more than one can be used. You may want to make two back ups of each database and store them at different locations (e.g., one at the office and one at home). While this may seem like overkill, it really isn't. It is cheap insurance, particularly if your second backup is on diskettes. You may also want to back up your databases by periodically printing hard copies of them.

▶ 10

Numerical Data Analysis

Computation is the application for which computers have been used the longest; the first ones were dedicated to this application. Consequently, they were referred to as computers because their intended function was to compute. While they had limited memory and relatively slow CPUs, they could perform calculations faster and more accurately than a mechanical calculator.

Numerical data analysis is still one of the main tasks for which computers (including microcomputers) are used. Five types of software—clinical index computation, calculator, spreadsheet, statistical analysis, and financial analysis—that you can use to analyze numerical data for administrative, clinical, and research purposes are described in this chapter.

CALCULATOR SOFTWARE

Any microcomputers can be programmed to simulate an electronic calculator. The machine language program needed for doing addition, subtraction, multiplication, division, square root, and most other arithmetic operations is a component of your computer's operating system software (see Chapter 3). The software described in this chapter enables you to access and use this component.

You probably already have calculator software. It may be a desk accessory that came with your computer or a component of a program that you presently have, such as a word processing program. A *desk accessory* program is one that you can access without having to "quit" the program you are using: You can switch back and forth between it and the desk accessory. The desk accessory usually is displayed as a "window" on the monitor screen. In Figure 10.1 a very basic calculator desk accessory is displayed as such a window. A key on the calculator can be "pressed" by placing the cursor on it (using the mouse) and pressing a button on the mouse.

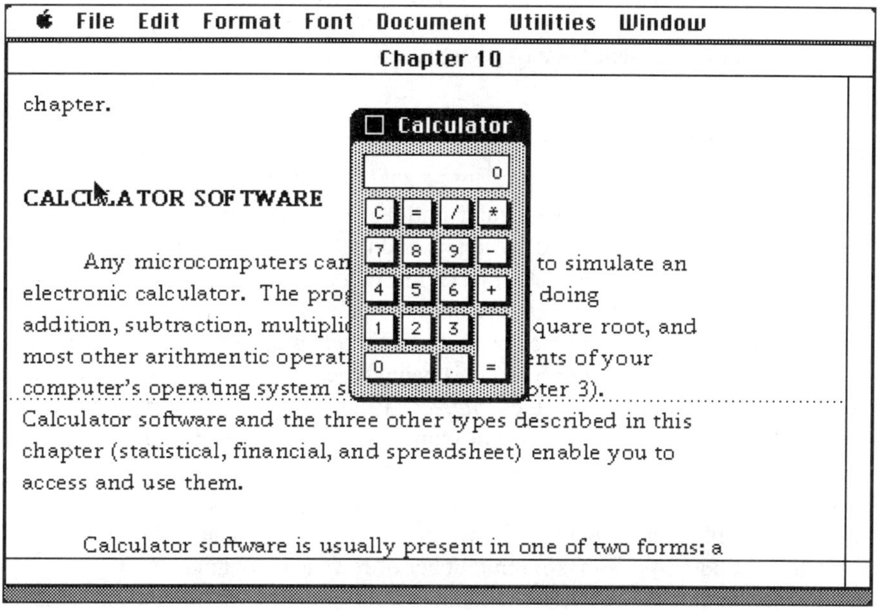

FIGURE 10.1 **A calculator desk accessory displayed as a "window" on a monitor screen.**

Some calculator desk accessories simulate a highly sophisticated, programmable, scientific printing calculator. They can do all of the computations that can be done with such a calculator. While you can use one to compute statistics, it is easier to do it with statistical analysis software (described elsewhere in this chapter) because you do not have to keyboard formulas. Furthermore, if you plan to compute several statistics from a set of data, with statistical analysis software you will only have to keyboard the data once.

You will also find calculator-type commands in programs that are not dedicated to analyzing numerical data (i.e., programs other than those discussed in this chapter). Most word-processing and database programs, for example, have commands that enable users to do at least basic arithmetic (i.e., addition, subtraction, multiplication, and division).

Numeric keypads (see Chapter 2) facilitate the data entry process for calculator software as well as the other types described in this chapter. Their rectangular layout of number keys makes possible more rapid data entry than their single line layout on the keyboard. Furthermore, they reduce errors by making it almost impossible to accidentally press character keys that are not number ones.

Audiologists, incidentally, have used calculator software clinically for analyzing data yielded by assessment tasks (Agnew, 1983).

SPREADSHEETS

A spreadsheet is a table—a rectangular grid—of rows and columns (Figure 10.2). The columns usually are labeled by letters and the rows by numbers (Figures 10.2 and 10.3). A spreadsheet can contain just a few columns and rows or hundreds (possibly even thousands) of them. An area one column wide by one row high is called a *cell.* A cell is a location—a particular row in a particular column—where something is typed. The cell in which information is being typed or from which information is being retrieved is referred to as the *active cell* (Figure 10.2). What is typed in a cell may be a number, a formula, or one or more words. Consequently, each cell would have a unique letter-number address—the address for the "active cell" in Figure 10.2 would be D8. Some cells in a spreadsheet will be empty (there will be nothing typed in them). The maximum numbers of rows and columns you can have in a spreadsheet is determined both by the maximum number of rows and columns the program can handle and the amount of RAM available in your computer. While the spreadsheet

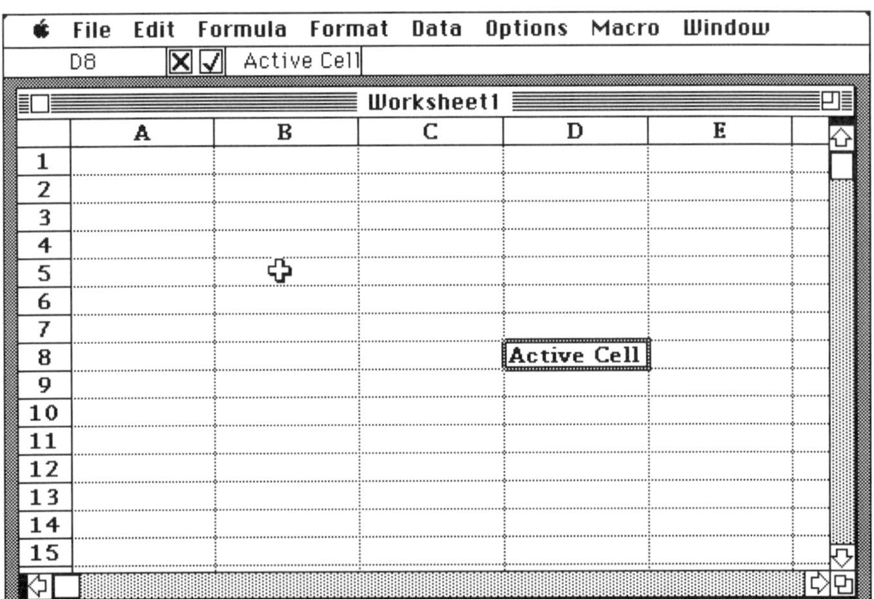

FIGURE 10.2 **The layout of rows, columns, and cells in a segment of a spreadsheet.**

File Edit Formula Format Data Options Macro Window

Y21 | Client

Thresholds (dB) for Left Ear

	Y	Z	AA	AB	AC	AD	AE
20							
21	**Client**	**500 Hz**	**1000 Hz**	**2000 Hz**	**3000 Hz**	**4000 Hz**	**6000 Hz**
22	Steve B.	5	10	0	5	5	5
23	Stacy C.	5	10	5	0	5	20
24	Sarah C.	3	10	0	-5	-5	20
25	Ryan C.	20	15	15	25	35	20
26	Ruth B.	15	10	-5	0	0	20
27	Mark C.	5	5	0	0	5	15
28	Kyle C.	15	15	10	5	20	5
29	Kori C.	5	0	15	15	20	5
30	Jody B.	10	5	10	15	20	30
31	Jason B.	10	10	10	10	20	5
32	Cathy T.	10	10	10	5	5	-5
33	Bob M.	10	5	5	10	-5	10
34	Ashley,C.	20	15	5	10	10	5
35	Adam C.	0	0	10	10	15	10
36	Aaron C.	20	25	20	20	10	15
37							
38							

FIGURE 10.3 **A segment of a spreadsheet in which are recorded hearing thresholds for pure tones.**

program I use can generate 256 columns and 16,384 rows, the amount of RAM in my computer isn't adequate to handle a spreadsheet this large.

A spreadsheet may be too large to display on a monitor screen. To view all of it you have to move (*scroll*) the spreadsheet both north and south (vertically) and east and west (horizontally). To visualize this process, imagine that the spreadsheet is printed on a scroll that can be moved in these four directions and that the monitor screen is an immovable window that is mounted in front of this scroll. As the scroll is moved, the portion of the spreadsheet that is visible in the window changes.

A spreadsheet may also be too large to print on a single sheet of paper. Such a spreadsheet would be printed in sections and the sheets on which the sections are printed could be taped together. The assembled spreadsheet could be taken to a copy shop and photocopied on a single large sheet of paper (with the type of machine used for photocopying architects' drawings).

Most spreadsheet programs can display and print numerical information in graphic as well as tabular form. They can generate almost any kind of graph from the information in a group of cells. The line graph in Figure 10.4, for example, was generated by the program from the cells that are "highlighted" in Figure 10.3.

Spreadsheets enable you to store, display, and manipulate numerical data. The value (number) in a particular cell may either be one that was keyboarded by you or the

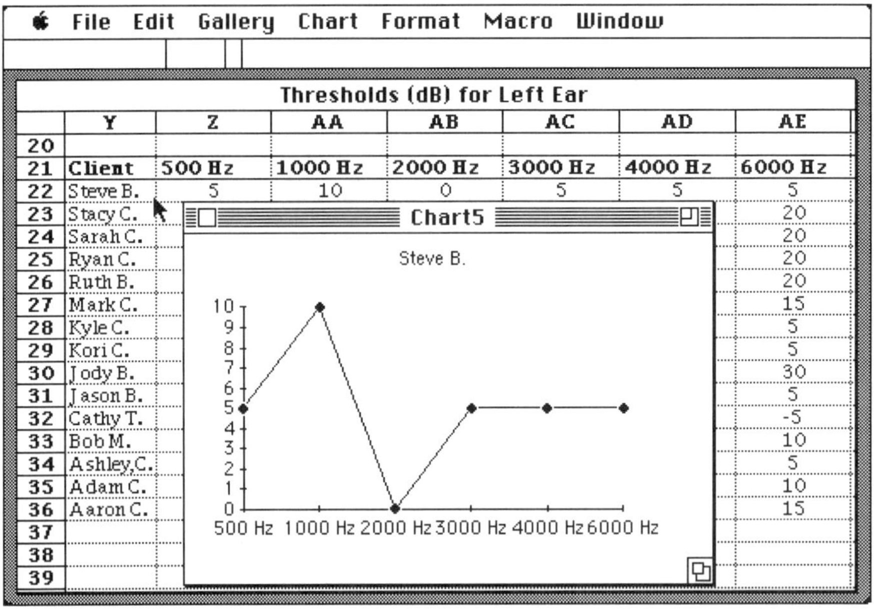

FIGURE 10.4 **A line graph generated by the program from the highlighted information in Figure 10.3.**

result of a calculation performed by the computer using the formula in that cell. The numbers used to compute a value for a particular cell are from other cells. The formula identifies them by giving their address—for example, C3 = A1 + B9 (Figure 10.5).

Spreadsheets that you intend to use more than once—for example, those for displaying and analyzing a client's audiometric test data—can be "locked" and saved as *templates*. The cells of a spreadsheet template contain only fixed values (constants), headings, and formulas. After "filling" the data cells in a spreadsheet template, you would save it under a name that differs from the one you gave the template. The purpose of "locking" the template is to keep yourself from absent-mindedly recording data in it.

The numbers in spreadsheet cells are interdependent. Changing the number in a cell causes all of the calculations involving that cell to be redone. For example, if the number in A1 in Figure 10.5 was changed from 25.5 to 20.1, the value displayed in C3 a fraction of a second later would be 50.6 rather than 56.

One application for which this cell interdependence is used is doing "what if" analyses. These analyses enable you to predict certain outcomes of decisions involving numbers. If you were considering purchasing a car, for example, you could do a "what if" analysis to determine the effect different interest rates would have on your monthly payments. When you changed the interest rate on the spreadsheet,

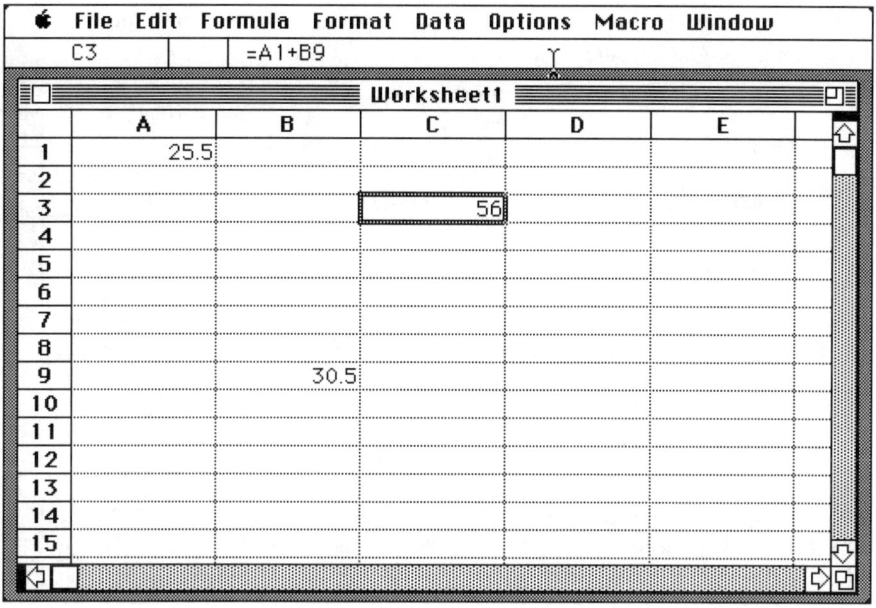

FIGURE 10.5 **A spreadsheet that calculates a value.**

the value in the cell displaying your monthly payment would change. You could also determine the effect of different purchase prices, down payments, and loan durations.

Speech-language pathologists and audiologists also use "what if" analyses for professional decision making. An audiologist in private practice who dispenses hearing aids may use one to determine how much he or she would have to charge for fitting them to be likely to have a yearly income of a particular size. And a speech-language pathologist in private practice may use this type of analysis for setting fees. Furthermore, practitioners in both fields who are considering establishing a private practice would be wise to use a spreadsheet to estimate how much income the practice is likely to yield before proceeding.

Spreadsheet software can also be used to create databases (see Chapter 9 for information about this application). For *flat-file* databases, the entire spreadsheet would be the *file*. For *relational* databases, the spreadsheet would be segmented into *two or more files*. Each row would be a *record* and each cell in it a *field*. The cells would contain *data entries* that are appropriate for the fields they designate (Figure 10.6). One of the main limitations of using spreadsheet programs for databases is that they tend to offer fewer options for laying out data-entry screen and reporting structures (see Chapter 9) than do database programs. However, if you do not require elaborate layouts and are not creating large, sophisticated databases that will be

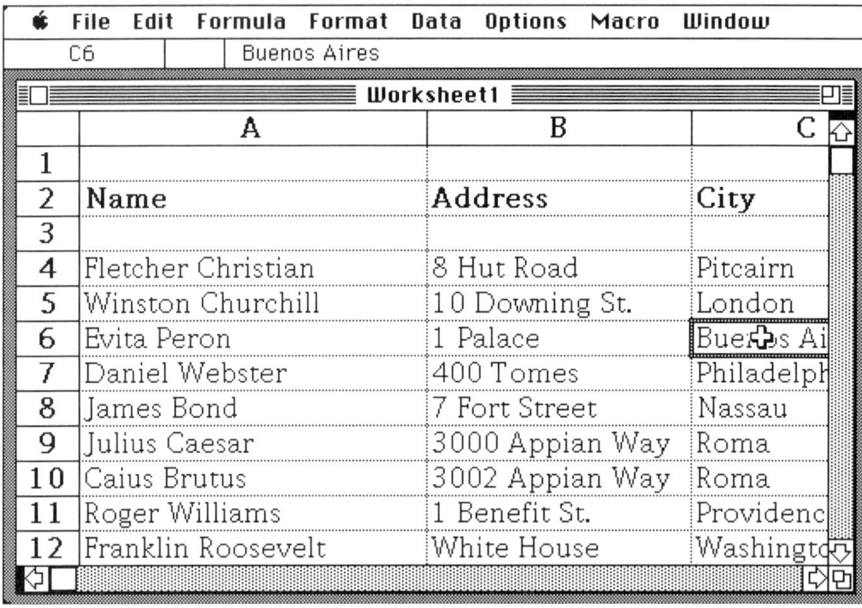

FIGURE 10.6 **Portion of a Rolodex-type database on a spreadsheet.**

accessed by other people, a spreadsheet program may be adequate for meeting both your spreadsheet and database needs.

Spreadsheet software can also be used for another purpose—drawing graphs. Most sophisticated spreadsheet programs—including Lotus 1-2-3 and Microsoft Excel—can draw most types of two-dimensional and three-dimensional graphs. The labels and numerical data needed to draw them are "communicated" to the computer by keyboarding or otherwise placing them in a spreadsheet. A graph drawn in this way can be *exported* to a paint or draw program (see Chapter 6) for enhancement before printing. Such enhancement could include adding or modifying text in a way that cannot be done with the spreadsheet program.

Practitioners in our field have used spreadsheets clinically for charting management progress (Owen & Owen, 1995). They have also used them clinically for analyzing data yielded by assessment tasks. They have used them, for example, to compute the Articulation Index (Korabic, 1993) and various hearing conservation program (HCP) performance indices (Simpson, 1994). They have also used them for analyzing attitude scale data, including that yielded by the *Communication Profile for the Hearing Impaired* (Korabic, unpublished manuscript). Furthermore, academicians in our field have used them to document student progress toward meeting requirements for ASHA certification (Harlan & Hasegawa, 1976).

STATISTICAL ANALYSIS SOFTWARE

You can use these programs, which are available for all microcomputers, to compute descriptive and inferential statistics. They have been used by practitioners in speech-language pathology and audiology to compute statistics for administrative and clinical purposes as well as research ones (see Anderson et al., 1991; Channell, 1990; Seaton, 1983, 1991b, 1991c, 1991d; Seaton & McVey, 1983; Simpson, 1994; Wynne, Friedman, Friedman, & Renshaw, 1993).

These are really spreadsheet programs that have built-in formula *templates* for computing various statistics. Some of these templates have cell linkage formulas that enable you to compute several statistics (e.g., the mean, median, range, and standard deviation) by issuing a single command.

Data are placed in the rows and columns of the program's spreadsheet (Figure 10.7). They can be keyboarded or imported from a spreadsheet that was created with another program. After the data have been entered into the statistical program's spreadsheet, you issue the appropriate command to perform a statistical analysis. The computer will then link the cells containing the data needed to compute the sta-

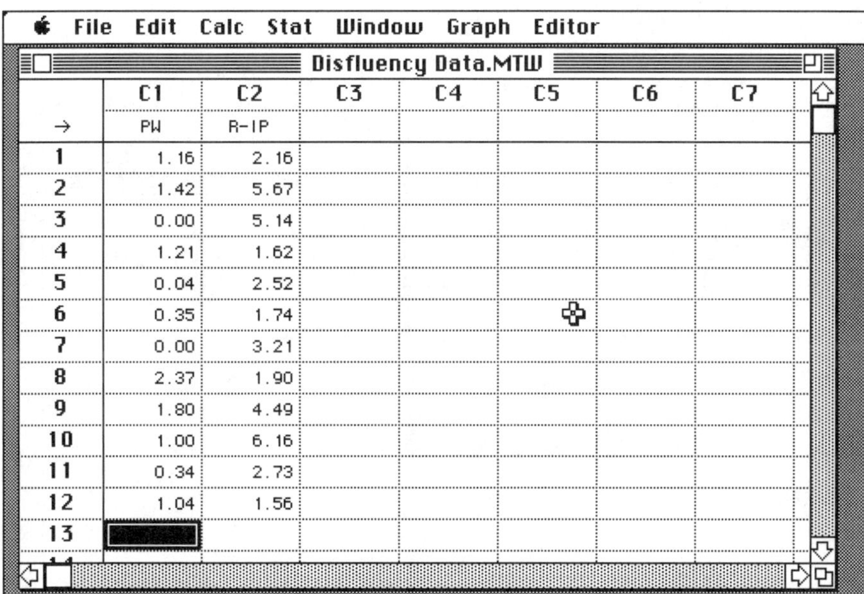

	C1	C2	C3	C4	C5	C6	C7
→	PW	R-IP					
1	1.16	2.16					
2	1.42	5.67					
3	0.00	5.14					
4	1.21	1.62					
5	0.04	2.52					
6	0.35	1.74					
7	0.00	3.21					
8	2.37	1.90					
9	1.80	4.49					
10	1.00	6.16					
11	0.34	2.73					
12	1.04	1.56					
13							

FIGURE 10.7 **An input spreadsheet from a statistical analysis program containing frequencies per 100 words of two types of speech disfluencies—part-word repetitions (PW) and revisions-incomplete phrases (R-IP)—for 12 children.**

tistic to the ones containing the formulas needed to do so and will display the value computed for the statistic on the monitor screen. The screen in Figure 10.8 displays some descriptive statistics that were computed from the data in Figure 10.7 by issuing a single command. These statistics are the number of items in the column (N), the mean, the median, the mean with the smallest 5 percent and the largest 5 percent of values trimmed (TRMEAN), the standard deviation (STDEV), the standard error of the mean (SEMEAN), the range (MIN and MAX), and the interquartile range (Q1 and Q3).

These programs can compute almost any statistic that an audiologist or speech-language pathologist is likely to need, including regression equations, correlation coefficients, parametric and nonparametric significance tests, and confidence intervals. They can even do multivariate statistical analyses, including multi-factor analyses of variance, multiple regression and correlation, discriminant function analysis, and factor analysis. Furthermore, they can create graphical displays, including scattergrams. For further information about the statistics and displays discussed in this paragraph, see Chapters 9 and 10 in Silverman (1993).

There are a number of statistical analysis programs for microcomputers, which vary considerably in both price and what they can do. If your present and anticipated future statistical analysis needs are modest—limited to descriptive statistics and uni-

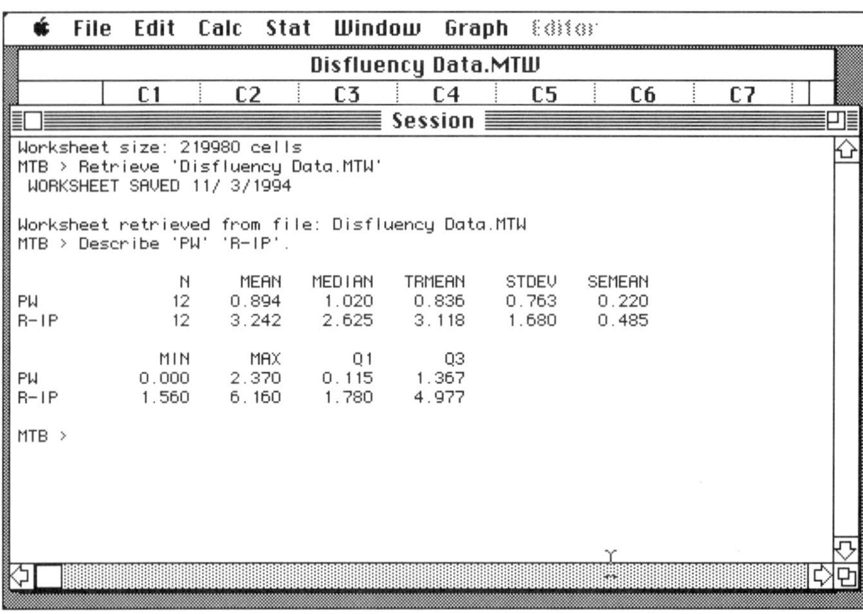

FIGURE 10.8 **Descriptive statistics that were computed from the data in Figure 10.7.**

variate parametric and nonparametric significance tests—a relatively low-priced program may meet your needs. Such a program, beside saving you money, is likely to consume less space on your hard drive and take less time to learn to use than a sophisticated one.

If you have access to a minicomputer or mainframe computer, you probably can use it for doing statistical analyses. Most, if not all, college and university centers have at least one statistical analysis software package installed on their minicomputers or mainframe computers. If you have a microcomputer at your office and/or home that can simulate a terminal for a minicomputer or mainframe computer (see Chapter 11), you will be able to do statistical analyses without having to go to the computer center.

FINANCIAL SOFTWARE

A clinical practice is a small business. It sells a service regardless of whether it is a for-profit or nonprofit entity. It is likely to have employees. It purchases products and services from others and keeps track of these expenditures. It has budgets for various purposes and has to monitor expenditures to stay within these budgets. It bills clients, insurance companies, and/or governmental entities for the services it provides. And it has to maintain certain types of financial records for tax and other purposes. There are several relatively inexpensive, easy-to-use financial analysis programs (for both IBM-compatible and Macintosh computers) that can help you to both track income and expenditures and generate financial records that are acceptable to the IRS and other government agencies (Kamara & Kamara, 1976; Prater, 1988).

Financial analysis programs, like statistical analysis ones, are actually spreadsheet programs that are "dedicated" to doing certain tasks. The templates that are built into them contain both formulas and layouts for input and reporting forms. These programs vary with regard to the level of knowledge of accounting practices they assume the user possesses.

You can do what a financial analysis program does with a spreadsheet program. However, since excellent financial analysis programs are available (such as Quicken) that are relatively inexpensive and do not assume a knowledge of accounting practices, it doesn't seem worth the effort to learn enough about these practices to set up a spreadsheet to do them.

Some financial analysis programs that are intended for persons who aren't accountants use an input screen layout that is similar to a checkbook register (Figure 10.9). For each transaction, you enter a description, the amount and type (payment or deposit), and a category. The category to which a transaction is assigned classifies it for tax, budgetary, and other analyses. For transactions that are payments by check, you also enter a check number. The computer enters the date and the current balance.

Information stored in the register can be used for a number of purposes. One is

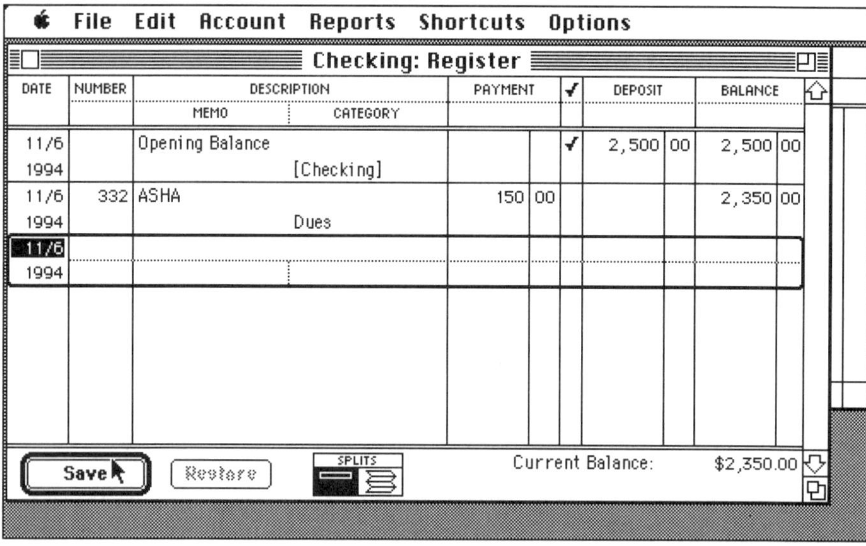

FIGURE 10.9 **The check register input screen for a financial analysis program.**

writing checks. After you fill in the check input form on the monitor screen (Figure 10.10), you print what you keyboarded on a check that is compatible with your printer.

Another way that you can use the information in the register is to monitor your operating budgets. The "categories" you would enter in the register are ones that designate budget accounts. The transactions involving any account and the balance in it can be displayed on a screen and/or printed. Detailed reports of expenditures during a specified time period can be created and printed by the software.

Another way you may be able to use this type of software—particularly if you are in private practice or do consulting—is keeping state and federal income tax records. The categories used in the register for classifying transactions would be ones needed for reporting business income and expenditures on income tax forms. After viewing these financial data on a screen or in a printout, you can "type" them on the forms. Alternatively, you can export these data to a *tax preparation* program. It can make the computations needed to complete both state and federal tax forms and print them.

The type of financial software that was discussed in this section is intended for persons who do not have any background in accounting. For persons who do have such a background, there are highly sophisticated programs available for both IBM-compatible and Macintosh computers. Some of these programs are sophisticated enough to maintain all the financial records for a company that has hundreds of employees and grosses millions of dollars a year.

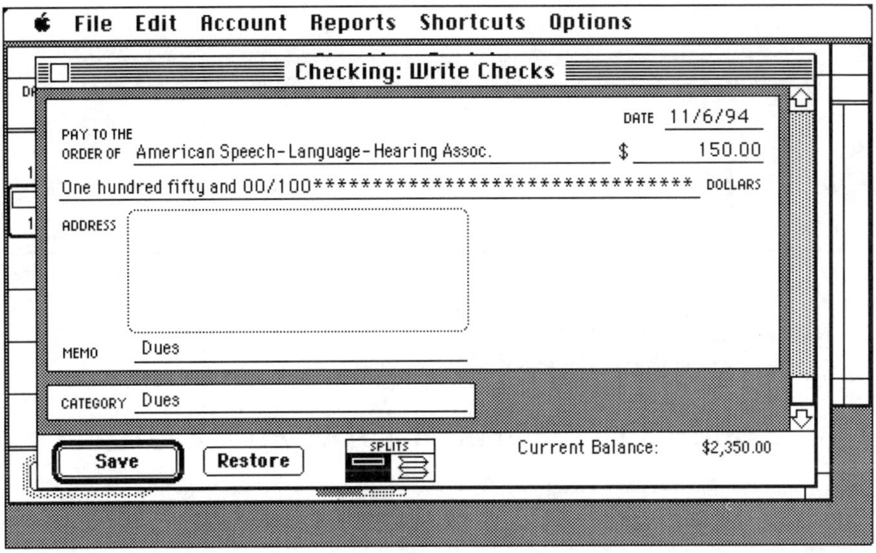

FIGURE 10.10 **The input screen for writing checks from information in the register in Figure 10.9.**

DEDICATED SOFTWARE FOR CLINICAL INDEX COMPUTATION

These are programs that compute specific indices from clinical data collected by speech-language pathologists or audiologists. For example, some compute indices from audiometric data that facilitate the hearing aid selection process (e.g., de Jong, 1985; Gans, VerHoef, & Berger, 1983). Most clinicians now use spreadsheet software (which is described elsewhere in this chapter) for computing such indices.

▶ 11

Literature Searching, E-Mail, Faxing, and Other Telecommunications Applications

For the applications that we have discussed thus far, the only computer it is necessary to control is your own. There are applications—that sometimes are referred to as computer-mediated communication ones—for which it is also necessary to control another computer, perhaps one thousands of miles away. It could be a microcomputer, a minicomputer, or a mainframe. You control it by linking it to yours. Since computers originally were linked by telephone lines (Figure 11.1), these applications became known as telecommunications applications. While most communication between computers still happens over telephone lines, for those that are a part of a *local area network*, or *LAN*, communication happens over special cables that connect them.

Three basic tasks can be performed by linking your computer to another:

1. *Gathering* information from the other computer
2. *Transferring* information to the other computer
3. *Processing* information in the other computer

Some of the ways in which the ability to do these tasks can facilitate your clinical functioning are described in this chapter.

HARDWARE AND SOFTWARE REQUIREMENTS FOR TELECOMPUTING

For two computers to communicate with each other by means of telephone lines, both must have a modem and communication software. However, they do not need to have the same disk operating system (see Chapter 3). Macintosh and IBM-compatible computers can communicate with each other in this way because information is

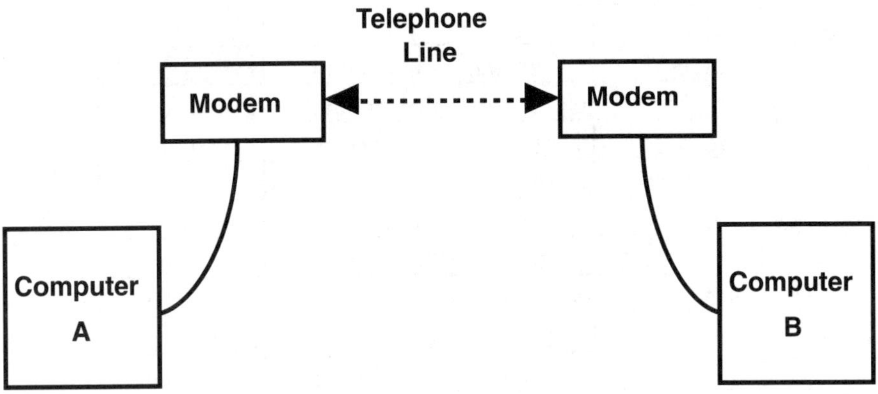

FIGURE 11.1 **Two computers linked by modems and a telephone line.**

exchanged in a standard code—usually ASCII (American Standard Code for Information Exchange). Each letter and digit has an ASCII equivalent consisting of a sequence of 1s and 0s (Figure 11.2). Punctuation marks and functions (e.g., spacing) also have ASCII codes.

When two computers that are a part of a local area network (LAN) communicate with each other, no modem is necessary because information is exchanged in digital form. It does not have to be transformed into analog form and then back into digital form as it does for telephone line exchanges. Both computers, however, must have communication software.

Another circumstance in which a modem is unnecessary is when the two computers that will be exchanging information are in the same room. They can be connected by a special cable known as a *null modem*. A regular modem isn't needed because data are exchanged in digital form (like they are in a LAN).

Modems

The word modem is a contraction of modulator/demodulator. The modem on the computer from which data are being transmitted modulates (converts) binary computer data (1s and 0s; Figure 11.2) into the electrical (analog) form that phone lines can carry. The modem on the computer from which data are being transmitted demodulates the analog signals coming through the phone line, converting them back into the binary form computers can understand. Computers and telephones use different languages to process data and the modem is the translator.

Some modems can transmit and receive faxes in addition to performing other telecommunication functions. Their hardware and software enables them to *emulate* a fax machine. You fax documents (files) by issuing commands that are comparable to those used for printing (Figure 11.3). These commands do, in fact, result in their

A 1000001	S 1010011	a 1100001	s 1110011
B 1000010	T 1010100	b 1100010	t 1110100
C 1000011	U 1010101	c 1100011	u 1110101
D 1000100	V 1010110	d 1100100	v 1110110
E 1000101	W 1010111	e 1100101	w 1110111
F 1000110	X 1011000	f 1100110	x 111100
G 1000111	Y 1011001	g 1100111	y 1111001
H 1001000	Z 1011010	h 1101000	z 1111010
I 1001001	0 0110000	i 1101001	. 0101110
J 1001010	1 0110001	j 1101010	, 0101100
K 1001011	2 0110010	k 1101011	? 0111111
L 1001100	3 0110011	l 1101100	) 0101001
M 1001101	4 0110100	m 1101101	{ 1111011
N 1001110	5 0110101	n 1101110	/ 0101111
O 1001111	6 0110110	o 1101111	& 0100110
P 1010000	7 0110111	p 1110000	+ 0101011
Q 1010001	8 0111000	q 1110001	- 0101101
R 1010010	9 0111001	r 1110010	= 0111101

FIGURE 11.2 **Examples of the seven-bit ASCII character code. Note that upper and lower case letters do not have the same code.**

being printed by either another computer (one that has been programmed to emulate a fax machine) or a fax machine.

Modems can be internal or external. Some newer computers—particularly laptops—have them built in as standard equipment. For further information about modems, see Chapter 2.

Computer Networks

Networks are groups of computers that are linked permanently by cables, rather than temporarily by modems and telephone lines. They can share files (e.g., programs and databases) and hardware resources—including printers and hard disks (that sometimes are referred to as *file servers*). One application for which a file server can be used is electronic mail (E-mail).

What are the advantages of having computers linked by cables rather than by modems and telephone lines? There are several. First, data can be transferred at a faster

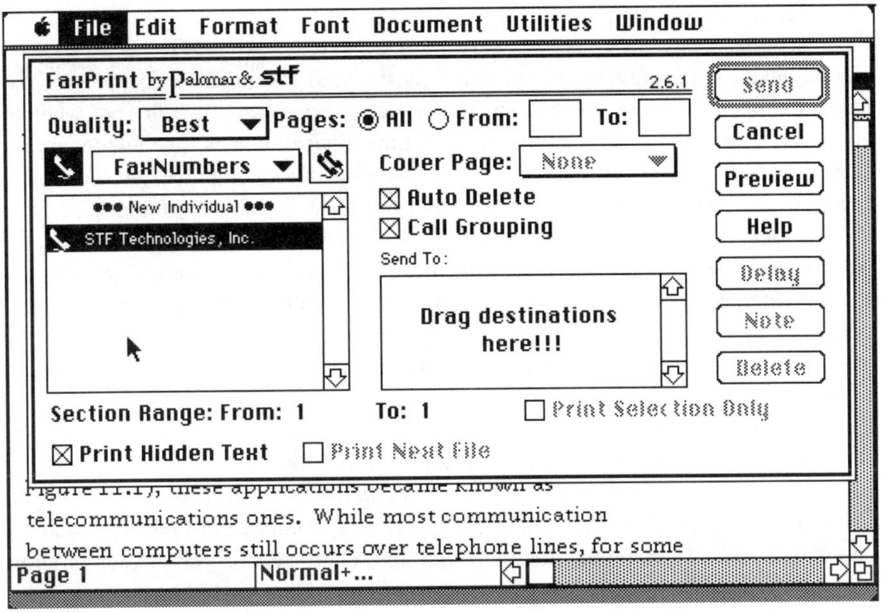

FIGURE 11.3 **A representative menu of commands for faxing documents—that is, printing them on another computer programmed to emulate a fax machine or on a fax machine.**

rate because it isn't necessary to translate it from digital-to-analog and analog-to digital form and the special cables that are used to link the computers in a network can transfer information more rapidly than can telephone lines. Also, some types of data—including photographs, drawings, and videos—that can be transferred reliably over such cables either cannot be transferred at all, or not as reliably, over telephone lines.

There are several cabling schemes that can be used to link computers into networks. One of the most popular of them is the *Ethernet* system. While the computers so linked are usually in the same building, they can be in different buildings. The buildings would be connected to each other by special cables. Computers in a number of university buildings, for example, could be linked to form a single network.

Local area networks (LANs) are almost always linked together by cables (Blache, 1985). Files and hardware resources in ones so linked can be shared by users in all of them. The *internet* consists of thousands of LANs that are linked in this way. Consequently, computers on the Internet can share files and utilize each other's hardware resources. While the internet can be accessed by a computer that is not a part of a LAN, all of its capabilities cannot be exploited by doing so. The internet is discussed further elsewhere in this chapter.

For further information about computer networks, including the internet, see Comer (1995).

Communication Software

Communication programs perform the tasks required to transfer information from one computer to another. You need a communication program regardless of whether your computer is linked to the other by telephone lines or cables. The telecommunication applications for which you plan to use your microcomputer determines the specific tasks your communication program has to be capable of doing. For some applications—such as directly transferring word-processor files from one microcomputer to another—almost any communication program can do them. For others—such as emulating a particular type of terminal to "control" a mainframe or minicomputer—this is not the case. Communication software is distributed as freeware (e.g., Kermit) and shareware (e.g., Procomm and Red Ryder) as well as commercially.

To successfully transfer information from computer to computer, both computers must communicate in the same language. Consequently, before calling another computer you must know what language (*communications protocol*) it expects you to use. If your computer is set up to use a different communications protocol than the one you are calling, you will either get "garbage" characters on your screen or nothing at all. Users have to set several parameters (Figure 11.4), including the following, to establish a communications protocol:

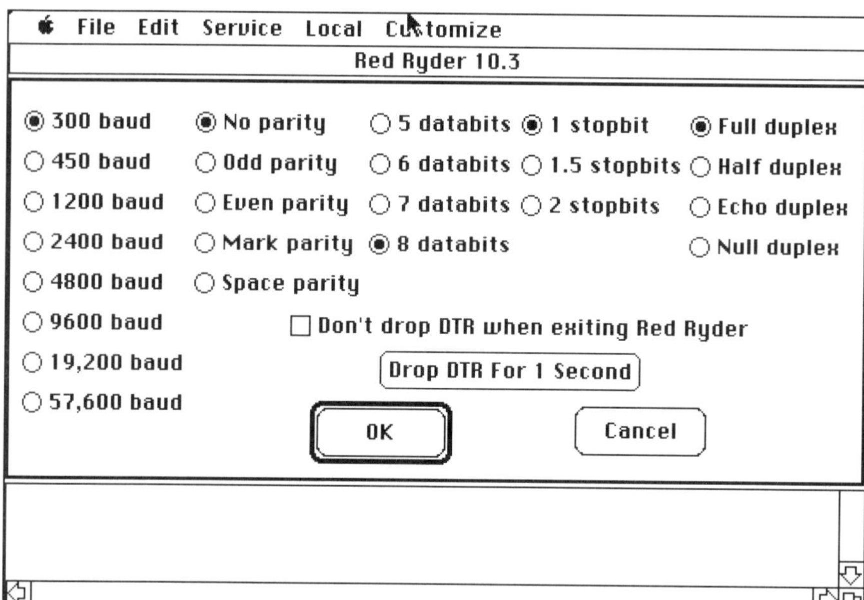

FIGURE 11.4 **A representative screen from a communication program for establishing a communications protocol.**

- **Baud rate:** This is how quickly the transmitting and receiving computers "speak" to each other. Both have to do so at the same baud rate (which is expressed in *bits per second* or *bps*). Some common baud rates are 300, 1200, 2400, 4800, 9600, and 14400 bps. Dividing the baud rate by 10 yields the approximate number of characters transferred per second—for example, at 2400 baud, approximately 240 characters are transferred per second. Almost all modems, incidentally, can function at baud rates slower then their maximums and will slow down automatically if the receiving computer is is set to communicate at one.
- **Parity checking:** This is a transmission error detection technique. A **0** or a **1** is appended (added) to the seven-bit machine code for a character (Figure 11.2) before it is transmitted. This extra bit (0 or 1) is referred to as the parity bit. If the user chooses NO parity, *parity bits* are not transmitted. This is the most common setting in microcomputer communication. With ODD parity, the transmitting computer always sends an odd number of 1 bits (bits with a value of 1). It adds a 1 bit to the codes for characters that contain an even number of 1 bits. With EVEN parity, the transmitting computer always sends an even number of 1 bits. It adds a 1 bit to the codes for characters that contain an odd number of 1 bits. If the receiving computer is not set to check parity in the same way as the transmitting one, it is likely to be confused by the parity bit and display garbage on the screen.
- **Data bits:** The number of bits (1s and 0s) the computer should use to code each character. This number has to correspond to that expected by the computer to which data are being transmitted. Otherwise, the receiving computer will not segment the string of 1s and 0s that it receives appropriately into characters and garbage will be displayed on the screen. Most computers use 7 or 8 data bits to code each character.
- **Stop bits:** Additional bits sent at the end of each character transmitted. If the number of stop bits the receiving computer expects to be added to character codes is not what the transmitting computer is adding to them, the receiving computer probably will not segment the string of 1s and 0s appropriately into characters. Consequently, garbage will be displayed on the screen. The most common number of stop bits added to character codes is 1.
- **Duplex:** There are two main types: FULL duplex and HALF duplex. FULL duplex transmits the characters to the receiving computer, which "echos" them back to yours. HALF duplex transmits the characters to your computer as well as to the receiving one. If you are using HALF duplex and see double characters ("HHEELLLLOO"), switch to FULL duplex.

What tasks can a communication program enable a computer to perform? There are many, including the following:

- Displaying incoming and outgoing data on a monitor screen.
- Automatically storing incoming data in the computer's RAM or on a disk for later use.

- Sending incoming data to the printer.
- Retrieving data for transmission from the computer's memory or from a disk.
- Automatically dialing numbers and answering the telephone.
- Preparing and/or editing files.
- Checking for and correcting transmission errors.
- Emulating a terminal for a mainframe or minicomputer (see Chapter 1).

Some of the ways that computers utilize these capabilities are described in the next section.

TELECOMPUTING APPLICATIONS

Tasks are described in this section for which speech-language pathologists and audiologists have used communication software and/or are likely to do so in the future.

Literature Searching and Other Types of Information Gathering

There is considerable clinically relevant information available in databases that you can access with your computer. Examples are library card catalogues (e.g., that of the Library of Congress) and professional literature databases, such as Medline.

There are four ways to access such databases. One is through a college or university LAN. The second is through *independent* bulletin board systems (BBSs). The third is through commercial computer networks (e.g., America Online), and the fourth is through national and international computer networks (e.g., the Internet).

If you are a student at a college or university, you should be able to access its LAN, using either a terminal that is cabled to it or a microcomputer and modem. One type of database you almost always will be able to access in this manner is a library card catalog. Figure 11.5 is a representative screen from such a database. Another type of database that you may be able to access in this manner is a literature database, such as Medline. Incidentally, colleges and universities that do not make literature databases available in this manner may do so on microcomputer-accessible CD-ROM disks at their libraries or computer centers. A CD-ROM disk may have several years of a literature database (such as Medline) recorded on it.

Independent bulletin board systems are maintained by individuals and organizations (Blache, 1985). They are accessed directly (by dialing their telephone number), rather than indirectly through a computer network. Their hardware usually consists of a microcomputer (with a hard drive and modem) that is never turned off. The main type of information available from them is answers to questions that you have asked or that have been asked by others. There usually is no charge for accessing bulletin boards—you pay only the normal fee for the telephone call. Thousands of independent BBSs were operating in the United States during the 1980s. Many organizations

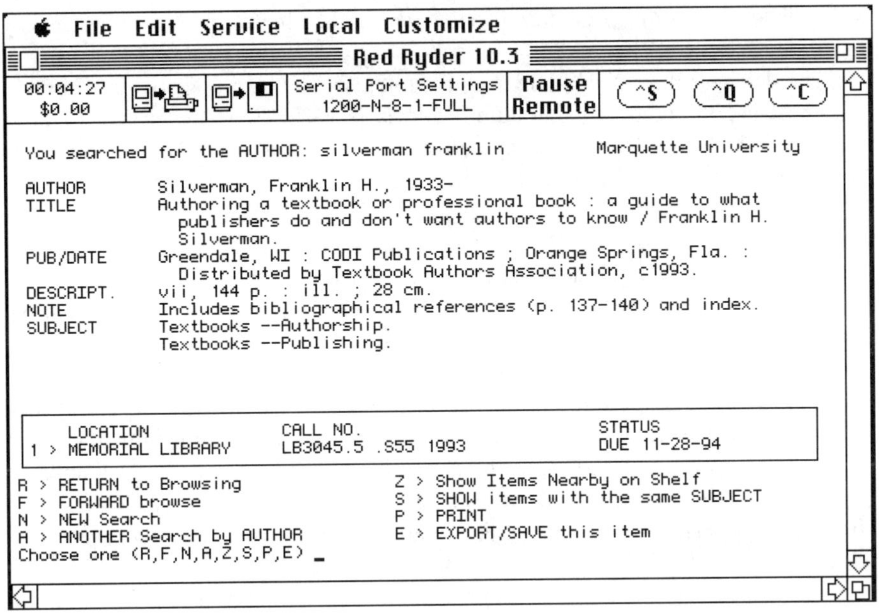

FIGURE 11.5 **A representative screen from a library card catalog database.**

that operate a BBS now do so on a computer network, such as America Online or the internet. One BBS, incidentally, on which you can share information about computer applications with other clinicians is that of the NCLIP (National Center to Improve Practice in Special Education Through Technology): Phone 617-969-4529 for information.

Almost all computer networks— including America OnLine, CompuServe, Delphi, and Prodigy—are commercial ventures. They charge users a fee. This fee could be a fixed monthly one and/or a per–minute connect-time charge. Connect-time charges tended to be higher during business hours than during the evening and on weekends when this chapter was written.

The *internet* is the largest computer network. It is international in scope and the de facto "information superhighway" (Comer, 1995; Kuster, 1995a, 1995b; Scherz & Kuster, 1995). While the internet is not primarily a commercial venture, you may have to pay to access ("surf") it and/or for some of the services that are available on it. Whether you will have to pay to access it depends on how you do so. If you access it through a commercial computer network (such as America OnLine, CompuServe, Delphi, or Prodigy), you probably will have to pay a fee. On the other hand, if you do it through a college or university computer center that is networked with the Internet, you probably will not have to pay one. You may, however, have to pay for certain services, such as accessing literature databases (e.g., Medline) and purchasing books (which would consist of computer files that you could, after retrieving, either display on a monitor or print).

The database that speech-language pathologists and audiologists probably will find most useful for doing literature searches is MEDLINE (Reiner & Ludlow, 1979a, 1979b, 1981). This is a computerized version of the *Index Medicus* abstracts journal. It can be used for doing literature searches that go as far back as the mid-1970s. Four other databases that can be quite useful when searching the communicative disorders literature are PsychLit (a computerized version of *Psychological Abstracts*), the Education Index, Articles First, and ERIC.

A search of a database such as Medline can yield several types of information. One is a bibliography of papers that deal with a particular topic. Such a bibliography can be displayed on a monitor screen, stored on a disk, and/or printed. The topic can be relatively broad (e.g., aphasia) or relatively narrow (e.g., use of Amer-Ind with aphasics). A search can be for a particular year or years or it can include the entire database. It can be limited to papers by particular authors or can include all authors.

A second kind of information you can obtain from a database such as Medline is abstracts of papers. You can instruct the computer to print abstracts of all the papers it locates on a particular topic or only certain ones.

For information about how to search a computer literature database, such as Medline, see Appendix A.

Electronic Mail (E-Mail)

A microcomputer with communications software and modem can be used for "mailing" letters and other printed materials (Dean & Pickering, 1991b; Sarachan-Deily, 1992), including coordination notes to members of a client's rehabilitation team (Clark, Wilson, Hass, & Olson, 1995) and messages to enhance clinician training (Van Vliet, 1995). This can be done in two basic ways. The first is to transmit them (via telephone) directly to the microcomputers of persons with whom you want to communicate. While this method is the most direct, it is often not the most convenient. Sending e-mail directly to another microcomputer requires that the person to whom it is being sent be at home or at least have his or her computer turned on and ready to accept a message.

The second way that you can send a letter to a person via computer is via his or her "electronic mailbox" on a networked computer (e.g., one that's part of the internet). This is how most people now send e-mail messages. An electronic mailbox is an addressable storage area on the hard disk of a computer that is part of a network. When a message arrives, it is automatically stored in the mailbox to which it is addressed. Each mailbox in a network has a unique address. While anyone can send a message to a mailbox, only the owner of the box (or someone to whom he or she has given the "password") can retrieve messages from it. You retrieve messages from your mailbox by accessing (with your computer) the computer in the network on which the mailbox is stored. There is software available that will notify you (e.g., by printing a message on the monitor screen) when an e-mail message arrives. Of course, to communicate with someone in this way it is necessary both that the person have an electronic mailbox and that you know its address.

Electronic mail services on networks such as the internet enable you to do more than just send text messages to individual recipients. For example, they enable you to send messages that contain voice (sound), video, and graphics as well as text. And they also enable you to send a single message (e.g., the announcement of a meeting) to a number of persons simultaneously (e.g., the members of an organization). One context in which this is done is LISTSERV. People subscribe to information about a particular topic by entering their e-mail address in a distribution list that is a computer file. (see Appendix B for some representative LISTSERVs). For further information about e-mail, see Comer (1995).

Professional Association, Class, and Interest Group Communication

Electronic bulletin boards have been established by professional organizations (including ASHA), classes (including undergraduate and graduate ones), and interest groups to facilitate internal communication and promote the rapid dissemination of information (Blache, 1985; Filter, Powell, & Campbell, 1994; Mitchell, 1986). They function much like the old-fashioned type—you post notes on them and read notes that were posted by others. After accessing a bulletin board you can do any of the following:

- Read notes (on your monitor) that were posted by others
- Post notes that are responses to what others have written
- Post notes for others to read and respond to

There are thousands of bulletin board discussion groups on the Internet. It would be difficult to think of a subject—no matter how "far out"—for which there wouldn't be at least one such group. Among them are those that provide information that can be helpful to you and your clients. The addresses of some are listed in Appendix B.

Clinical Consulting (Asking and Answering Questions)

If you are like most clinicians, you sometimes seek a second opinion about the nature and/or management of a client's disorder. One way that you may be able to get one if you can't from someone at your facility is to post a query on the bulletin board of a discussion group in which there are persons who are knowledgeable about the disorder. The query would consist of relevant background information about the client and the questions you want answered. There is a listing of internet bulletin boards on which you could consider posting such a query in Appendix B.

Incidentally, it is likely that you will learn quite a bit by becoming a regular participant in such a discussion group. And by responding to other clinicians' queries, you will enable clients other than your own to benefit from your training and experience.

Conferencing

Computer bulletin boards sometimes are referred to as computer conference services because they can be used for this purpose. Computer conferencing has been used in our field for a number of purposes, including clinician training (Mower, 1995).

There are two types of computer conferences: delayed time and real time. To participate in a delayed-time conference, you post your comments on a bulletin board. Others read what you have written and you read their contributions. One advantage of delayed-time conferencing is that participants have plenty of time to ponder each other's comments before replying.

A real-time computer conference—which sometimes is referred to as a CHAT mode conference—is structured similarly to a conference telephone call. All participants are on-line at the same time. When one participant keyboards a comment, the others see it on their monitor screen and can immediately post replies.

Participants in a computer conference can consult, listen, learn, nurture, clarify, announce, share, and explore. Unlike attending a traditional face-to-face conference, they do not have to be in the same place at the same time. They can even be in different countries. Participants can keep in constant touch with each other without a need for expensive and time-consuming travel.

Most computer conferences in which speech-language pathologists and audiologists were participants when this chapter was written were of the delayed-time type. What would your participation in a typical session of such a conference be like? Upon entering the conference, you would be informed about any items you hadn't seen and new responses to items you had already seen. At this point you could look at any new items or new responses to old items and/or enter new items or responses to old ones. When you finished, you would hang up the phone. After a period of time (e.g., a week) you would access the conference again and repeat the process. The conference would continue for as long as you and your group needed to communicate with each other.

Coauthoring

Telecommunications network technology can facilitate the coauthoring of reports and other documents. The document would be stored on the hard drive of a computer that can be accessed by its coauthors via modem.

The drafting-editing process can proceed in two ways. The first is to draft and edit the document on the computer on which it is stored. This computer, of course, would have to have word-processing software. Coauthors can be alerted to modifications in several ways, including saving lines in which changes occur in a different font. The lines would be changed back to their original font after the modifications were approved by the coauthors.

The second way that the process can proceed is downloading (copying) the document file from the hard drive of the computer on which it is stored and modifying it with your computer. You would then upload the revised file. That is, you would either replace the file of the document on the hard drive with the revised one or you would save your revised document file on this hard drive and not delete the original one. If both files are available on the hard drive, your coauthor(s) can use a *file comparison program* to identify revisions. These programs compare two versions of a word-processing file and indicate words that have been added to and deleted from the most recent version.

Electronic Publishing

Documents can be published and distributed as computer files. They can be sent via modem or cable to the computers of persons who request them (e.g., LISTSERV documents and E-journals—see Appendix B) or they can be downloaded by persons who want them from the hard drive of a computer they can access—for example, one in their LAN. Those acquiring a document in one of these ways can print it with their word processing or desktop publishing software. A number of publishers, incidentally, are selling books on the internet as computer files that you can download after paying for them with a credit card. Documents distributed as computer files have the same copyright protections as those that are distributed in printed form (see Silverman, 1992a).

Purchasing

You can purchase almost anything from an on-line shopping service, including copies of journal articles. These shopping services are found on all of the national computer networks. You can even to make your own airline reservations. Payment is almost always by credit card.

Utilizing Minicomputers and Mainframe Computers

You can use your microcomputer to control (i.e., function as a *terminal* for) a mainframe or minicomputer if there is one at your institution that you can access. You enter the data you want to process into the host computer's (mainframe's or minicomputer's) memory. After it is processed, you could either download it or send it to one of the host computer's output devices.

There are several reasons why you might want to use a microcomputer as a terminal for a larger one, including the following:

- Having access to greater disk *storage* capacity than that your microcomputer has available

- Having access to types of *software* you don't have available for your microcomputer
- Having access to *output devices* that you don't have available for your microcomputer
- Having access to *programming languages* that you don't have available for your microcomputer
- Being able to *store information* at a central location
- *Accessing networks* such as the internet

These are discussed below.

Greater Storage Capacity. Minicomputers and mainframes almost always have larger hard disks than microcomputers. If a particular task (e.g., maintaining a large database for client records) requires greater disk storage capacity than your microcomputer has available, it may be possible to use an institutional minicomputer or mainframe for doing it.

More Software. You can increase the amount of software to which you have access by using your computer as a terminal for a minicomputer or mainframe. You will have access to both the programs for your computer and those for the other. Some of the latter may enable you to do tasks that you can't do with your computer.

More Output Devices. By using your microcomputer as a terminal for a minicomputer or mainframe, you have access to a greater variety of output devices. You may find doing so particular advantageous if you do desktop publishing and your institutional computer can access a very high quality printer, such as a 2400 dot-per-inch laser one.

More Programming Languages. There are more programming languages available for minicomputers and mainframes than for microcomputers. Using your microcomputer as a terminal for a larger institutional computer can give you access to a programming language either unavailable for it or for which you have not purchased the necessary software.

Central Information Storage. There are certain applications for which storing data in a mainframe or minicomputer could be advantageous. Public school speech-language pathologists in a large school system, for example, could maintain client records in this way. The records of all of the children they are serving would be stored on the hard drive of a mainframe or minicomputer that they could access from their office or home.

Accessing Computer Networks. You access a computer network—such as the internet—by programming your microcomputer to function as a terminal for the mainframe and/or minicomputers in the network. There is special communication software available that automates the process of accessing and "navigating" some computer networks.

Exchanging Software: Freeware, Shareware, and Templates

You can download copies of programs from BBSs with your computer. Of course, the programs you download must be written in the dialect of a language that your computer understands and be compatible with your computer's disk operating system (DOS) to be usable. Consequently, one Macintosh user can exchange software with another, but not with a user of an IBM-compatible computer.

Programs that are not copyrighted—which are referred to as *public domain* software or *freeware*—can be legally distributed in this way. Some programs that are copyrighted—known as *shareware*—can also be legally distributed in this way. The author of a shareware program allows you to try it without paying a fee. However, if you like the program and decide to use it, you are requested to pay him or her a fee. For all other programs that are copyrighted, it is a violation of U.S. copyright law to distribute them in this way. Downloading one is engaging in *software piracy* and could result in your being sued by the copyright owner (see Silverman, 1992a). Doing so is also a violation of professional ethics (see Langford, 1995).

Treating Clients

Telecommunication can be helpful to clients in several ways. One is as an adjunct to therapy. Clients who have some communicative disorders (including aphasia), for example, benefit from daily stimulation. One possible way to provide it is via an interactive telecommunication link between the client and the clinician's computer (Fitch & Cross, 1983).

A second way that telecommunication can benefit clients is providing them with a self-help/support group. A number of such groups—for example, STUTT-L for stutterers (see Appendix B)—can be accessed through the internet.

A third way that telecommunication can benefit clients is providing them with a source for language stimulation. Aphasics, for example, have been provided with language and memory stimulation by encouraging them to spend time "surfing" the internet (Rickard, Shuler, & Jackson, 1995).

Telecommunication Relay Services

You may occasionally need to communicate by telephone with a client who is severely hearing and/or speech impaired. If the client has a telecommunication device for the deaf (which is actually a "dedicated" microcomputer) or a microcomputer and a modem, you can do so by means of a telecommunication relay service.

There are telecommunication relay services (TRSs) in all fifty states. Their establishment was mandated by Title IV of the Americans with Disabilities Act, which was passed by the Congress in 1990. They enable persons who are severely speech impaired and have either a microcomputer and modem or a telecommunication device for the deaf (TDD) to initiate and receive telephone calls. They also enable those who have dedicated augmentative communication devices that contain a microcomputer and modem to do so.

Relay services operate 24 hours a day, 365 days a year. Telephone calls made through them cost no more than regular ones. Most can be used for both long-distance and local calls. Full confidentiality is maintained and no records of the contents of calls are retained by the TRS.

A user usually contacts a TRS by dialing an 800 number. When the operator (referred to as a communication assistant, or CA) answers, the user types the telephone number that he or she wants to call. The CA dials this number and when the party answers, the user types the first thing that he or she wants to say. The CA "voices" this to the party and when the party responds, the CA types what was said. This interaction can go on for as long as the people want to "talk." If the person initiating the call can talk, he or she would dial the same 800 number and would tell the CA the number of the speech or hearing impaired person whom he or she wants to contact.

A speech-impaired user who has normal hearing can hear the contacted person's responses (rather than having to have them typed by the CA) if he or she has a TDD and the TRS offers *hearing passthrough*. Unfortunately, hearing passthrough is not possible with a microcomputer if the user has a single telephone line.

Information about accessing the TRS in your state can be obtained from your local telephone company. TRSs also exist in Canada and other countries; they are run in some countries by volunteer organizations rather than government agencies. Information about their availability can be obtained from local associations for the deaf.

If a client is going to be accessing a TRS with a microcomputer, you may want to encourage him or her to purchase a fax modem rather than a regular one. These modems, in addition to enabling a client to access a TRS, can augment his or her ability to communicate by "mail."

▶ 12

Measurement and Control of Instrumentation

You can program a computer to measure almost anything and to control almost any electrical device. You can, for example, use one to measure the fundamental frequency of a client's voice or to turn several lights in your home on and off while you are out of town at times that aren't predictable. You can even program a computer to integrate its measurement and control capabilities—one clinical application for which you could to this is EMG (electromyography) biofeedback. The electrical signals that would be *measured* contain information about the presence or absence of muscle action potentials in a particular group of muscle fibers. The microcomputer could be programmed to use this information to *control* the frequency of the tone generated by a pure-tone oscillator. The client would use the frequency of the tone to monitor the level of electrical activity in the muscle fibers that he or she is trying to learn to tense or relax—for example, the greater the level of such activity, the higher the frequency of the tone. For examples of other clinical applications of EMG biofeedback as well as other types of feedback for measurement and/or control, see Dalston and Keefe (1987), Fox (1993), Gulian, Hinds, and Nimmo-Smith (1986), Schwartz, Brogan, Emond, and Oleksiak (1993), and Volin (1989, 1993a).

Applications also are discussed in this chapter in which the information the computer uses for measuring or controlling electrical devices is not abstracted by it from electrical signals, such as muscle action potentials. Rather, the information is generated directly or indirectly by manual switch activations (e.g., Lehnhardt, Battmer, & Becker, 1980; Mills, 1986e; Stach & Jerger, 1986). An example would be a client who is severely motorically impaired using the switching mechanism of a microcomputer-based environmental control unit to turn a television set on and off (see Chapter 8 in Silverman, 1995).

Our focus in this chapter is not solely on the use of devices regarded as microcomputers for measurement and/or control. The "brain" of a microcomputer is a microprocessor chip (see Chapter 2). Many devices other than microcomputers contain microprocessor chips that are used for measuement and/or control. Examples are automobile engines, audiometers, and augmentative communication devices. The programs that enable them to perform these functions are "burnt" into PROM or EPROM chips (see Chapter 2). These chips, with their accompanying circuitry, function as single-application (dedicated) microcomputers. Incidentally, microcomputers—with appropriate software and peripherals—can mimic any of these dedicated devices.

INTERFACES USED FOR CONNECTING MEASUREMENT AND CONTROL DEVICES TO MICROCOMPUTERS

Interfaces are electronic circuits that make it possible for computers to receive data from and send data to external devices (Figure 12.1). The interface that you need for a particular application may or may not be built into your computer: If it is not built-in, you will connect it to your computer with a cable. The devices from which you are receiving signals for measurement and/or to which they are being sent for control are connected to the interface by cables. Such devices can range in complexity from simple on-off switches to sophisticated audiometers and instruments for measuring air flow during speech.

The data sent to the microcomputer (via the interface) may or may not be processed immediately. If it is processed immediately and the processed data is sent immediately (through the interface) to an external device, the application is referred to as a *real-time* one.

The functioning of the interface is controlled by software. The software does whatever is necessary to translate data being sent from an external device to a microcomputer into the form the microcomputer can process (i.e., *digital*) and/or it does whatever is necessary to translate processed data being sent from the microcomputer to an external device into a form that can be used for controlling it (i.e., electrical or *analog*).

Data in digital form consists of sequences of 1s and 0s. Data in analog form consists of fluctuations in the strength of an electrical signal. The process by which an interface converts analog data into digital form is described in the next section.

Converting Analog Data into Digital Form

The process by which an interface translates analog data into digital form is illustrated in Figure 12.2. The analog signals containing the data may or may not be electrical . Examples of analog signals that are electrical are muscle action potentials and audio and video signals generated by videotape recorders (see Mills, 1991). And an example of an analog signal that isn't electrical is the mechanical movement (from center) of the shaft of a joystick.

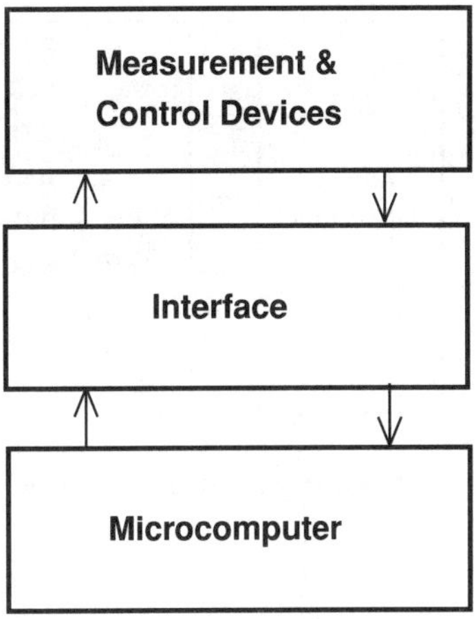

FIGURE 12.1 **An interface consists of electronic circuits that connect one or more measurement and/or control devices to a microcomputer. Signals flow in both directions through the interface.**

If the analog signal containing the data isn't an electrical one, it must be converted into an electrical signal before it can be processed. A *transducer* is used to do this. Transducers are devices that convert energy from one form into another—for example, air pressure (Blood, 1994) or degree of sway (Cavette, Battani, Smith, & Heidlauf, 1993; Cavette, Wiley, & Marion, 1993) to an electrical signal. One transducer with which all speech-language pathologists and audiologists are familiar is the microphone. Microphones transduce acoustical ("vibratory") energy into electrical energy. If the analog signal containing the data is an electrical one, it can be sent directly to the interface for processing (Figure 12.2).

The circuitry of most interfaces contains three types of components: signal conditioners, analog multiplexers, and analog-to-digital converters. *Signal conditioners* take analog electrical signals and condition (modify) them so that they are in the form that the analog-to-digital converter circuitry requires for processing. If the signals are too weak, the signal conditioner circuitry will amplify them to the necessary level. And if the signals contain extraneous information ("noise") that could produce errors during the analog-to-digital conversion process, circuitry within the signal conditioner will filter out (eliminate) this information.

The signals that are processed by a computer at a particular point in time do not have to come from a single source (Figure 12.2). A microcomputer can be configured to access information in real-time simultaneously from a number of sources, and the kinds of information being processed can be different. A speech-language pathologist, for example, could attach electrodes to several sites on a stutterer's body, thereby making it possible for the microcomputer to process information about sequences of muscle contractions during moments of stuttering. If he or she wanted to integrate this information with information about the stutterer's speech (i.e., acoustic data), the system could be configured to allow the microcomputer to also process speech-related analog signals from a microphone. The microcomputer in

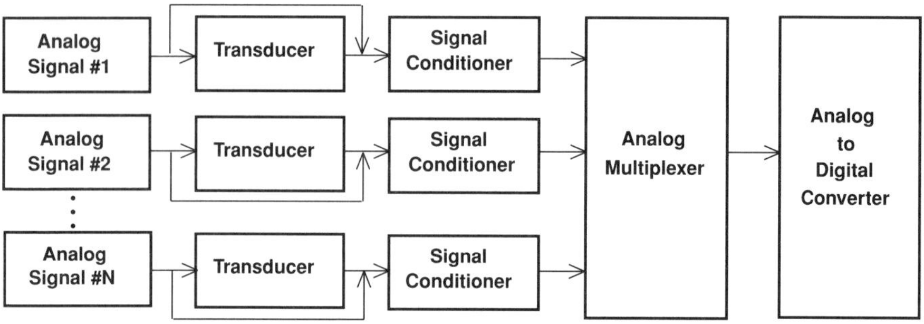

FIGURE 12.2 **Block diagram of an interface for translating analog data into digital form.**

this example would be processing two types of data—physiological and acoustical—simultaneously in real-time.

The interface circuit that is responsible for controlling the flow of information from various sources is known as an *analog multiplexer*. This is a switching device that connects multiple analog input signal points, one at a time, to a microcomputer via an analog-to-digital converter. A computer program determines which analog signal the multiplexer will input into the computer (via the analog-to-digital converter) at any given point in time. The multiplexer may switch from signal to signal very rapidly. The signal from a particular conditioner may be sampled for a fraction of a second every second that the program is run. The analog multiplexer also has a second function. It makes it possible to use a single analog-to-digital converter. If there were no multiplexer circuit in the interface, it would be necessary to have a separate analog-to-digital converter for each input signal source.

The *analog-to-digital* converter generates a digital signal (consisting of sequences of 1s and 0s) that is equivalent to the analog (electrical) signal sent to it by the multiplexer (Figure 12.2). That is, it *translates* the information in the analog (electrical) signal into a form that the computer can understand—a digital one. It can make many thousands of such conversions per second (Mahaffey, 1975). The "translated" information is then sent to the computer where it is processed.

Converting Digital Data into an Electrical Analog Form

The process by which an interface translates digital data into electrical (analog) data is diagrammed in Figure 12.3. Data in digital form are sent from the computer to a *digital multiplexer* if more than one output device is needed to perform a task. These data consist of instructions for controlling the output devices. If only one output device is needed, the data are sent directly to a *digital-to-analog converter*. There is one attached to each output device. The digital multiplexer can direct instructions to

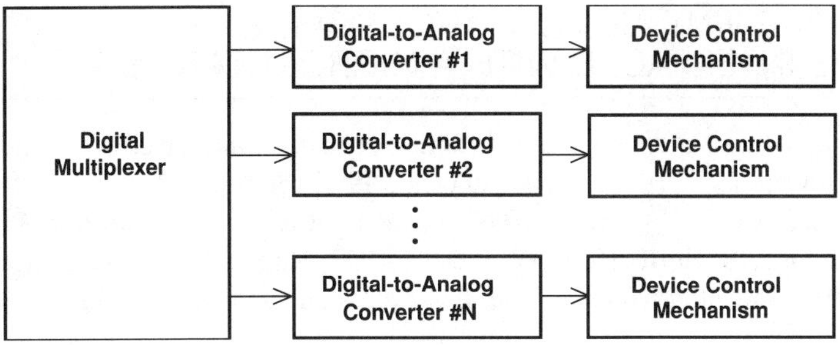

FIGURE 12.3 **Block diagram of an interface for translating digital data into analog form for controlling devices.**

one device at a time or to several simultaneously. The devices to which the digital multiplexer directs signals can change rapidly—for example, every fraction of a second.

The digital-to-analog converter translates the instructions into an analog (electrical) signal that contains the same information as the digital one entering it. The translated instructions are sent from the digital-to-analog converter to the control mechanisms of the various output devices.

The function that the control mechanism of an output device performs can be quite simple. If a microcomputer is merely being used to turn a device on and off, the control mechanism can be a relay. A *relay* is a type of switch that can be turned on and off by an electromagnet. An electromagnet consists of a coil of wire wound around a piece of iron. When an electrical signal (current) passes through the coil of wire, it causes the piece of iron around which it is wound to become magnetic. If an electromagnet is mounted under the two contacts of a switch and a small piece of iron is attached to the top contact, it will cause the top contact to lower and touch the bottom one thereby closing the switch and turning "on" the electrical device attached to it. The switch will remain closed until the computer stops sending an electrical signal to the relay. When this happens, the piece of iron will no longer be a magnet and consequently, the top contact will rise to its original position, thereby turning "off" the electrical device.

Some application require both analog-to-digital and digital-to-analog converters. One such application would be to adjust the output of a device if certain events occur. If, for example, you wanted to use a microcomputer to control or simulate a pure-tone audiometer, the presence or absence of a switch activation after a tone is presented could be fed back to the microcomputer and used by it to set the intensity of the next tone that is presented to the client (Fausti, Frey, Henry, Knutsen, & Olson, 1990; Hashimoto, Murata, Minami, Taniguchi, & Katayama, 1977; Jerivall, Dryselius, & Arlinger, 1983; Levitt, 1980; Lutman, 1983).

MEASUREMENT AND CONTROL DEVICES THAT CAN BE INTERFACED WITH A MICROCOMPUTER

Many types of measurement and control devices can be interfaced with a microcomputer (see Campbell, 1974; Espinoza-Varas, 1992; Ferrero, et al., 1993; Friedman, 1989; Hancock, 1986; Herman, 1989; Kennedy et al., 1991; Lauridsen & Nielsen, 1981; Osredkar & Horii, 1991; Pratt et al., 1993; Rubin, 1987; Ryalls et al., 1991; Zara, 1993). Some that you may find useful clinically are described in this section.

Measurement Devices

Measurement devices abstract information from an event (e.g., a speech sample) about the presence, absence, or magnitude of one or more of its attributes. Any attribute of an event that is an electrical signal or can be transduced into an electrical signal can be measured in this manner. Attributes of events that you can measure in this way include physiological, acoustical, and mechanical ones.

Attributes of Physiological Events. Attributes of almost any bodily process that is directly or indirectly associated with speech, language formulation, or hearing can be measured. Instruments that can be interfaced with a microcomputer for doing so include the following:

- **Electromyographs.** These devices detect the presence or absence of contractions of groups of muscle fibers through one of two types of electrodes: surface or needle. *Surface* electrodes are temporarily "glued" to the skin over the muscle fibers being monitored. *Needle* electrodes are inserted through the skin into these muscle fibers. The electrodes detect the weak electrical signals—muscle action potentials—that cause the fibers to contract. Most electromyographs have more than one channel; the number of channels determines the maximum number of sites at which muscle action potentials can be monitored simultaneously.
- **Electroencephalographs.** These devices are used to monitor electrical activity (e.g., the alpha rhythm) in the brain, particularly that in the cerebral cortex. Surface electrodes are attached to the skin over each site at which brain wave activity is to be monitored. Most of them have more than one channel and consequently, they can monitor brain wave activity at several sites simultaneously.
- **Psychogalvanometers.** These devices monitor a client's anxiety level indirectly by monitoring changes in skin resistance. Surface electrodes are attached to the client's skin, usually on an arm. If the client's anxiety level increases, he or she will perspire more profusely, which will change the resistance of his or her skin to the flow of an electrical current.
- **Pneumotactographs.** These devices are used to monitor the flow of air (or momentary interruptions in this flow) in the oral and nasal cavities (Charpied, 1994a). They transduce air flow information into electrical (analog) signals.

Attributes of Acoustical Events. These devices use a microphone to transduce acoustical (vibratory) signals into electrical (analog) ones. They enable you to monitor (measure) attributes of speech and other acoustical events—for example, the presence of hypernasality (Kataoka, Mayo, Zajac, Kataoka, & Warren, 1995). With them, your computer can emulate an acoustical display/measurement device such as a Visipitch or Sonograph.

Attributes of Mechanical Events. These are mechanical movements, such as the movement of the shaft on a joystick. Such movements have to be transduced into electrical signals before the information in them can be processed by a computer. For information about how this is done with switching mechanisms, see Chapter 5 in Silverman (1995).

Control Devices

These devices enable you to control an instrument (e.g., an audiometer) with a microcomputer. They do it by manipulating the switches on the instrument. The manipulating can be done by a person following instructions generated by a computer (e.g., Fritze, 1978) or directly by a computer. There are several devices that a computer can use to manipulate switches. One of these—the relay—is described elsewhere in this chapter. Two other devices that a computer can use for this purpose are the solenoid and the integrated circuit.

Solenoids, like relays, are electromagnetic devices. They differ in that they manipulate (e.g., push) switches rather than function as switches. A solenoid, for example, could be mounted below each key on a manual typewriter in a manner that when the electromagnet in it was activated, the key would be pulled down and type a character.

Integrated circuits (ICs), like solenoids and relays, can function as switches. However, they control instruments electronically rather than by manipulating the switches on them with devices containing electromagnets. An IC is particularly likely to be used instead of a solenoid and relay for applications in which a switch has to be manipulated—turned on and off—more than once a second.

There are several ways that microcomputers can send electrical signals from their digital-to-analog converters to control devices. The most common (particularly if the computer and control device are in the same room) is through a *cable* that runs from the converter to the control device.

A second way that this can be done if the computer and control device are in the same room is by the computer directing an *infrared light* beam at the device. This is the technology, incidentally, that most remote controls for television sets and VCRs use.

A third way this can be done if both the computer and control device are located in the same building is *through the building's wiring*. The signals would enter the wiring through an electrical outlet near the computer and would be detected by a special module attached to an outlet near the output device. A microcomputer can be programmed to control more than one device in this manner. It can, for example, be programmed to turn lamps in different rooms on and off at different times. A separate module would be needed for each device.

If the computer is not located in the same building as the control device, the signals can be sent via *radio waves*. The electrical signals from the digital-to-analog converter would be sent to a radio transmitter. A radio receiver would detect the signals and activate the switching mechanism. This strategy, incidentally, is used for controlling model airplanes.

A fifth way the signals could be transmitted if the computer and control device were not in the same room would be by *telephone lines*. It would be necessary with this approach to have a second computer in the same room as the control device and for both computers to have modems (see Chapter 2).

Emulation Software for Measurement and Control Instrumentation

Software is available for microcomputers that enables them to emulate many clinical instruments that speech-language pathologists and audiologists (particularly the former) use for measurement and control. With this software, for example, you can emulate a Visipitch, a Sonograph, and an EMG or other type of biofeedback unit. These programs—which tend to be less expensive than the equipment they emulate—include **LabView** (Espinoza-Varas, 1992; Titze et al., 1995), **SoundWave** (Chaney, 1992), **SoundEdit Pro** (Chaney, 1992), and **MacSpeech Lab** (Hancock, 1986; Herman, 1989; Rubin, 1987; Scherz, 1993b) for the Macintosh and **Lab Windows** (Espinoza-Varas, 1992), **Dr. Speech Science** (Huang, et al., 1992), and **IBM SpeechViewer** (Ferrero et al., 1993; Friedman, 1989; Kennedy et al., 1991; Osredkar & Horii, 1991; Pratt et al., 1993; Ryalls et al., 1989; Ryalls et al. 1991; Zara, 1993) for IBM-compatibles.

▶ 13

Authoring Assessment, Management, and Learning Aids Using HyperCard and Similar Programs

Our discussion thus far of ways to utilize a computer clinically has focused on tasks done with existing software. No knowledge of computer programming is required for doing them. There are times, however, when you may need a program for promoting the welfare of clients or their families that either is not available or is available but not affordable. Such programs can sometimes be created by connecting blocks of computer code in much the same way that a child creates a toy by connecting the blocks in a Lego set. Programs that create software in this way are referred to as *authoring* programs. The prototype for these programs and the one that has been most widely used by persons in our field is HyperCard (Ambron & Hooper, 1990; Apple Computer, 1989; Beekman, 1992; Bluestone, 1992a; Bull & Cochran, 1992; Daniels & Mara, 1988; Goodman, 1988, 1990; Horton, 1990; Winkler & Kamins, 1990; Winkler & Knaster, 1990). Others available for the Macintosh include **SuperCard** and **HyperStudio** (Mizuko, 1995). Comparable authoring programs (e.g., Toolbook) are available for IBM-compatible microcomputers that use the Windows operating system (Bull & Cochran, 1992; Hadjian, Drumm, & Hanes-Drumm, 1994) and for the Apple IIGS (Leeper, 1992c).

WHAT IS HYPERCARD?

HyperCard, according to its creator Bill Atkinson, "is an authoring tool and an information organizer" (Goodman, 1990, p. 851). As an authoring tool, it is used to write computer programs that are referred to as *HyperCard stacks*. They are referred to as stacks because they can be conceptualized metaphorically as being comparable to stacks of file cards that are linked to each other.

The HyperCard Stack

Cards. A HyperCard stack is a collection of "cards" that can be thought of as being a document. Several representative "cards" from such stacks are illustrated in Figure 13.1. The number of cards in a stack can be in the thousands. A HyperCard stack card, like one in a stack of index cards, can contain text, drawings, and photographs in black-and-white or color. However, unlike one in a stack of index cards, it can also contain sound (including speech), animation, and movies. Furthermore, HyperCard stack cards can contain more information than can be displayed on the screen at one time—text and graphics can be viewed in segments through a "window" in the same manner that word-processor documents are viewed (Figure 13.1c). All of the cards in a HyperCard stack may have the same form printed on them—for example, the pages of an appointment book (Figure 13.1b). HyperCard stacks can be linked together to form new stacks. Also, cards in one HyperCard stack can be copied and utilized in another.

A

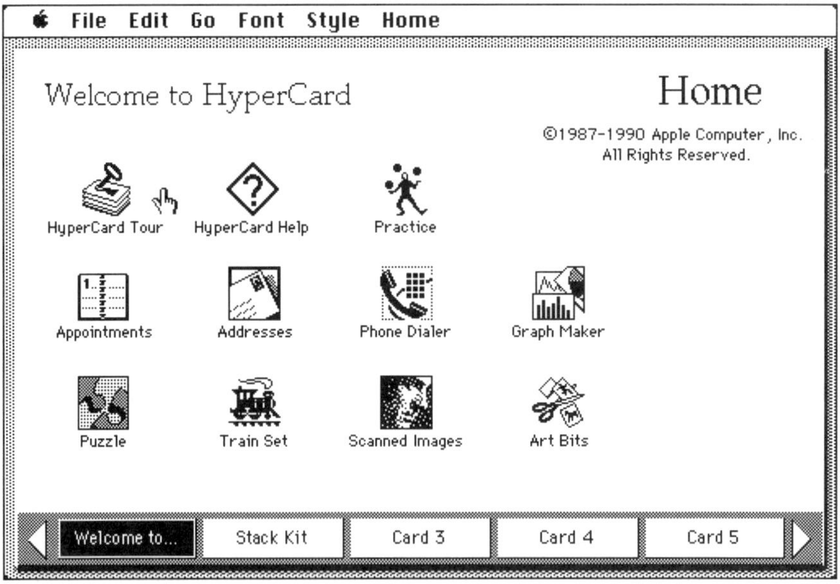

FIGURE 13.1 **Three representative "cards" from HyperCard stacks.**

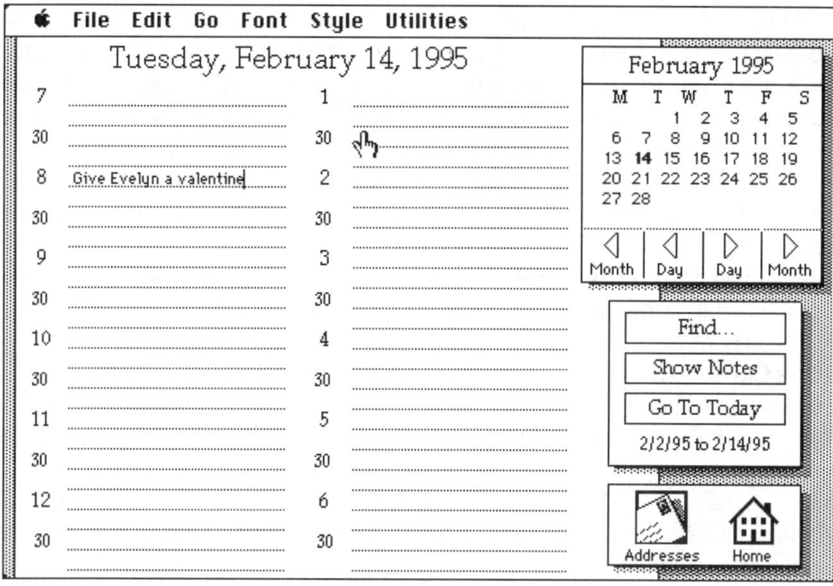
File Edit Go Font Style Utilities
Tuesday, February 14, 1995
7
30
8 Give Evelyn a valentine
30
9
30
10
30
11
30
12
30
1
30
2
30
3
30
4
30
5
30
6
30
February 1995
M T W T F S
1 2 3 4 5
6 7 8 9 10 11 12
13 14 15 16 17 18 19
20 21 22 23 24 25 26
27 28
Month
Day
Day
Month
Find...
Show Notes
Go To Today
2/2/95 to 2/14/95
Addresses
Home

B

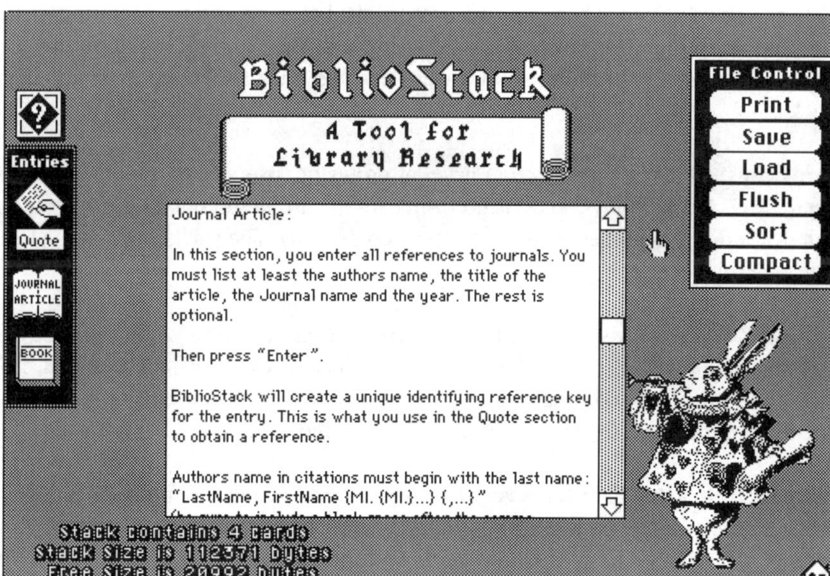
BiblioStack
A Tool for
Library Research
Entries
Quote
JOURNAL ARTICLE
BOOK
Journal Article:
In this section, you enter all references to journals. You must list at least the authors name, the title of the article, the Journal name and the year. The rest is optional.
Then press "Enter".
BiblioStack will create a unique identifying reference key for the entry. This is what you use in the Quote section to obtain a reference.
Authors name in citations must begin with the last name: "LastName, FirstName {MI. {MI.}...} {,...}"
File Control
Print
Save
Load
Flush
Sort
Compact
Stack contains 4 cards
Stack Size is 112371 bytes
Free Size is 20992 bytes

C

Buttons. Almost all of the cards in HyperCard stacks contain buttons. Buttons are procedures that link the cards in a stack. You "browse" through a stack—that is, move from card to card in one—by "pressing" buttons. Consequently, you don't move from card to card in a stack in a fixed (linear) sequence as you do from page to page in a book. To "press" a button, you place the little hand icon (Figures 13.1a, b, and c) on it by moving the mouse and then clicking (pressing the button on) the mouse. All eleven icons in Figure 13.1a are buttons as are the seven rectangles and triangles at the bottom of the card. Each date on the calendar in Figure 13.1b is a button as are all of the icons, rectangles, and triangles on the card. And all of the icons, rectangles, and arrows on the card in Figure 13.1b are buttons.

Home Card. The first card that you will usually see when you start the HyperCard program is the home card (Figure 13.1a is a representative home card). The home card contains icons (that are buttons) for the HyperCard stacks that your computer can access. You access ("open") a stack by moving the small hand to its icon (with the mouse) and then clicking the mouse. Most (if not all) of the cards in the stack will have an icon on them depicting a home. By clicking this icon, you quit the stack and return to the home card.

User Level Settings

The user level setting in a HyperCard stack determines the ways in which its contents can be modified. There are five user levels: browsing, typing, painting, authoring, and scripting. The "lowest" is browsing and the "highest" is scripting. Each level incorporates everything from lower ones and adds new options for modifying stacks.

Browsing. If a stack's user level is set at browsing, users cannot modify the stack in any way. All that they can do is go from card to card in the stack by either clicking buttons or doing searches (using the "find" command). The stacks for some tutorials are set at this level.

Typing. If a stack's user level is set at typing, users can browse through the stack and make changes to text (add, delete, or modify). They could, for example, fill in the appointment calender page in Figure 13.1b. This is the *default* user level—the one the program sets the stack at if it isn't instructed otherwise.

Painting. If a stack's user level is set at painting, users can browse through the stack and manipulate both text and graphics (see Chapter 6). Manipulation of graphics includes both creating them on cards and transferring them to cards from other sources. Graphics can be transferred that were either created with a paint-type program or scanned. Both drawings and photographs can be transferred to cards after being scanned.

Authoring. If a stack's user level is set at authoring, users can do all of the above plus assemble programs from "standard components." Such components—which are referred to as HyperCard *objects*—include buttons, fields, cards, backgrounds, and stacks. These objects are connected to create programs in much the same way as the bolts and metal pieces of an erector set and the plastic blocks of a Lego set are connected to create toys.

The standard object component kit for *buttons* offers an number of options. You can make a button either visible or invisible. You would choose the invisible option for buttons over text or graphics. For example, the buttons over each of the twenty-eight dates in the calender in Figure 13.1b are invisible ones. For visible buttons, you have options concerning shape, size, icon, placement, and functions.

Fields on HyperCard stack cards, like those on forms in databases (see Chapter 9), are places where you type text. Each of the time slots on the appointment book page in Figure 13.1b is a field. The standard HyperCard component kit offers a number of options for laying out fields on cards. It also enables you to make a field editable or locked and to determine the visual characteristics of both the text in the field (the font and size) and the field itself (e.g., transparent or opaque, lined or unlined, and scrolling or nonscrolling).

There are a number of *card-related* "tools" in the standard HyperCard component kit, including ones that enable a stack's author to generate cards and arrange them in the appropriate sequence. There also are tools that enable users to add, delete, and rearrange cards (if the stack's author wants them to have these options).

There are a number of tools and components in the standard HyperCard kit for creating *backgrounds*. Backgrounds consist of pictures, fields, and buttons that are shared by a number of cards. A background picture, for example, would consist of text and graphics that are shared by at least some of the cards in a stack. The times and lines on the appointment calendar in Figure 13.1b are elements of the background picture for the cards ("pages") in that stack. And the home icon in the lower right corner of the card in Figure 13.1b is a background button for the cards in that stack.

A *stack* is a group of cards based on the same theme (e.g., an appointment calendar). There are tools in the standard HyperCard kit that enable you name and rename a stack, learn the number of cards in a stack and the amount of space (memory) a stack uses, and read the name of the folder and disk the stack resides on.

Scripting. If a stack's user level is set at scripting, users can do all of the above plus write and edit scripts. A script is a series of commands that are associated with an object (e.g., a button, a picture, or a field). Scripts are written in *HyperTalk*, HyperCard's built-in language (for a description of this language, see Goodman, 1990; Martin & Lieberth, 1992a; Winkler & Kamins, 1990). All of the objects in the standard HyperCard kit were created by such scripts. If an object needed for a stack is not in the standard kit, it can be created by writing a script for it with HyperTalk.

You may be able to create an object that you need without having to know how to write HyperTalk scripts. If you can locate a stack that contains such an object, you can copy the script for the object from it. The script may be usable as is or with minor modification. HyperTalk, incidentally, is easier to learn than most computer languages because it has an English-like vocabulary and syntax (Goodman, 1990).

If the objects that you need for a stack cannot be created with HyperTalk, they can be created with another computer language—such as assembly language (see Chapter 3)—and interfaced with the stack by a HyperTalk script. These sub-programs are known as *XCMD*s (external command). Using them, you can create a HyperCard stack for doing almost any task.

The objects you will need to assemble most of the types of stacks that you are likely to find useful for clinical purposes will be in the standard HyperCard kit. Consequently, you will not have to know how to write the scripts or XCMDs for objects.

HOW HAVE SPEECH-LANGUAGE PATHOLOGISTS AND AUDIOLOGISTS USED STACKS CREATED WITH HYPERCARD-TYPE AUTHORING PROGRAMS?

Speech-language pathologists and audiologists have used stacks created with HyperCard and similar authoring programs clinically in a number of ways, including facilitating:

- Accent reduction with non-native speakers of English (Ferrier, Blackmer, DiGiacomo, & Walsh, 1993; Ferrier, Clough, Reid, & Walsh, 1994)
- Analysis of clinical test data (Palmer, 1992)
- Aphasia therapy (Dressler, 1992; Pitts, 1991)
- Augmentative communication and other activities for persons who are severely communicatively impaired (Harlan, 1988; Mervine & Ziegler, 1994; Mizuko, 1992, 1995; Mizuko & Erickson, 1994; Mizuko & Hornstadt, 1992b; Mizuko, Hornstadt, & Erickson, 1993; Scherz, 1995; Vanderheiden, 1990)
- Aural rehabilitation (Lieberth, 1992; Smaldino & Smaldino, 1991)
- Communication by infants with cerebral palsy (Fell, Ferrier, Hariklia, & Peterson, 1994)
- Controlling a videodisc player for presenting drill-practice stimulus material (Ott-Rose & Cochran, 1992; Pickering, 1992)
- Counseling clients and their families—for example, providing them with information about the communicative disorder with which they have to cope (Parker, Arnett, & Eldred, 1993; Wynne, Martin, & Matt, 1995)
- Development of clinical treatment materials (Leeper, 1992a, 1994), including those that utilize videotape (Nelson, 1993) and interactive multimedia (Valentine, 1995b)
- Enhancing the ability of classroom teachers to determine whether the commu-

nicative behaviors they observe warrant referral for evaluation (Cuda, Wynne, & Sawyer, 1992)

- Occupational hearing conservation (Bradley, 1994)
- Proper articulatory placement and sound awareness for isolated speech sounds (Clarke & Kneil, 1990)
- Teaching manual sign language (Lieberth & Martin, 1992)
- Therapy for children and adolescents with language-learning disabilities (Fischer, 1991a, 1992b, 1993)
- Voice therapy (Bless,et al., 1992)

Speech-language pathologists and audiologists have also used HyperCard stacks to create tutorials on and databases for a number of aspects of clinician training, including the following:

- Aphasia (Beckman, 1994)
- Aspects of anatomy/physiology (Leeper, 1991a)
- Audiology (de Jonge, 1992; Kuster, 1995b)
- Clinical process (Beckman, 1994; Shadden & Aslin, 1992)
- Hearing science concepts (Khoo & Allington, 1993)
- Phonological processes (Kneil, et al., 1991)
- Recording clinical practicum hours (Bradley & Krumm, 1995)
- Statistics (Anderson et al., 1991)
- Strategies for reading journal articles with good comprehension (Beckman, 1994)
- Syndromes in speech and hearing (Brorson, Chlopan, Grimmett, Humphries, Murphy, & Kneil, 1995)
- The decibel scale (Kneil, 1991)
- The international phonetic alphabet (Beckman, 1994)
- Voice disorder identification and treatment (Wiepsuj et al., 1992)
- Voice disorders in singers (Bernstorf, Kneil, & Burk, 1991)

The papers that are cited in this section provide convincing evidence that HyperCard-type authoring programs can enhance our ability to be helpful to both clients and students.

A FINAL COMMENT

Software is available for doing many of the tasks that you are likely to find clinically useful. Consequently, it probably would not be a good use of your time to create software for doing such tasks—that is, to "reinvent the wheel." There are clinical tasks, however, for which software is not available—for example, programs that would enable your computer to manipulate the controls on certain instruments that were interfaced with it in the specific ways that you desired (Birk & Stewart, 1991) or programs that would "drill" your clients on the specific vocabulary, concepts, or linguistic rules on which they are working. It is likely that the software needed to do such tasks could be created from HyperCard-type objects. I strongly recommend, therefore, that you learn how to use HyperCard or a similar program at the "authoring" level. When doing so, there are some papers in our literature that may be helpful (see Allen, 1992b).

You can copyright the HyperCard stacks you create and distribute them as freeware, shareware, or commercial products (see Chapter 3). No royality or licensing fee had to be paid to Apple Computer (the publisher of HyperCard) when this chapter was written. Be aware, however, that this may not be true for stacks created with HyperCard or HyperCard-type programs when you produce one. The manual for the software will indicate whether there are any restrictions on the distribution of stacks created with it.

▶ 14

Time and Project Management

Our professional and personal responsibilities sometimes require us to maintain a complex schedule and/or manage aspects of several projects. The more responsibilities that we have, the more difficult it becomes to *remember* to do what has to be done when it has to be done. There are several categories of software that can help us to manage our time and projects. These programs—which include alarm clock, calendar generating, personal scheduling, group scheduling, meeting scheduling, to-do list, project management, and time-billing ones—are described in this chapter.

The fact that these tasks are described singly does not necessarily mean that a program can do only one of them. Some can do several—for example, maintain both personal appointment schedules and to-do lists. These are referred to as *personal information managers*, or PIMs.

The use of computers for time and project management has received very little attention in the speech-language pathology and audiology literature. Perhaps the reason is, in part, that few clinicians are aware of these programs and/or how they could use them to help manage their responsibilities. The discussion in this chapter will, hopefully, help to alleviate this situation.

ALARM CLOCK PROGRAMS

The operating system files of most microcomputers contain a few mini-application programs. These may be referred to as *desk accessories* (DAs). One that is usually included simulates an alarm clock (Figure 14.1).

Most contemporary microcomputers have a built-in clock and calender (usually battery operated) that functions even when the computer is turned off. Both are accessed by alarm clock DAs.

The alarm clock is active whenever the computer is turned on. When the alarm

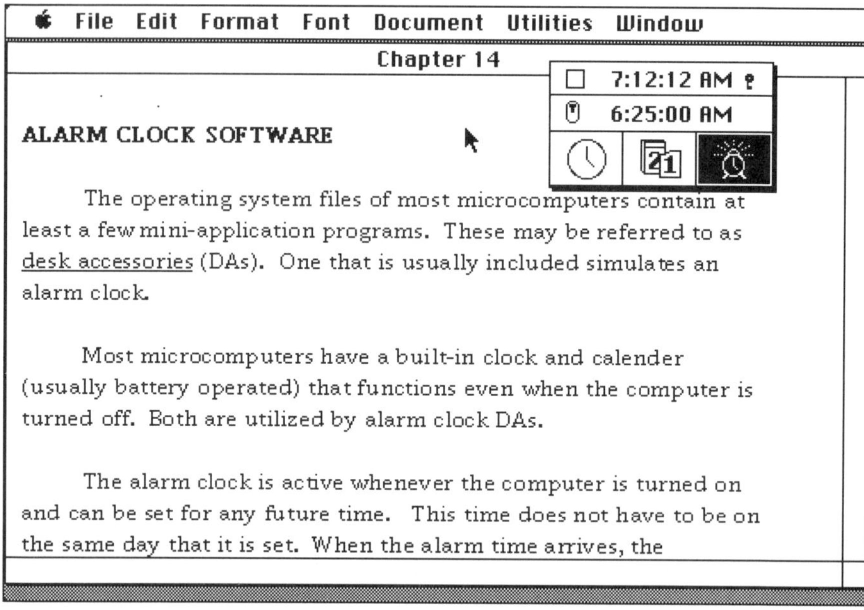

FIGURE 14.1 **An alarm clock desk accessory (DA).**

time arrives, the computer "beeps" and/or an icon is flashed on the screen (see the clock icon in the upper left corner in Figure 14.2). If the computer is turned off when the alarm time arrives, you get the beep and/or screen icon when it is turned on. The amount of time that it takes to set the alarm is usually less than a minute.

An alarm clock DA can be used by clinicians in several ways. One way is to signal both the clinician and the client when a therapy session is over. Such a signal can be particularly helpful with clients who often try to extend their session beyond its termination time—they may regard the computer "saying" that the session is over as being more authorative than the clinician's doing so. Another way that clinicians can use alarm clock DAs is to remind them of appointments, including therapy sessions.

CALENDAR-GENERATING PROGRAMS

These programs print monthly calendar pages. Most can generate them for a wide range of months. (The one that I use can do so for any month between 1905 and 2030.) Pages can be printed with all of the day spaces blank (Figure 14.3) or with information typed in some of them. Small drawings (icons) can also be inserted in these spaces. For example, you could put a small drawing of yourself in the space for

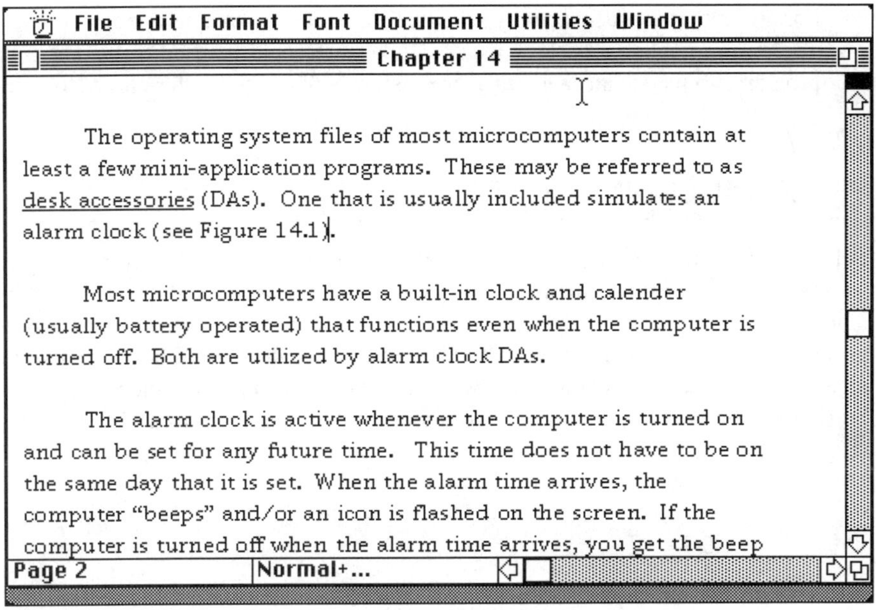

FIGURE 14.2 **The flashing alarm clock icon in upper left corner of the monitor screen signals that the alarm time has arrived.**

each day that a client is scheduled for therapy on a monthly appointment-reminder page that you would give him or her. You may also be able to insert drawings or scanned photographs on the tops of calendar pages (which could enable you to desktop publish picture calendars that have formats similar to commercial ones). Furthermore, you can print daily and weekly appointment calendar pages with some of these programs.

Most calendar programs enable you to print pages in almost any size, either vertical or horizontal. They can be made small enough to fit into a wallet or large enough to cover a wall. Pages that are larger than letter size would be printed in sections and taped together.

You probably can use pages that are generated by a calendar program to facilitate your professional activities in at least one of the following ways:

- As appointment reminders for clients and their families
- To produce wall and desk calendars for yourself and your staff (you'll never have to purchase a calendar again)
- As monthly reminders for staff of meetings, task deadlines, and other professional activities

- For presenting monthly activity schedules in organizational newsletters
- To desktop publish a desk or wall calendar that could be used to market your programs to physicians and other professionals who could refer clients to them

PERSONAL SCHEDULER PROGRAMS

Personal scheduler programs enable you to book activities—usually referred to as *events*—by assigning them to blocks of time on specific days. Some, like alarm clocks, are desk accessories. Figure 14.4 shows a window for such a program set to display a work week. Alternatively, the window could be set to display a day, a full week, or as many as six weeks. The days displayed in the window can be changed by clicking the buttons (triangles) at the top and bottom of the display (Figure 14.4).

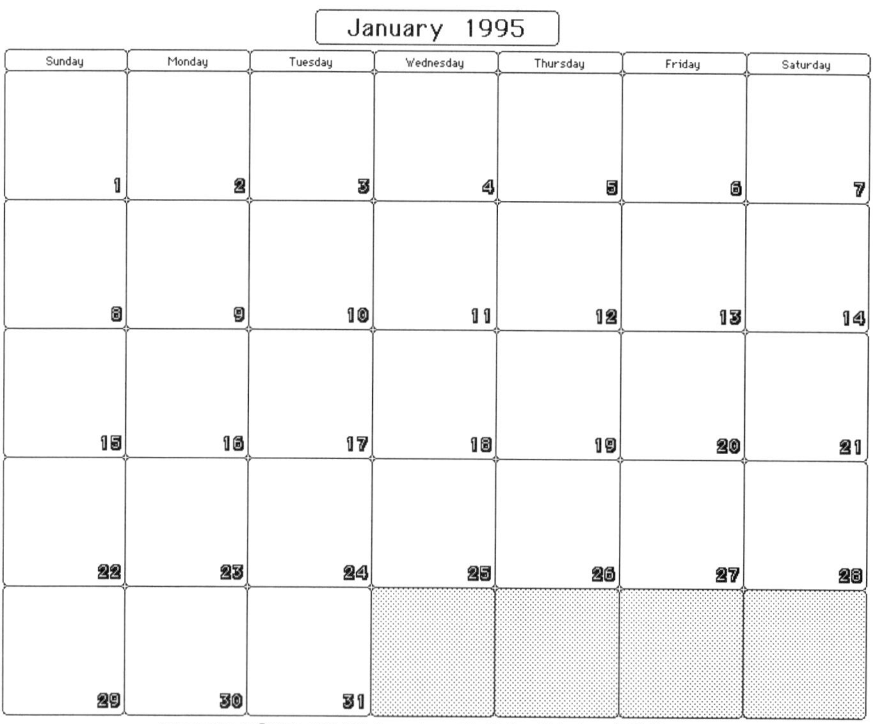

FIGURE 14.3 **A monthly calendar page with all of the day spaces blank.**

A new event may be added to the schedule by responding to items in a dialog box; the dialog box in Figure 14.5 is representative. It allows you, among other things to describe the event (and record information related to it such as names, addresses, and/or telephone numbers) and to enter the date the event occurs and when it begins and ends. Furthermore, it allows you to assign events to professional categories such as client appointments, meetings, phone calls (e.g., for periodic case follow-ups), and report deadlines, as well as personal events such as birthdays and the like. Once assigned, they can be retrieved by both categories and dates. For example, you could retrieve all report deadlines between specified dates. Events can be booked months or years in advance.

When booking an event, you can program the computer to remind you when it needs attention. It will do so by sounding an alarm and/or displaying a message on the monitor screen (Figure 14.6). Most of these programs will alert you when the alarm time arrives regardless of whether you are using it or another program. If the computer is turned off when an alarm time arrives, you will be alerted the next time that you turn the computer on.

One limitation of a software scheduler is that you can't have it available to use all of the time unless you have a laptop computer. However, since most of these pro-

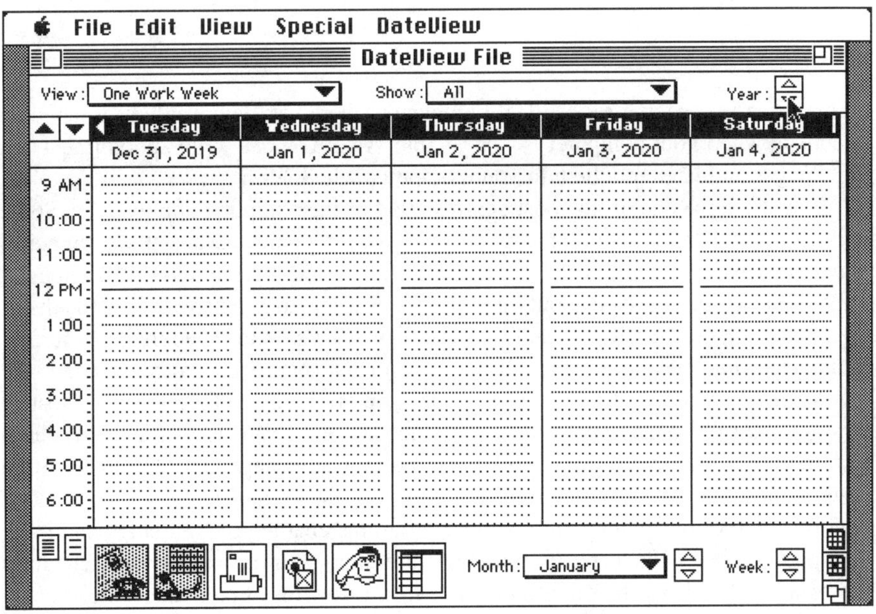

FIGURE 14.4 **A grid display for a personal scheduler (calendar) program.**

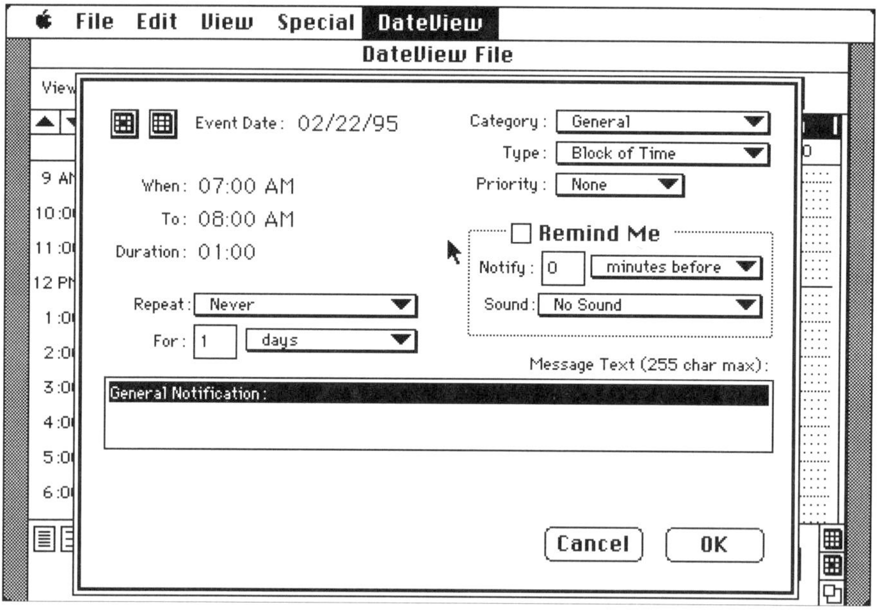

FIGURE 14.5 **A dialog box for adding a new event to the calendar of a personal scheduler (calendar) program.**

grams can print pages for loose-leaf organizers/schedulers, you can have a schedule to consult when your computer isn't available. Also, you can write appointments on these pages and later add them to your computer scheduler file.

Scheduling is one of the most controversial of the computer applications. Some persons believe that scheduling software is a waste of money because they can maintain their schedule as well with an inexpensive notebook-style appointment calendar. Those who are enthusiastic about these programs argue that they have several advantages over notebook-style schedulers. First, they allow you to schedule items further in advance than notebook schedulers—even many years in advance. Second, the reminders nag you about items in the future you are likely to forget. Since most of these programs also maintain to-do lists (which are discussed elsewhere in this chapter), they feel that this is a particularly important advantage. Third, you have the space to describe items more completely than you do in most notebook schedulers. And fourth, the files maintained by these programs enable you to archive and track your past activities. You can export information every year or two from the scheduler file to an archival one to keep the former from growing to unmanageable proportions. These programs, incidentally, all have "find" commands that enable you to

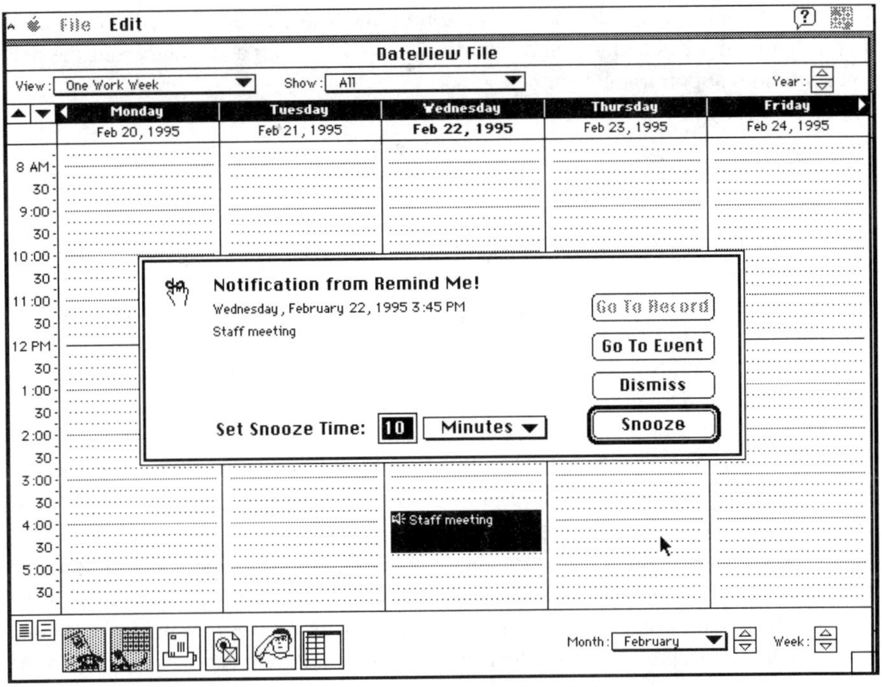

FIGURE 14.6 **An alert dialog box for a personal scheduler (calendar) program.**

quickly locating words (e.g., client names) in schedule records. It certainly is easier to locate information in such records if they are in a computer file than it is if they are written on pages that are stored in a box or filing cabinet.

GROUP SCHEDULER PROGRAMS

This is the type of software that is used at clinics (for example, medical and dental offices) and other facilities to maintain appointment schedules for groups of persons. The scheduling software and files are maintained on a computer at the facility that can be accessed by other computers. The other computers may be linked to it by a local area network (LAN), telephone lines and a modem, or both (these options are discussed in Chapter 12). Almost all of these programs offer the option of password protection for maintaining security and confidentiality.

The value of group scheduler software, unlike the personal scheduler variety, is not controversial. Few, if any, clinics or other facilities would choose to trade their appointment scheduler software for an appointment book because with it appointments can be made, changed, and monitored easily by both a secretary and the person for whom appointments are being made.

MEETING SCHEDULING PROGRAMS

These programs identify possible times for a meeting by examining the personal scheduler files of participants. They will identify the first date and time that all participants should be free to attend. These programs tend to be most practical when the computers of possible participants (e.g., all of the professional and support staff employed by a facility) are linked by a local area network. They, of course, are only effective if all participants keep their personal scheduler file up to date.

After the software compares the participants' personal scheduler files and identifies a possible date and time for a meeting, it sends a message to the computer of each participant in the meeting inquiring whether the meeting time proposed is acceptable. Each participant responds to the message with a *yes*, *no*, or *will decide later*. A message usually is sent immediately to computer of the person arranging the meeting when a participant says no. The computer then identifies another possible meeting time. The proposing-messaging process continues until a time is found that is acceptable to all participants. Most of these programs will send a message to the arranger's computer after all participants have accepted.

TO-DO LIST PROGRAMS

Most clinicians have professional obligations that extend beyond treating clients and attending meetings. They have tasks to do for which there are deadlines. Such tasks could include drafting reports and making telephone calls. While some clinicians maintain their to-do task list in their head, others don't trust their memory and write the items in it on slips of paper. There is software available for maintaining such lists that can enable you to do a better job of meeting deadlines than slips of paper. This software can be a separate program or a module of another, such as a personal scheduler or personal information manager (PIM) one.

Software to-do lists have at least one big advantages over paper ones. The items (events) in them can have reminders attached that will alert you to deadlines. When you add an event to the list you can specify the date (and possibly also the time) that you want to be alerted about it. If the computer is not turned on at this time, the reminder message will be displayed the next time that the computer is turned on.

After you complete a to-do item, you enter this information into the computer. If you do not complete an item by the date/time you specify, it will be added to your to-do list for the next day (or for some other date that you specify). Seeing a reminder about a item displayed day after day motivates (nags) you to complete it.

Most of these programs allow you to prioritize to-do list items. Consequently, by using the program's "find" function, you can quickly identify items that have to be completed by a certain date if you don't have time to do them all.

You can use this type of software in another way if your computer is networked with those of your secretary and/or other assistants. Rather than telling them to do something, you can add it to their to-do list, along with a priority. They probably are more likely to meet your deadlines if you do this instead of just telling them.

PROJECT MANAGEMENT PROGRAMS

These programs generate a type of to-do list. The tasks that appear on the ones they generate differ in several ways from those discussed in the previous section. First, all of the tasks that appear on them are related to a single project—they indicate what has to be done for the project to be completed successfully. And second, a resulting to-do list may not be a personal one—some of the tasks that appear on it may be assigned to (i.e., done by) other persons. Programs of this type that were available when this chapter was written include **FastTrack Schedule, MacProject Pro, Micro Planner Manager, Microsoft Project**, and **Project Scheduler**.

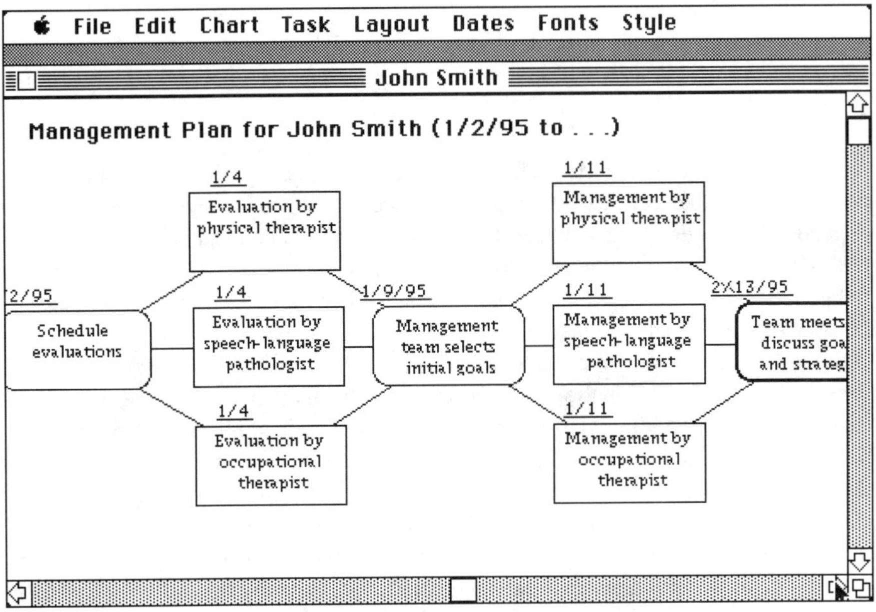

FIGURE 14.7 **Schedule view of a portion of a rehabilitation plan for a child who has cerebral palsy.**

Such software could help you to plan and organize a number of types of projects, including the following:

- Management plans for clients (Figure 14.7)
- New clinical programs
- In-services, continuing education courses, open houses, conferences, conventions, and workshops
- Grant applications (proposals)
- Remodeling rooms in clinical facilities
- Weddings and other complex social functions (The applications mentioned in this book hopefully will facilitate your personal activities as well as your professional ones.)

Note that all of these projects are multi-task ones that are likely to involve the efforts of more than one person and take weeks or months to complete.

Project management programs generate schedule charts (Figure 14.7). These charts—which indicate tasks that have to be done to achieve milestones, or goals—contain four basic elements:

- Boxes that represent *tasks* (the rectangular ones in Figure 14.7)
- Boxes that represent *milestones*, which can be either goals or subgoals (the ones with rounded corners in Figure 14.7)
- *Lines* connecting the boxes that indicate how tasks are related to milestones
- *Dates* by which tasks will hopefully be begun and/or completed and milestones will occur

The manner in which these elements are used to map a project is as follows. The boxes for tasks that have to be completed before others can be begun—tasks that are dependent on others—are arranged from left to right and connected by lines. In Figure 14.7, the alignment of boxes indicates that there have to be evaluations before initial goals can be established and management can begin. The boxes for tasks that can be done during the same time interval—tasks that are independent—are aligned vertically and not connected to each other by lines. In Figure 14.7, the alignment of the three task boxes for "evaluation" and the three for "management" indicates that in this case the clinical activities of speech-language pathologists, physical therapists, and occupational therapists are independent of each other. The dates above the task and milestone boxes are the earliest ones that the activity specified in them can begin.

Perhaps the application for which project management software can be most helpful to clinicians is developing and communicating management plans for clients. Schedule charts for this purpose can be created quickly with such software and modified and added to easily. To speed up the drawing process, you could create a template that contains the task and milestone boxes that appear in most of your management plans. Then, when you needed to develop a management plan for a client, you wouldn't have to start from scratch. These charts can help you to communicate to clients and their families what is being planned and what it is hoped will be accomplished. They can also help to communicate these to the members of the management team and to third-party payers. Furthermore, they can help to convey an image of professionalism and competence to the latter.

Most project management programs can be used to plan, schedule, and otherwise manage projects that are far more complex than client management plans. One could be used, for example, to plan a project as complex as an ASHA convention. A schedule chart containing the task and milestone boxes for such a project would be likely to cover a large wall.

TIME-BILLING PROGRAMS

If you are speech-language pathologists or audiologists who are not employed by the public schools, it is likely that you charge by the hour for your clinical and/or consulting services. There is software available that can help you to both track and bill for your time. Time-billing software maintains a database of your billable activities and uses this information to generate invoices.

To set up a time-billing program, you have to input the following information:

- A list of the services that you render (referred to as *activities*) and the hourly rate for each
- The names and addresses of persons to whom you render services (referred to as *users*)
- The names and addresses of persons and organizations who are billed for the services that you render (referred to as *clients*)

If a person is billed for the services he or she receives, the person is listed as both a user and a client.

These programs usually refer to their database records as *time slips*. With most of them, you create a screen for adding time data to a time slip by selecting a *client* (the person or organization who will be billed), a *user*, and an *activity* (service). When the input screen is displayed, you enter the time data manually or activate the program's timer. Most of these programs have built-in timers that you can start when you begin a billable activity (e.g., a therapy or consulting session) and stop when it ends. All time-billing programs allow you to annotate time slips with comments. You can decide for each such comment whether you want it printed on the bill that is sent to the client.

These programs can generate invoices that summarize the services performed for which clients are financially responsible and show the amounts due. Alternatively, time slip data can be exported to an accounting program, and it can be used to generate invoices.

The types of software that are described in this chapter probably are not the only ones that can facilitate your ability to manage your time and projects well. Furthermore, you may be able to use them to manage these in ways other than those suggested. The use of computers for time and project management appears to have received little attention from clinicians in our field—perhaps too little considering its potential for benefiting them and their clients.

▶ 15

Microcomputer-Related New Technologies

A microcomputer does not have to be labeled a microcomputer to be one. There are a number of electronic devices that sometimes are labeled *new technologies* that, although not referred to as such, actually are microcomputers. Several that could be useful in the management of communicative disorders are described in this chapter.

PERSONAL DIGITAL ASSISTANTS (PDAS)

The first of the personal digital assistants (PDAs) was the Apple Newton MessagePad, which was available for purchase in 1993 (Bortman, 1993; Lu, 1993). These devices can be held comfortably in one hand—they are about the size of a trade paperback book and usually weigh less than a pound. They can be powered by either penlight batteries or rechargable NiCad ones.

PDAs have a touch-sensitive LCD (light conducting diode) screen that is used as both an input and output device (Figure 15.1). The screen on most is a little smaller than a 3-x-5 inch card turned sideways. You input information by writing or drawing on the screen with a special stylus (or another device that has a dull point). PDAs have software built in that recognizes both cursive and printed handwriting and translates it into print that it can display on the screen. They also have software built in that can "clean up" symmetrical shapes (such as circles and rectangles) in drawings. If you prefer to enter text with a keyboard, you can display one on the screen and activate keys by touching them with the stylus.

The hardware and software of PDAs, like that of desktop and laptop microcomputers, can be expanded. Additional memory (RAM) and a fax modem can be added. Furthermore, the built-in software can be supplemented by programs that can transform a PDA into such devices as a sophisticated calculator, a drawing tablet, an out-

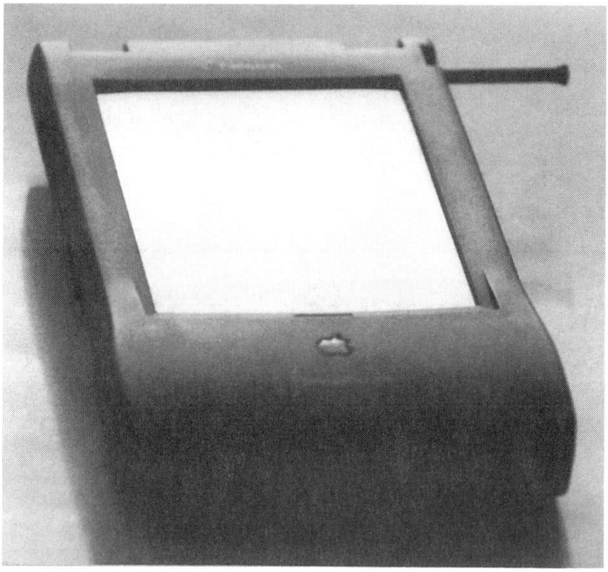

FIGURE 15.1 **A personal digital assistant.**

liner, a billable hour tracker (i.e., time-billing database), a flat-file database manager, a terminal for telecommunication, and a prompter for presentations.

Information that is stored in a PDA can be transferred to a microcomputer. That stored in the Apple Newton MessagePad, for example, can be transferred to either a Macintosh or an IBM-compatible microcomputer. Also, information that is stored in a microcomputer can be transferred (with a cable) to a PDA.

PDAs do tasks that could facilitate your clinical activities in a number of ways, including the following:

- **Making to-do and progress notes during clinical sessions.** You would keep a PDA close at hand while you are with clients and write your clinical notes on it. The notes would be stored in the PDA until they are printed or transferred (exported) to your clients' computer files. Any to-do items could be added to the list that you maintain on your PDA or microcomputer. Most PDAs come with the software needed to maintain a to-do list (see Chapter 14).
- **Maintaining your appointment schedule.** Most PDAs come with the software needed to maintain personal appointment schedules (see Chapter 14). They are about as convenient to carry and use as appointment books. You can either view your appointments on the screen or print them. And you can attach reminder signals to them (see Chapter 14). Furthermore, you can import appointment data

from other sources (e.g., your secretary's computer) and export your appointment schedule to other computers (e.g., your secretary's).

- **Maintaining an address file for clients and professional contacts.** Most PDAs have software built in for maintaining this type of database. Records can include other information, such as telephone numbers. If you are going to maintain this type of database, you probably would find it more useful to so on a device that you can always have with you rather than on one that you keep at your home or office.
- **Sending e-mail messages and faxes and receiving pager-type messages when you are away from your office.**
- **Tracking billable hours.** Invoices can be printed with the PDA or the data can be exported to a microcomputer and invoices can be printed with its accounting or time-billing program.

ELECTRONIC ORGANIZERS

These devices look like sophisticated pocket calculators (Figure 15.2). They have keyboards and display screens. The layout that they use for alphanumeric character keys—which are calculator size or a little larger—is the same as that on a computer keyboard. The screen may be capable of displaying as many as 20 lines of text. It

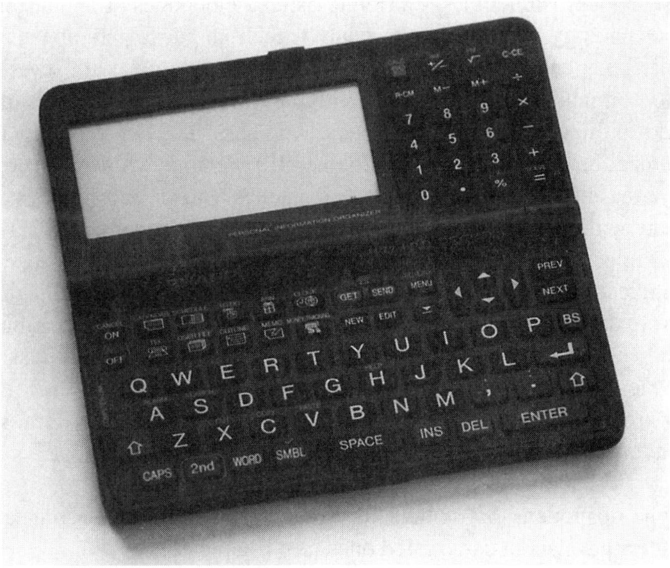

FIGURE 15.2 **An electronic organizer.**

may also be capable of displaying drawings. Some can export data to and import data from a microcomputer.

You can perform many of the clinical tasks mentioned in the section on personal digital assistants (PDAs) with these devices. You can maintain personal schedules, to-do lists, and address files with all of them. Furthermore, with some of the more expensive ones you can send faxes and e-mail messages and do the word processing necessary for progress notes.

These devices differ from PDAs in several ways. First, they use a keyboard rather than a touch screen for data entry. Second, they are less versatile—the only programs that almost all can run are the ones that are built-in. And third, they tend to be less expensive.

One of the main concerns that I initially had about using these devices for progress notes and other applications that require extensive typing was the size of the keys. While I found that the alphabet character keys were too small for touch typing, I could place my fingers over them in the approximate positions they would be in for touch typing and type at an acceptable rate of speed—definitely a more acceptable option than using only on one finger. However, I would not want to type an evaluation report or other long document on one of these.

TELECOMMUNICATION DEVICES FOR THE DEAF (TDDs)

While these devices, sometimes referred to as text telephones (TTs), historically are not a new technology, they are one to many speech-language pathologists and some audiologists. They enable persons who are deaf and some who are severely speech impaired to communicate by telephone (Figure 15.3 for a photograph of a TDD). They can do so directly with another person who has a TDD or indirectly by using a telecommunication relay service (see Chapter 12). Persons who are severely speech impaired for reasons other than being deaf (e.g., ones who are severely dysarthric) can communicate with them if they are sufficiently intact motorically to use a keyboard.

TDDs are actually dedicated microcomputers with built-in monitors, modems, and communication software. Some also have a built-in printer. *Dedicated* means that they were designed for doing a single task—telephone communication. Because they contain only the components that are needed for doing this task, they are smaller and less expensive than standard microcomputers.

TDDs are not all designed the same. Their features differ in several significant ways, including the following:

- The type of modem that is built-in. Some TDDs have direct-connect modems and others have acoustic-coupled ones (see Chapter 2).
- The code(s) they use. Some TDDs—particularly older ones—can only send and receive messages in the *Baudot code*. This code—which was developed in the

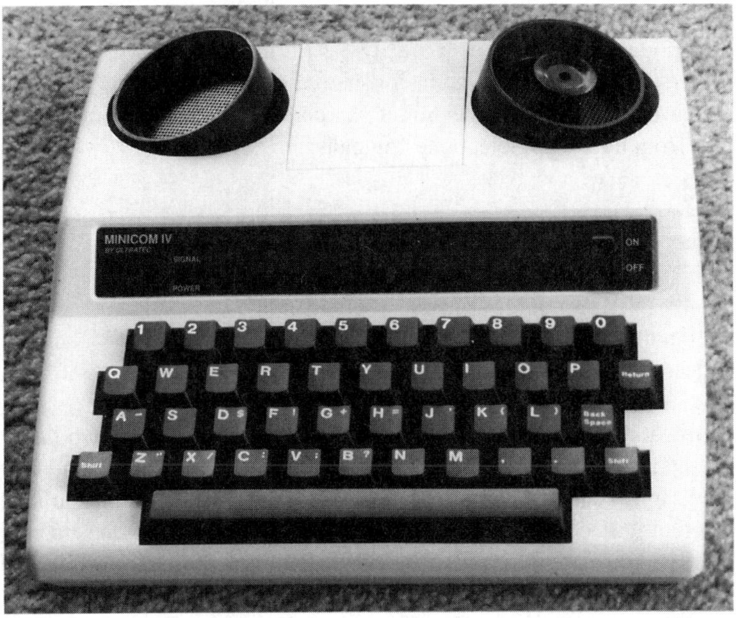

FIGURE 15.3 **A Telecommunication Device for the Deaf (TDD) with an acoustic coupler.**

late 19th century by Emile Baudot—was one of the first standards for international telegraphy. It was adopted for TDDs because it was the language used by teletypewriters. Many deaf persons used teletypewriters for telephone communication before TDDs became available and affordable. The Baudot code enabled persons who used TDDs to communicate with ones who had teletypewriters.

Some TDDs manufactured now use the *ASCII code* for sending and receiving messages instead of—or in addition to—the Baudot one. This is the code that computers use for encoding characters (see Chapter 3) and, as such, it enables them to communicate with computers without translation (Lynn, 1991). It also permits messages to be transmitted more rapidly than does the Baudot code.

- Their size. Some are relatively large units that are intended to be used on a table or desk and others are relatively small—about the size of a personal digital assistant or an electronic organizer.

A client may be able to get a TDD without having to purchase it. TDDs usually can be leased for a monthly fee from a local telephone company. This is a particularly good option for clients who only need one for a short time—e.g., those who have vocal nodules and are on "vocal rest". Furthermore, some states distribute TDDs to persons who are deaf and, in some cases, also to ones who are severely speech impaired. Clients or their families can obtain information about such distribution plans from their local telephone company.

VIRTUAL REALITY TECHNOLOGY

Virtual reality (VR) technology enables users to create and explore events in a computer-generated world (Wilson & Fox, 1993). What it is and what it can enable you to do are described succinctly below:

> Virtual reality is a breakthrough technology the allows you to step through the computer screen into a 3-D simulated world. You can look around, move around, and interact within computer worlds every bit as fantastic as the wonderland Alice found down the rabbit hole. All you have to do is to put on the special video goggles, and then almost anything is possible—you can fly, visit exotic lands, play with molecules, swim through the stock market, or paint with 3-D sound and color. (Pimentel & Teixeira, 1995, p. xvii)

Virtual reality technology differs from the others mentioned in this chapter in that it utilizes a computer. However, since it is referred to as a new technology and some of the devices it utilizes contain microprocessors, it seems appropriate to include a discussion of VR here.

Virtual reality is a technology for simulating visual, auditory, and tactile attributes of an event. The event simulated could be one that you could experience or one that it would be impossible for you to do so. An example of the former would be walking from your car to your office. An example of the latter would be walking from your car to your office in a building that has been planned, but not yet built.

Various devices are used to create sensory (i.e., visual, auditory, and/or tactile) attributes of a simulated event. These devices serve as tools for either creating sensory output or inputting information about the user's actions into the computer. These actions cause the computer to manipulate the sensory output devices that are interfaced with it in a manner that creates the visual-auditory-tactile aspects (attributes) of the simulated event. The input devices are *switching mechanisms* and the output devices are *displays* (see Chapter 5 in Silverman, 1995).

The input devices—switching mechanisms—that are used in VR for controlling a computer are of many kinds. One of the most common is *wired clothing*—particularly gloves. These devices track, or monitor, the position and orientation of key hand or other body parts. A glove, for example, could be wired so that it would detect the hand and finger movements you are making while typing with a computer-generated image of a keyboard—that is, a simulated keyboard.

Another type of input device that is used for VR simulations is a *wand* (i.e., "magic" wand). You can use a wand like a mouse to select objects (see Chapter 2). You point the wand at an object you see and want to select and press a button. You can also use a wand to navigate. You point the wand in the direction that you want to move and press a button.

A third type of input device that is used for VR simulations is a *biosensor*. These are electrode-based devices that detect electrical activity within the body—for example, muscle action potentials. Changes in the level of the electrical activity being monitored change one or more aspects of how an event is perceived.

A fourth type of input device that is used for VR simulations is a *speech-recognition* one. The user controls the virtual environment, in whole or part, by giving voice commands.

A number of types of output devices—displays—have been used for VR simulations. The type that probably has been used most often is referred to as *video goggles*. This device is also referred to as a *head-mounted display*. All that a person wearing one can see are the images that the computer creates on one or two miniature video monitors that are built into the device. If two monitors are built-in, their images will be fused into a single 3-D image (like those seen through a viewer for Viewmaster reels). These devices may also have built-in stereo headphones. They both attenuate environmental sound and generate the auditory attributes of the event being simulated.

The technology for simulating tactile attributes of events is not as highly developed as that for simulating visual and auditory aspects of them. One approach utilizes a special glove (Pimentel & Teixeira, 1995). When a person touches an object in a simulated visual environment, he or she experiences something that is somewhat similar to touching the actual object.

For descriptions of other input and output devices that are used for experiencing, manipulating, and navigating in VR environments, see Chapter 8 in Pimentel & Teixeira (1995).

How might speech-language pathologists and audiologists use VR technology to facilitate their clinical activities? This question is difficult to answer because of the paucity of reports by them of attempts to apply it to our field. The suggestions below are mostly based on applications that have been made of VR in other fields.

- Training persons who are severely communicatively impaired to use augmentative communication devices. Both the device and communication situation could be simulated. The switching mechanism that the person would use to control the communication device could be either a real or a simulated one (Colan, 1994). The technology needed to create such a simulation exists (and has for a while).
- EMG biofeedback training. A VR environment can be created that is controlled by the activity level of an EMG biosensor (Colan, 1994). Such an approach may be usable for relaxation training. Environments could be simulated in which a

client would have a great deal of difficulty remaining relaxed and the client could be provided with continuous feedback about his or her relaxation level while in them.

- Systematic desensitization. This is a technique that is used for reducing the extent to which a person responds to a stimulus—an event—with anxiety (Wolpe, 1958). The person is repeatedly exposed to the stimulus in a controlled way while he or she remains relaxed. This is usually done by either having the person repeatedly imagine experiencing the stimulus (event) or by repeatedly having him or her actually experience the event. VR may be a better way to simulate some feared events than having clients imagine them because it gives the clinician more control. Its use may be particularly practical for events that cause large numbers of clients anxiety, such as the telephone situation for stutterers (see Silverman, 1996).
- Language assessment and intervention (Colan, 1994; Wilson & Fox, 1993). Children are likely to consider such activities—if they are well designed—to be arcade-type videogame. They could incorporate auditory as well as visual stimuli and utilize speech recognition technology as a response mode.
- "Front ends" (displays) for computer-simulated audiometric and other clinical instrumentation. Software and hardware are available that enable a microcomputer to simulate most of the electronic instrumentation used by audiologists and speech-language pathologists (see Chapter 12). The ways in which controls are manipulated, however, is usually not the same as on the actual instrument. VR technology could be used to simulate both a visual image of an instrument and the tactile feedback that the user experiences when manipulating controls on it.
- Switching mechanisms for augmentative communication devices (Colan, 1994). Components used for VR can have other applications. Some of the input/tracking devices that were developed for it may be usable for interfacing clients with augmentative communication devices (see Chapter 5). These include gloves containing sensors that can detect very small movements, mechanisms for tracking eye movements, and biosensors.
- Helping clients and their families understand anatomical and physiological abnormalities of the speech and hearing mechanism. This is usually done now with anatomical diagrams. A VR trip into the part of the mechanism that is abnormal should convey the information more effectively. Similar VR simulations, incidentally, could be used to augment traditional instruction in anatomy and physiology courses. Students, for example, could take a trip down the pharynx into the larynx to look at the structures and their functions. They could also dissect the head and neck of a virtual cadaver.

For further information about virtual reality technology and how it has been utilized, see Burdea and Coiffet (1994), Carr and England (1995), Colan (1994), Larijani (1993), and Pimentel and Teixeira (1995).

▶ APPENDIX A

Searching the Literature with Online, Interactive Computer-Based Information Retrieval Systems

This appendix is a "how to" supplement to the discussion of literature searching with online, interactive computer-based information retrieval systems found in Chapter 11. These systems are referred to as being *online* because the user is in direct communication with the computer containing the database through a terminal or a microcomputer that has been programmed to function as one. And they are *interactive* because the user and computer engage in a "conversation" in which the computer responds quickly.

There are several computer databases that can be used with online, interactive information retrieval software for searching portions of the international communicative disorders literature. The one that probably has been used most often for this purpose by speech-language pathologists and audiologists is MEDLINE. This database indexes papers in more than 3000 journals (including those of the American Speech-Language-Hearing Association) dealing with medicine and related subjects from 1966 to the present. It is available in two forms: one that is stored on tape and requires the use of a mainframe or minicomputer (e.g., a VAX minicomputer) to access and one that is stored on CD-ROM disks (see Chapter 2) and can be accessed with a microcomputer. A single compact disk can store as many as 275,000 pages of typed information. While the 3000+ journals indexed by this database include most that publish papers on communicative disorders, it does not include them all. The *Journal of Fluency Disorders*, for example, was not indexed when this appendix was written. Other databases that index a portion of the communicative disorders literature are described in Chapter 11.

Planning the Search

Before performing a search using a computerized database it is necessary to decide the following:

- The keywords that will be included in the search and the manner in which they will be "linked." Ways in which they can be linked are discussed in the next section.
- The database(s) that will be searched.
- The range of years that will be included in the search.

COMPUTER SEARCH REQUEST—MARQUETTE UNIVERSITY LIBRARIES

DATE ______________________
Name ______________________
School or Dept. ______________________
Address ______________________
Phone Day ________ Night ________
(In case further information is needed)

FACULTY ___ STAFF ___ GRADUATE ___
UNDERGRAD ___ ID NUMBER ________

____ Dissertation/thesis
____ Coursework
____ University research
____ Other (specify)

SEARCH TOPIC Please explain in sentences exactly what you want covered. Be specific! Define terms that have special meanings. Feel free to attach another page.

SUGGESTED KEYWORDS/DESCRIPTORS

Which indexes or abstracts have you searched? Which subject headings were useful?

Please list a few recent relevant articles or books (authors, titles, journals, dates).

How many citations do you need?

___ A few relevant articles (under 25)
___ An exhaustive search which may retrieve a substantial number of irrelevant citations
___ Something in-between

Can you think of an ideal journal article title on the subject?

Time period to be covered

___ Current (last 2–3 years)
___ All years possible
___ Other time period (specify)
___ English ________ All languages
___ Other languages (specify) ____________

FIGURE A.1 **A representative search request form.**

FIGURE A.2 **A single keyword search strategy.**

- Whether the search should be limited in any way(s), such as English language only, children only, females only, human subjects only, or review articles only.
- Whether abstracts, if available, will be printed.

After these have been decided the search can be performed by either a research librarian or the end user (You!). If a database to be searched is on CD-ROM disks or on tape at one of the college or university's computer facilities, it should be possible for the end user to do the search himself or herself. However, if the database is on a computer that does not belong to your college or university, the search may have to be performed by a research librarian. If this is the case, then information defining the search usually will be communicated to the librarian on a special form (Figure A.1).

Search Strategies

Most computer databases are searched in a similar fashion—through the use of keywords and the Boolean logic connectors AND, OR, and NOT. [Boolean logic was named after the mathematician who invented it, George Boole.] The manner in which this is done is illustrated in Figures A.2 through A.9. Let's represent the keywords "hearing loss," "otitis media," and "children" by A, B, and C respectively. The strategy diagrammed in Figure A.2 is one in which we are searching for all references containing a particular keyword (which can consist of more than one word). We would use this strategy, for example, if we were interested in retrieving from a database all references containing the keyword "hearing loss."

The strategy diagrammed in Figure A.3 is one in which we are searching for all references containing two keywords. We could use this strategy, for example, if

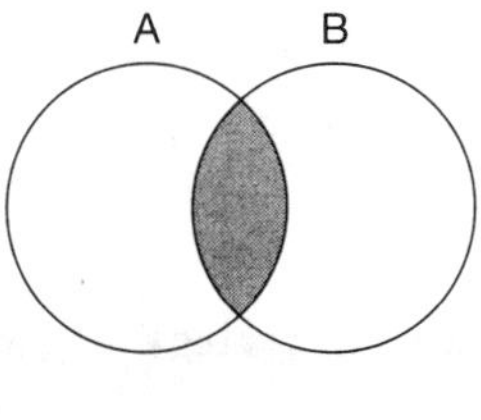

FIGURE A.3 **A single AND search strategy.**

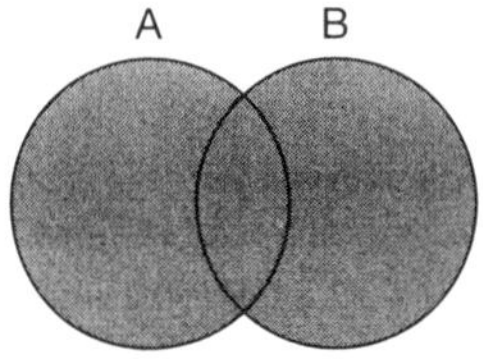

FIGURE A.4 **An inclusive OR search strategy.**

we were interested in retrieving from a database all references containing the keywords "hearing loss" AND "otitis media." That is, we would use it if we were only interested in retrieving references dealing with hearing loss resulting from otitis media.

The strategy diagrammed in Figure A.4 is referred to as the *inclusive* OR strategy because it not only will retrieve references containing one of two keywords, but also those containing both of them. We could use this strategy, for example, if we were interested in retrieving from a database all references containing the keywords "hearing loss" OR "otitis media" OR both of these. All such computer databases support an OR search strategy that functions in this manner.

Some databases also support an *exclusive* OR search strategy (Figure A.5) which will not retrieve references containing both keywords. Because you usually would not want to exclude such references, the *inclusive* OR strategy is used far more often than this one. An example of where you might want to use the *exclusive* OR strategy is for retrieving references dealing with "dysarthria without aphasia" and "aphasia without dysarthria: The two keywords here would be dysarthria and aphasia.

The AND NOT search strategy is illustrated in Figure A.6. (In some systems it may be referred to as the NOT or BUT NOT one.) It will retrieve references that mention one keyword that do not mention a second keyword. It can be used, for example, to retrieve all references on hearing loss that do not mention otitis media. This strategy should be used with caution because it will eliminate all references that mention the excluded keyword, including those that only do so in passing.

A search strategy can involve more than two keywords. A multiple AND search strategy that involves three keywords is illustrated in Figure A.7. It can be used for retrieving references in which three keywords are mentioned. It could be used, for

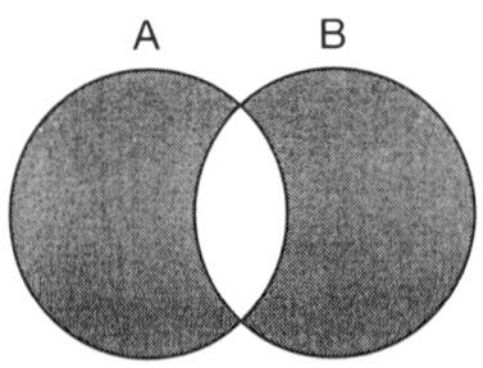

FIGURE A.5 **An exclusive OR search strategy.**

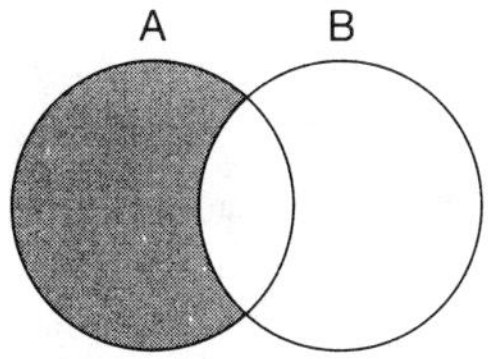

FIGURE A.6 **An AND NOT search strategy.**

example, for finding papers dealing (at least in part) with "hearing loss" in "children" resulting from "otitis media." This search strategy—which can use more than three keywords—is one of the most useful ones.

Another type of search strategy that involves more than two keywords combines the AND and AND NOT logical connectors (Figure A.8). It can be used for retrieving references that mention two keywords that do not mention a third. It could be used, for example, for finding papers dealing with "hearing loss" in "children" that do not mention "otitis media." The problem mentioned in the discussion of the AND NOT search strategy affects this one also.

A third type of search strategy that involves more than two keywords combines the AND and OR logical connectors (Figure A.9). When using it, two keywords are connected to each other by OR and these in turn are connected to another keyword by AND. This strategy could be used, for example, to locate papers dealing with "children" in which either "otitis media" or "hearing loss" is mentioned.

CONDUCTING THE SEARCH

If a database you decide to search is one that can be searched at your institution by an end user, you can begin the search after you have formulated a strategy for doing so. The first step in the process is "logging on," or "signing on," to the computer on which the database is stored. If the database is stored on CD-ROM disks on a microcomputer, you would log onto that computer.

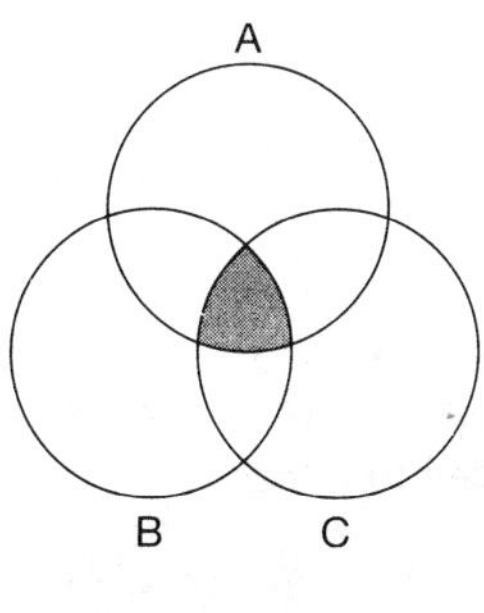

FIGURE A.7 **A multiple AND search strategy.**

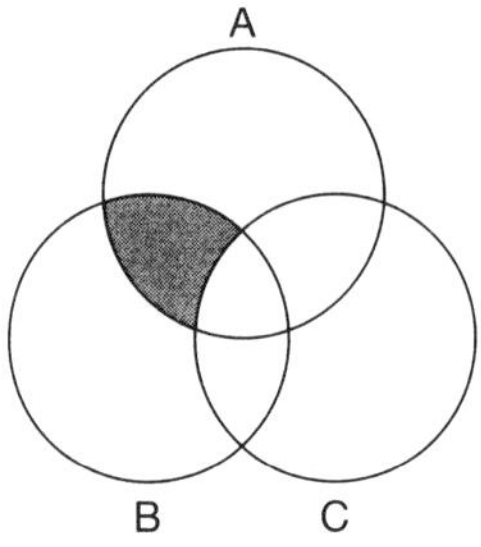

FIGURE A.8 **A compound AND and AND NOT search strategy.**

If the database is stored on a mainframe or minicomputer at your institution's computer center, you would log onto it using a computer terminal or a microcomputer that was programmed to simulate one. Most logon procedures involve keyboarding your name and a password when requested to do so. For security reasons, the password, which probably would be issued by your institution's computer center, probably will not be displayed on the screen while it is being keyboarded.

When the logon procedure is completed, you are given access to the database's main menu (Figure A.10). This menu may also give you access to a tutorial that provides basic information about the commands and procedures used for searching that database. It is a good idea to go through the tutorial at least once, particularly if you do not have access to a manual that provides this information.

The second step in the process is actually executing the search. This is done by selecting the appropriate item from the main menu (it would be "search for information" in Figure A.10) and by sending commands to the computer. Commands may be sent by activating single keys or combinations of ESCAPE or CONTROL keys and other keys. For example, X may be used for highlighting an option on a menu (Figure A.10), CONTROL J (abbreviated as ^J) for instructing the computer to browse through a set (Figure A.11) , and ESCAPE E for instructing it to move to the last line of a citation. Unfortunately, the commands used for accessing databases have not

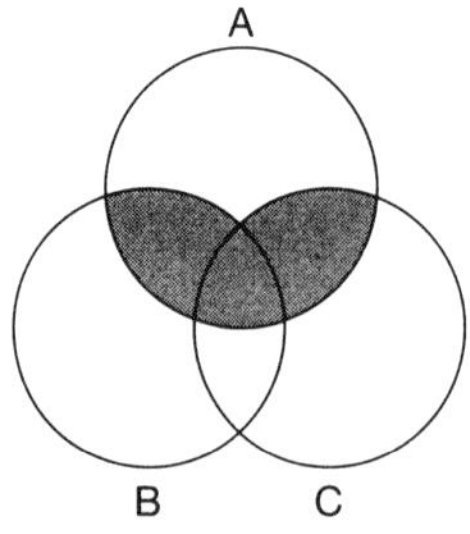

FIGURE A.9 **A compound search strategy in which two keywords are connected to each other by OR and these in turn are connected to another keyword by AND.**

	Options	
	Search for information Review search results File management Print or copy search results Maintenance functions Introduction Tutorial Copy tutorial and editor Exit	
	Use ^ or v to position cursor. Press 'x' to highlight an option,. then press ENTER to select that option.	

FIGURE A.10 **A representative main menu screen for a computer database intended for enduser searching.**

been standardized. The same command may be used in two databases, but have a different meaning in each.

The search is initiated by entering the "string" containing the keywords you are using for it (Figure A.11). The string entered for the example diagrammed in Figure A.2 would be the following:

hearing loss

After searching, the computer will indicate whether there are any items in the database that can be indexed by the string, and if so, how many. If there are many, it may indicate ways that you can eliminate some (i.e., narrow the search) by focusing more

Number	**Search Sets**	**Results**
	Enter subject, then press ENTER ___. hearing loss	

FIGURE A.11 **A representative screen for entering the subject of a search.**

	Medical Subject Headings Line 1 of 10	
	hearing loss, sensorineural hearing loss, noise-induced hearing loss, partial hearing disorders cochlea neomycin evoked potentials, auditory audiometry, evoked response occupational disease middle age	
	Press 'x' to mark the single most relevant subject heading, then press ENTER. Or press ENTER to pick no heading, or ^A for help.	

FIGURE A.12 **A representative screen menu of subject headings for limiting a search by adding a Boolean AND and a keyword.**

directly on the specific information you want. It may do this by adding a Boolean AND and keyword to the search. For example, it may permit you to limit the items selected to those dealing with partial hearing loss or hearing loss occurring during middle age (Figure A.12). After you have made a decision about whether you are interested in all the items or a more limited set, you will be informed how many items there are and possibly given the opportunity to limit the search further by restricting it to articles in which the keyword (index term) is a main focus (Figure A.13). After making this decision you may be presented with another menu of subheadings that will allow you to further limit (focus) the search if you want to do so (Figure A.14). After you respond to this menu, the number of items in the search set is indicated and you are given the opportunity to "browse" through them (Figure

	Index Term Selected	
	*hearing loss, partial	
	565 articles contain the above index term. In 456 articles this term is the focus of the article. Restrict to focus? Enter 'y' or 'n', then ENTER___.	

FIGURE A.13 **A representative screen for limiting a search by restricting it to articles in which the keyword (index term) is a main focus.**

	Subheadings	Line 1 of 20	Results
	chemically induced		33
	complications		15
	congenital		7
	diagnosis		69
	drug therapy		9
	epidemiology		11
	etiology		113
	genetics		16
	history		1
	immunology		1
	The subheadings shown above may be applied to refine your search. Press 'x' to mark as many as are relevant, then press ENTER. To restrict to no particular subheading, simply press ENTER.		

FIGURE A.14 **A representative screen menu of subheadings for limiting a search by adding a Boolean AND and a keyword.**

A.15)—that is, to view them one at a time on the screen (Figure A.16). If you want an item included in the printout, you can issue a command (e.g., ^*E*) after viewing it (Figure A.16).

If the computer indicates that there are no items containing the keywords you selected, the reason may be that you have chosen the wrong keywords. Each database has a printed thesaurus, as a reference tool, which lists the keywords to which it will respond—that is, ones that are in its index.

The final steps in the search process are printing relevant items and logging off. You may be given choices about the format in which you want the bibliography printed, including whether you want abstracts included, if available. If you are using a microcomputer as a terminal, you probably will be given the option of download-

Number	Search Sets	Line 1 of 1	Results
01	*hearing loss, partial		456
	Mark set to browse, then press ENTER. Press ENTER to browse last set.		

FIGURE A.15 **A representative screen for selecting a search set to browse.**

Citation 4 of 56

Unique Identifier
91073233
Author
Hasegawa S.
Title
Hearing and language ability in mild and moderate hearing impaired children [Jpn]
Institution
Department of Otolaryngology, Nagoya University School of Medicine.
Journal
Nippon Jibiinkoka Gakkai Kaiho [JC:jjz] 93(9): 1397–409, 1990 Sep.
Abstract
102 children (mean age–7 years 9 mo.) with mild and moderate perceptive hearing impairment who had neither any auditory training nor had used a hearing aid were studied. Mean hearing level was 51.9 dB. Our findings: (1) Speech discrimination score (SDS) correlated with the hearing level at 2, 4 and 1 kHz, in that order. In all patients SDS gradually worsened to 60 dB

FIGURE A.16 **A representative screen when citations are being browsed. You could have the remainder of the abstract displayed by typing a command.**

ing the bibliography to it for saving as a file that can be edited and printed with a word-processing program. After the bibliography is printed or transferred to the microcomputer and saved as a file, you are expected to log off unless you plan to do another search immediately. Doing so usually involves sending a command indicating that you want to quit and possible keyboarding a sequence of characters such as LO (for "logging off").

Some computerized databases support searches other then keyword topic ones. For example, they may allow you to identify items by a particular author or those published by authors at a particular institution.

APPENDIX B

Resources on the Internet

There are a several ways that information can be gleaned from the internet. These include mailing lists, newsgroups, gophers, World Wide Web, and FTP resources. All of these have addresses. Those listed were obtained from a number of sources, including Kuster and Kuster (1995).

MAILING LISTS

Being a subscriber to a mailing list results in information about a particular topic being sent automatically from the computer on which the information is stored to the computer on which you receive e-mail—that is, the computer designated by your e-mail address. You subscribe by sending an e-mail message to the person who manages the mailing list. Subscribing is usually free.

There are two types of "publications" that are distributed by mailing lists: listservs and E-journals. *Listserv* subscribers receive copies of the messages in their e-mail "boxes" that are posted by other subscribers on a bulletin board (see Chapter 11). Messages sent to the listserv address for posting are automatically relayed to all subscribers. Anyone can join the discussion by sending comments or questions to the listserv address. The following are the e-mail addresses of some of the listservs that were active when this appendix was written:

- ads-l@uga.cc.uca.edu—English as a second language
- aging-dd@ukcc.uku.edu—gerontology issues
- alzheimer@wubios.wustl.edu—Alzheimer's disease
- asha-aud-headlines-request@postman.ncm.com—audiology (ASHA)
- audiol-l@uxa.ecn.bgu.edu—audiology
- autism@sjuvm.bitnet—autism
- c-palsy@sjuvm.bitnet—cerebral palsy

- cdmajor@kentvm.kent.edu—students and faculty in training programs
- cnet-dil@listserv.arizona.edu—neurogenic communication disorders
- commdis@rpitsvm.bitnet—communication disorders
- deaf-l@siucvmb.bitnet—deaf culture, education, medical advances
- deafblnd@ukcc.uky.edu—persons who are both deaf and blind
- ecenet-l@uiucvmd.bitnet—early childhood disorders
- gopherjewelslist-request@tpis.cactus.org <subscribe>—gopher sites where information on communication disorders can be found
- grndrnds@wvnvm.wvnet.edu—grand rounds in communicative disorders
- morse2000@trace23.waisman.wisc.edu—use of Morse Code for augmentative communication
- my-face@sjuvm.stjohns,edu—orofacial disorders (support group)
- prosody@msu.edu.—rhythm, intonation, and phrasing
- stroke-l@ukcc.uky.edu —cerebrovascular disease
- stut-hlp@bgu.edu—persons who stutter and their families (support group)
- stutt-l@templevm.bitnet—stuttering
- stutt-x@asuvm.inre.asu.edu—research on fluency disorders
- tbi-sprt@sjuvm.bitnet—traumatic brain injury and neurological disability

E-journals are automatically sent by e-mail to all subscribers. Submissions are welcome. Articles may or may not be peer-reviewed. The following are the e-mail addresses of some of the E-journals that were active when this appendix was written:

- *The Achiever Report*—discusses mental and emotional problems that interfere with learning, memory, and achievement. To subscribe, send e-mail to MoreMind@aol.com with message <sub ar subs>
- *Deaf Magazine*—a weekly deaf magazine. To subscribe, send e-mail to deaf-request@clark.net with message <sub deaf firstname lastname>
- *foNETiks*—a monthly newsletter for those studying and working in areas of phonetics, phonology, and speech science. Request the newsletter from R34334@uqam.bitnet
- *Handicap Digest*—contains articles about all types of issues affecting persons with disabilities. To subscribe, send e-mail to wtm@bnker.shel.isc-br.com

NEWSGROUPS

These are bulletin boards that function similarly to listserv ones except that new messages "posted" on them are not forwarded to e-mail addresses. The host computer—the one on which the bulletin board is located—accepts messages sent in, stores them for a short time (usually only a few days), and then throws them away. Consequently, the contents of such boards are constantly changing. Anyone can access them at any time, browse the messages that are currently posted, add a comment or a question, and then leave. The following are the addresses of some of the newsgroups that were active when this appendix was written:

- alt.education.disabled—education of the disabled
- comp.speech—computer speech generation and recognition
- alt.human.brain—neurology
- alt.support.stuttering—stuttering (support group)
- alt.science.physics.acoustics—acoustics
- alt.handicap—handicaps, including those associated with communicative disorders
- alt.support.cerebral-palsy—cerebral palsy (support group)
- k12.ed.special—special education for K-12
- alt.support.tinnitis—tinnitis (support group)

GOPHERS

Gophers provide access to information pertaining to a particular topic or field that is on computers linked to the internet worldwide. You are presented with a series of menus, from which you make choices that lead to other menus, until finally you reach the information you seek. The information can be read onscreen or downloaded to your computer. The following are the addresses of some of the gophers that were active when this appendix was written:

- gopher://burrow.cl.msu.edu/msu/dept/deaf—"deaf gopher" at Michigan State University
- gopher://dixson.sinsw.gov.au:70/11/DRA—Australian Deafness and Hearing Impaired Organizations as well as providing links to many other resources about deafness
- gopher://ericir.syr.edu—Eric Clearinghouse documents
- gopher://ieeir.unh.edu—International Exchange of Experts and Information on Rehabilitation (a project of the National Institute for Disability and Rehabilitation Research)
- gopher://mankato.msus.edu/communication disorders/stuttering—fluency disorders gopher (see Internet, 1995)
- gopher://refmac.kent.edu/departmental gopher servers at Kent State/speech path and audiology electronic library (ELSA)—Diversity University Virtual School of Speech Pathology and Audiology gopher (see Mitchell, McComas, McClowry, & Prichard, 1995)
- gopher://trace.waisman.wisc.edu/trace publications and reprints—Trace Center at University of Wisconsin documents concerning persons who are severely communicatively impaired
- gopher://una.hh.lib.umich.edu/inetdirsstacks/commdis. Judith Kuster—Internet Guide for Communication Sciences and Disorders lists many pertinent gopher sites, listservs, and e-journals

- gopher://val-dor.cc.buffalo.edu—Cornucopia of Disability Information (CODI) is intended to serve as a community resource for disability-related information

WWW (WORLD WIDE WEB)

The Web provides access to text and graphic resources throughout the world by means of hypertext links. Clicking certain words in one document "opens" other documents to which it is linked. Consequently, documents so linked function like cards in a hypercard stack (see Chapter 13). The difference is that the documents do not have to be on the same computer to be linked in this way. They only have to be on computers that are a part of the internet. The documents can, in fact, be on computers in different countries.

Addresses on the Web are designated by URLs (Universal Resource Locators). The following are some URLs that were active when this appendix was written:

- URL http://biomed.nus.sg/DF/databases.html—University of Singapore's Web server for the deaf and hearing impaired
- URL http://lethe.leeds.ac.uk—speech laboratory in the Department of Psychology at Leeds
- URL http://www.psych.indiana.edu—contains Indiana University's program to foster interdisciplinary research efforts, which includes speech and hearing science

FILE TRANSFER PROTOCOL (FTP) RESOURCES

FTP enables you to locate and download files (text, programs, graphics) from computers around the world that are linked to the internet. While some such resources can only be retrieved by persons who have the appropriate account and password, others can be retrieved by anyone. Freeware and shareware programs can be downloaded using FTP. Documents of various types (with or without illustrations) can also.

Files that can be retrived using FTP (known as *FTP resources*) are stored in a variety of formats. Consequently, before downloading a file, you must identify its format and then set your computer to receive it in the same format. You may have to process a file further after receiving it before it will be compatible with your computer.

ARCHIE (for searching ARCHives of files) is the indexing service to FTP resources and their addresses. Using a terminal emulation program, you would contact an Archie site (such as archie.sura.net) and login as archie. You would then type the keyword for the file(s) you seek, which will start the search.

The following are the addresses of some FTP resources that were available when this appendix was written:

- handicap.shel.isc-br.com—contains files and/or programs for all types of disabilities
- mac.archive.unich.edu—contains Joe Williams' and Clifford Guren's HyperCard stack to teach finger spelling
- orion.oac.uci.edu—contains Michael Williams' *Neuroanatomy Foundations Hypercard—Introductory Atlas to the Human Brain*

For further information about gleaning information from the internet and other networks, see Comer (1995).

APPENDIX C

Publishers of Clinical Software for Managing Communicative Disorders

This directory should be regarded as being a "first approximation." It was compiled mainly from advertisements and software reviews in the *Asha* journal. All of the software that could be useful to you clinically probably was not mentioned in the issues I searched. Also, some listings are not complete because an address was not included in the advertisement or review—only a telephone number and/or an e-mail address. The programs listed for a firm may not be the only ones that it publishes. If you're in the market for clinical software, you'll probably want to request catalogues from these publishers.

Aphasiaware, Inc.
24 Old Milford Road
Brookline, NH 03033
Aphasia software

Audiologic Software, Inc.
10407 Greentop Road
Cockeysville, MD 21030
1-800-666-9390
Audiologic report writing software, etc.

AVAAZ Innovations, Inc.
P.O. Box 8040
1225 Wonderland Road North
London, Ontario N6G 2B0, Canada
1-519-472-7944

avaaz@hookup.net
Computerized Speech Research Environment; Speech Assessment and Interactive Learning System

Don Johnston, Inc.
1-800-600-7808
Talk:About and other software for augmentative communication

GW Instruments
35 Medford Street
Somerville, MA 02143-4237
1-617-625-4096
SoundScope software for speech/voice analysis

IBM
1-800-426-4832
Computer-aided therapy tools

ideaBASE inc.
5005 Lakeland Circle
Waco, TX 76710
1-800-867-4332
ideabase@AOL
Sound Therapy Professional software for assessment, therapy, and administrative tasks

Kay Elemetrics Corporation
2 Bridgewater Lane
Lincoln Park, NJ 07035-1488
1-802-289-5297
Nasometer software, etc.

Laureate Learning Systems, Inc.
110 East Spring Street
Winooski, VT 05404
1-802-655-4755
Language software for children and adults

Micro Video
P.O. Box 7357
Ann Arbor, MI 48107
1-800-537-2182
Video Voice Speech Training System

Prentke Romich Company
1022 Heyl Road
Wooster, OH 44691
1-800-262-1933
Augmentative communication software

Psychological Corporation
555 Academic Court
San Antonio, TX 78204-2498
1-800-228-0752
PictureGallery, etc.

Salient Systems Technology, Inc.
1-800-344-1778
Augmentative communication software

Speech Bin
1965 Twenty-Fifth Avenue
Vero Beach, FL 32960
1-800-4-SPEECH
Articulation therapy software

Tiger Electronics, Inc.
P.O. Box 85126
Seattle, WA 98145
1-206-499-5757
Dr. Speech software for speech/voice assessment and training

Trinity Software
P.O. Box 960
Campton, NH 03223
1-800-352-1282
Speech Works accent reduction software

References and Bibliography

This is both a reference list and a bibliography of papers dealing with computer applications in speech-language pathology and audiology and software intended for practitioners in these fields. It is a comprehensive bibliography of the communicative disorders computer literature through October 1995. Because I wanted it to be a resource that would facilitate your exploring all aspects of this literature, I included both items that are and are not referred to in the text. A number of sources were consulted when compiling it, including convention programs of the American Speech-Language-Hearing Association. At the end of almost every ASHA convention presentation listing there is a reference to the October issue of Asha that contains a short abstract of it. You can usually obtain longer abstracts (about 150 words), handouts, or sometimes even a copy of the entire presentation by writing to the presenter(s). Mailing addresses can be obtained from the abstract or from the *Membership Directory of the American Speech-Language-Hearing Association.*

This list includes computer programs and reviews of them. Bibliographical information about almost all the programs was obtained from the reviews or from publishers' catalogues. Unfortunately, the copyright year was not mentioned in many of them. The year given for such programs was that preceding the review or the one that the catalog was published.

A copy of the Macintosh Word 4.0 file for this bibliography (that can be "indexed" using your word processor's FIND command) can be obtained by sending a check for $10.00 to CODI Publications, P.O. Box 261, Greendale, WI 53129.

Adams, B. C. (1992). *My House: Language Activities of Daily Living* [Computer program]. Winooski, VT: Laureate Learning Systems.

Agnew, J. (1983). The role of the small computer in hearing aid fittings. *Hearing Instruments*, 34, 7.

Ahead Designs (1987). *Spide Attack* [Computer program]. Tucson, AZ: Communication Skill Builders.

Aitken, S., & Bianco, C. (1985). Computerized instruction for hearing-impaired preschoolers. Presentation at the annual meeting of the American Speech-Language-Hearing Association, Washington, DC. [Abstract in *Asha*, 27(10), 89.]

Alberti, P. W., & Hyde, M. L. (1983). A computer data bank system for otolaryngologic and audiologic data. *Archives of Otolaryngology*, 109(4), 245–251.

Aldham, L. J., Rochefort, S. L., & Warling, A. R. (1987). Evaluation of CAST: A computerized method for lipreading training and assessment. Unpublished undergraduate thesis, Department of Industrial Engineering, University of Toronto, Ontario, Canada.

Aleksandrovsky, I. V., McCullough, J. A., & Wilson, R. H. (1993). Development of Russian word-identification material. Presentation at the annual meeting of the American Speech-Language-Hearing Association, Anaheim, CA. [Abstract in Asha, 35(10), 173.]

Allen, B. (1990). Video and word processing meet re-invention. *Journal for Computer Users in Speech and Hearing*, 6(1), 50–53.

Allen, B. (1993). Computerized Language Error Analysis Report (CLEAR) [Review of computer program]. *Asha*, 35(5). 68–69.

Allen, G. D. (1992a). Phonetics world—The second generation. Presentation at the annual meeting of the American Speech-Language-Hearing Association, San Antonio, TX. [Abstract in Asha, 34(10), 166.]

Allen, G. D. (1992b). Problems and solutions with large exploratory hypertexts: Lessons learned from Phonetic Symbol Guide-Electronic Edition. *Journal for Computer Users in Speech and Hearing*, 8(1,2), 79–93.

Allen, G. D. (1993). Introduction to multimedia with QuickTime. Presentation at the annual meeting of the American Speech-Language-Hearing Association, Anaheim, CA. [Abstract in *Asha*, 35(10), 195.]

Allen, G. D., & Harper, V. P. (1991). Prosody training workstation. Presentation at the annual meeting of the American Speech-Language-Hearing Association, Atlanta, GA. [Abstract in *Asha*, 33(10), 193.]

Allen, G. D., Orlikoff, R. F., Barlow, S. M., Jamieson, D. G., Keller, E., Milenkovic, P. H., McCabe, S. J., Renck, R. E., & Taylor, P. A. (1989). Speech analysis systems for personal computers. Presentation at the annual meeting of the American Speech-Language-Hearing Association, St. Louis, MO. [Abstract in *Asha*, 31(10), 142.]

Allen, G. D., Pullum, G. K., & Ladusaw, W. A. (1991). An electronic edition of Phonetic Symbol Guide. Presentation at the annual meeting of the American Speech-Language-Hearing Association, Atlanta, GA. [Abstract in *Asha*, 33(10), 193.]

Almenoff, P. (1985). *Spelltronics* [Computer program]. Freeport, NY: Educational Activities, Inc., P.O. Box 392.

Almqvist, B., & Aursnes, J. (1978). Computerized pure tone audiometry. *Scandinavian Audiology*, 8,193–196.

Ambron, S., & Hooper, K. (1990). *Learning with Interactive Multimedia: Developing and Using Multimedia Tools in Education*. Redmond, WA: Microsoft Press.

Amerine, K. L. (1991). Buying the "correct" computer system for the hearing health care office. *Journal for Computer Users in Speech and Hearing*, 7(1), 61–64.

Ames, M. (1990). Cue-Write [Review of computer program]. *Asha*, 32(8), 74.

Ames, M. (1991). Early Emerging Rules [Review of computer program]. *Asha*, 33(12), 105–106.

Ames, M. (1992). First Categories and First Verbs [Reviews of computer programs]. *Asha*, 34(12), 91–92.

Anderson, E. (1985). Keyboarder, PICAPAD, Understanding Questions [Review of computer programs]. *Journal for Computer Users in Speech and Hearing*, 1(2), 149–152.

Anderson, P. (1986). Holiday [Review of computer program]. *Asha*, 28(9), 77.

Anderson, P. J., Kneil, T. R., & Burk, K. W. (1991). A HyperCard decision tree for inferential statistics. Presentation at the annual meeting of the American Speech-Language-Hearing Association, Atlanta, GA. [Abstract in *Asha*, 33(10), 187.]

Apple Computer (1989). *HyperCard Stack Design Guidelines*. Reading, MA: Addison-Wesley.

Armstrong, C. L. (1984). SPEAK-EASY: Computer software to mediate communication dysfunction. *Cognitive Rehabilitation*, 2, 34–36.

ASHA Committee on Educational Technology (May 1984). Coming soon!! Computer software reviews for clinical materials. *Asha*, 26, 67.

Ashbaugh, J. A. (1988). Drawing phonetic symbols on the Macintosh 512K computer. *Journal for Computer Users in Speech and Hearing*, 4(2), 113–119.

AudioPro 2 [Computer program]. Somerset, NJ: Oticon.

AUDIOS-Direct [Computer program] (1994). Cockeysville, MD: Audiologic Software. [Advertisement in *Asha*, 36(10), 184.]

Awan, S. N. (1993). Computation of vocal area in phonetograms. Presentation at the annual meeting of the American Speech-Language-Hearing Association, Anaheim, CA. [Abstract in *Asha*, 35(10), 133.]

Bacon, M. J., & Shearer, W. M. (1989). Computer assisted or traditional report writing—A comparative evaluation. Presentation at the annual meeting of the American Speech-Language-Hearing Association, St. Louis, MO. [Abstract in *Asha*, 31(10), 75.]

Bade, P., Engebretson, A., Heidbreder, A., & Nielmoller, A. (1984). Use of a personal computer to model the electroacoustics of hearing aids. *Journal of the Acoustical Society of America*, 75, 617–620.

Baker, M. O., & Dietrich, G. L. (1991). *Thinkanalogy Puzzles* [Computer program]. Pacific Grove, CA: Critical Thinking Press and Software, P. O. Box 448.

Baker, P. C., et al. (1985). A comparison of live, videotaped, and computer-assisted instructional methodologies. Presentation at the annual meeting of the American Speech-Language-Hearing Association, Washington, DC. [Abstract in *Asha*, 27(10), 155.]

Baker, R. G., Downton, A. C., King, R. W., & Damper, R. I. (1986). Television and video technology in the education of deaf children. *British Journal of Audiology*, 20, 101–113.

Baker-van den Goorbergh, L., & Baker, K. (no date). *Computerized Language Error Analysis Report (CLEAR)* [Computer program]. United Kingdom: Far Communications, Ltd., 5 Harcourt Estate, Kibworth, Leics.

Baker-van den Goorbergh, L. (1990). Computerized language error analysis report. *Clinical Linguistics and Phonetics*, 4, 285–293.

Bakker, K., Arkebauer, H. J., & Boutsen, F. R. (1993). Computer-assisted determination of diadochokinetic rate and variability. Presentation at the annual meeting of the American Speech-Language-Hearing Association, Anaheim, CA. [Abstract in *Asha*, 35(10), 109.]

Ball, L. L., Anderson, C. D., & Schweitzer, C. (1986). Microcomputers in office management of speech and hearing facilities. In J. L. Northern (Ed.), *The Personal Computer for Speech, Language, and Hearing Professionals*. Boston: Little, Brown, pp. 243–250.

Balthazor, R. J., & Cavette, M. J. (1979). Computer processing of clinical experiences in speech pathology and audiology. Presentation at the annual meeting of the American Speech-Language-Hearing Association, Atlanta, GA. [Abstract in *Asha*, 21(10), 748.]

Baquet, G. M., & Tobin, H. (1991). A computer learning approach to audiologic habilitation. Presentation at the annual meeting of the American Speech-Language-Hearing Association, Atlanta, GA. [Abstract in *Asha*, 33(10), 187.]

Bardzik, Jr., P. P. (1985a). Planning Individualized Speech and Language Intervention Programs: Computer Software Adaptation [Review of computer program]. *Asha*, 27(6), 75–76.

Bardzik, Jr., P. P. (1985b). Wizard of Words [Review of computer program]. *Asha*, 27(11), 74.

Bardzik, Jr., P. P. (1986). Computer Managed Articulation Diagnosis [Review of computer program]. *Asha*, 28(2), 74–75.

Barratt, S. E., & Bakker, K. (1994). Interactive phonetics teaching system. Presentation at the annual meeting of the American Speech-Language-Hearing Association, New Orleans, LA. [Abstract in *Asha*, 36(10), 174.]

Barron, T. P., & Hamill, T. A. (1991). Implementation of a personal computer-based auditory evoked potentials system. *Journal for Computer Users in Speech and Hearing*, 7(1), 65–69.

Barsella, D. F., & Silverman, F. H. (1986). An expert system for clinical decision making with the neurologically impaired. Presentation at the annual meeting of the American Speech-Language-Hearing Association, Detroit, MI. [Abstract in *Asha*, 28(10), 146.]

Basham, C. H. (1994). The essence of effective presentations. Presentation at the annual meeting of the American Speech-Language-Hearing Association, New Orleans, LA. [Abstract in *Asha*, 36(10), 174.]

Basham, C. H., & Basham, R. L. (1994). Creating a computerized slide show. Presentation at the annual meeting of the American Speech-Language-Hearing Association, New Orleans, LA. [Abstract in *Asha*, 36(10), 107.]

Beck, K. (1987a). Aphasia VI: Vocabulary by Definition [Review of computer program]. *Asha*, 29(11), 65–66.

Beck, K. (1987b). Language Stimulation Software #4, Associative Naming: Mixed Cues [Review of computer program]. *Asha*, 29(5), 75–76.

Beckman, S. L. (1994). Diversifying instruction: The computer as tutor in pre-service training. Presentation at the annual meeting of the American Speech-Language-Hearing Association, New Orleans, LA. [Abstract in *Asha*, 36(10), 107.]

Beekman, G. (1992). *HyperCard 2 in a Hurry*. Belmont, CA: Wadsworth.

Benguerel, A.-P., & Pichora-Fuller, M. K. (1988). Design of a computer-aided speechreading training system. *Annual Bulletin of the Research Institute of Logopedics and Phoniatrics*, 22, 105–116.

Benguerel, A.-P., & Pichora-Fuller, M. K. (1989). MIMILLE: une methode interactive microinformatisee de labio-lecture [MIMILLE: An interactive computer-aided method of speechreading]. *Audiology*, 28, 284–194.

Benjamin, B. J. (1985). Computerized Assessment of Intelligibility of Dysarthric Speech [Review of computer program]. *Asha*, 27(3), 72–73.

Benjamin, B. J. (1987). Phonemic Symbols [Review of computer program]. *Asha*, 29(5), 74–75.

Benjamin, B. J. (1988). Slow Speech: Rate Drill for Dysarthric Speakers [Review of computer program]. *Asha*, 30(5), 79.

Benjamin, B. J. (1991). Message Maker-Keyboard [Review of computer program]. *Asha*, 33(8), 68–69.

Bergsma, K. E., & Rushakoff, G. E. (1984). Issues in microcomputer based therapy for preschool aged children. Presentation at the annual meeting of the American Speech-Language-Hearing Association, San Francisco, CA. [Abstract in *Asha*, 26(10), 185.]

Bermejo, J. (1984). Computer-assisted instruction in communication disorders: An investigation of the effects of interactive and passive instructional methods upon student achievement in basic electronics. Unpublished doctoral dissertation, Ohio University, Athens, OH.

Bermejo, J. J. (1985). Computer-assisted instruction for communication disorders. *Journal for Computer Users in Speech and Hearing*, 1(1), 17–28.

Bernstein, L. E. (1989). Computer-based speech training for profoundly hearing-impaired children: Some design considerations. In N. McGarr (Ed.), *Research on the Use of Sensory Aids for Hearing-Impaired People*. Washington, DC: Alexander Graham Bell Association for the Deaf, pp. 19–28.

Bernstein, L. E., Goldstein, Jr., M. H., Kewley-Port, D., Mahshie, J. M., Maki, D., & Watson, C. S. (1987). Computer-based speech training for the deaf. Presentation at the annual meeting of the American Speech-Language-Hearing Association, New Orleans, LA. [Abstract in *Asha*, 29(10), 152.]

Bernstorf, E. D., Kneil, T. R., & Burk, K. W. (1991). HyperCard instructional program for voice disorders in singers. Presentation at the annual meeting of the American Speech-Language-Hearing Association, Atlanta, GA. [Abstract in *Asha*, 33(10), 187.]

Berryman, J., Johnson, R., & Toman, T. (1984). *Planning Individualized Speech and Language Intervention Programs: Computer Software Adaptation* [Computer program]. Tucson, AZ: Communication Skill Builders.

Beukelman, D. R., Garrett, K., Lange, U., & Tice, R. (1988). *Cue-Write* [Computer program]. Tucson, AZ: Communication Skill Builders, 3830 East Bellevue.

Beukelman, D. R., Naranjo, C., & Yorkston, K. M. (1979).Computer analysis of word and phrase "vocabularies" in non-vocal adults. Presentation at the annual meeting of the American Speech-Language-Hearing Association, Atlanta. [Abstract in *Asha*, 21(9), 775.]

Beukelman, D. R., Traynor, C., Poblete, M., & Warren, C. G. (1984). Microcomputer-based communication augmentation system for two nonspeaking, physically handicapped persons with severe visual impairment. *Archives of Physical Medicine and Rehabilitation*, 65(2), 89–91.

Beukelman, D. R., Yorkston, K. M., & Tice, R. L. (198•). *Pacer/Tally for Pacing and Tallying Responses* [Computer program]. Tucson, AZ: Communication Skill Builders.

Beukelman, D. R., Yorkston, K. M., & Traynor, C. (1984). *Computerized Assessment of Dysarthric Speech.* Austin, TX: PRO-ED.

Beyer, N. L. (1988). *BOSTON* [Computer program]. Centertown, MO: Hearing and Speech Care, Inc., Rural Route 1.

Bickley, C., Hunnicutt, S., & Lamel, L. (1993). Alternative strategies for creating autocad drawings. In Björn Granström, Sheri Hunnicutt, & Karl-Erick Spens (Eds.), *Speech and Language Technology for Disabled Persons* (Proceedings of an ESCA Workshop, Stockholm, Sweden, May 31-June 2, 1993), pp. 103–106.

Biomedical Laser Industries (1986). *SpeechMaster* [Computer program]. Salt Lake City, UT: BioMedical Laser Industries, Educational Division, 64 East 6400 South.

Birch, M., & Birch, J. (1990). *Communication Board Builder* [Computer program]. Solana Beech, CA; Computerade Products.

Birk, J. D., & Stewart, D. L. (1991). It always tastes better if it's grown at home. *Journal for Computer Users in Speech and Hearing*, 7(1), 70–71.

Blache, S. E. (1984). *BLACHE Phonemic Inventory* [Computer program]. San Diego, CA: College-Hill.

Blache, S. E. (1985). Computer networking, information transfer, and the communication disorders specialist. *Journal for Computer Users in Speech and Hearing*, 1(1), 29–35.

Blache, S. E., & Friend, C. M. (1985). Using microcomputers to generate graphic clinical materials for language therapy. Presentation at the annual meeting of the American Speech-Language-Hearing Association, Washington, DC. [Abstract in *Asha*, 27(10), 59.]

Black, H., & Black, S. (1991a). *W.O.R.D. Benders Complete the Phrase* [Computer program]. Pacific Grove, PA: Critical Thinking Press & Software, P. O. Box 448.

Black, H., & Black, S. (1991b). W.O.R.D. Benders Definition [Computer program]. Pacific Grove, PA: Critical Thinking Press & Software, P. O. Box 448.

Bless, D. M., Canfield, R. A., Emerich, K. A., Leddy, M., Poburka, B., & Ramos, C. A. (1992). HyperCard applications for voice therapy. Presentation at the annual meeting of the American Speech-Language-Hearing Association, San Antonio, TX. [Abstract in *Asha*, 34(10), 101.]

Blinn, J. (1985). Articulation Error Analysis (AEA) Software [Review of computer program]. *Asha*, 27(5), 73.

Blissymbolics Communication International (1992a). *BlissProcessor* [Computer program]. Toronto, Ontario, Canada: Blissymbolics Communication International, 1630 Lawrence Ave. West, Suite 104.

Blissymbolics Communication International (1992b). *AccessBliss Talker* [Computer program]. Toronto, Ontario, Canada: Blissymbolics Communication International, 1630 Lawrence Ave. West, Suite 104.

Block, F. K. (1991). *SunTool.* Speech/Language IEP Writer + Version 3.0 for use with the Apple Macintosh Computer [Review of computer program]. *Asha*, 33(8), 69–70.

Block, M. G. (1983). Computer applications in acoustic reflex research. Miniseminar presented at the annual meeting of the American Speech-Language-Hearing Association, Cincinnati, OH. [Abstract in *Asha*, 25(10), 59.]

Blockcolsky, V. D., Frazer, J. M., & Frazer, D. H. (1988). *40,000 Selected Words* [Computer program]. Tucson, AZ: Communication Skills Builders, 3830 E. Bellevue.

Bloem, D. F. (1991). The eyes have it: Microcomputers dramatically enhance the power of ENG. *Journal for Computer Users in Speech and Hearing*, 7(1), 72–78.

Bloise, C. G. R., & Tompkins, C. A. (1989). Evaluation of microcomputer software for aphasia therapy. Presentation at the annual meeting of the American Speech-Language-Hearing Association, St. Louis, MO. [Abstract in *Asha*, 31(10), 166.]

Blood, G. W. (1991). Efficacy of voice therapy: Computer-assisted feedback (CAFET) with relaxation. Presentation at the annual meeting of the American Speech-Language-Hearing Association, Atlanta, GA. [Abstract in *Asha*, 33(10), 108.]

Blood, G. W. (1994). Efficacy of a computer-assisted voice treatment protocol. *American Journal of Speech-Language Pathology*, 3(1), 57–66.

Bluestone, R. (1991). The Macintosh in rehab: HyperCard to the rescue. Presentation at the annual meeting of the American Speech-Language-Hearing Association, Atlanta, GA. [Abstract in *Asha*, 33(10), 122.]

Bluestone, R. (1992a). Integrating computers into daily practice: The clinical potentials of HyperCard. Presentation at the annual meeting of the American Speech-Language-Hearing Association, San Antonio, TX. [Abstract in *Asha*, 34(10), 133.]

Bluestone, R. (1992b). Memory Challenge! Improving Spatial Memory Skills [Review of computer programs]. *Asha*, 34(5), 93.

Bluestone, R. (1992c). Thinkanalogy Puzzles [Review of computer program]. *Asha*, 34(5), 94–95.

Bluestone, R. (1992d). Training the trainers: Integrating computer technology into a rehabilitation setting. Presentation at the annual meeting of the American Speech-Language-Hearing Association, San Antonio, TX. [Abstract in *Asha*, 34(10), 111.]

Bluestone, R., & Lefkowitz, N. G. (November 22, 1993). Computers and aphasia: Beyond the looking glass. *ADVANCE for Speech-Language Pathologists and Audiologists*, 6–7.

Bluestone, R., Lefkowitz, N. G., & Boole, K. V. (1994). Evolution and clinical application of a commercial database: Filemaker Pro. Presentation at the annual meeting of the American Speech-Language-Hearing Association, New Orleans, LA. [Abstract in *Asha*, 36(10), 175.]

Bluestone, R., Lefkowitz, N. G., Violock-Boole, K., McLean, S. N., & O'Neil-Pirozzi, T. M. (1993). Managing documentation: A cost-effective computerized model. Presentation at the annual meeting of the American Speech-Language-Hearing Association, Anaheim, CA. [Abstract in *Asha*, 35(10), 227.]

Bluestone, R., Shugarts, D. D., & Lefkowitz, N. G. (1989). Computer assisted treatment: Unexpected results of a national survey. Presentation at the annual meeting of the American Speech-Language-Hearing Association, St. Louis, MO. [Abstract in *Asha*, 31(10), 132.]

Boothroyd, A. (1987). CASPER: A computer-assisted system for speech-perception testing and training. *Proceedings of the 10th Annual Conference of the Rehabilitation Society of North America*, 734–736.

Boothroyd, A., Archambault, P., Adams, R., & Storm, R. (1975). Use of a computer-based system of speech analysis and display in a remedial speech program. *Volta Review*, 77, 178–193.

Boothroyd, A., Hanin, L., & Waltzman, S. (1987). Development of speech perception skills in cochlear implantees. *Proceedings of the 10th Annual Conference of the Rehabilitation Society of North America*, 428–430.

Boothroyd, A., & Hnath-Chisolm, T. (1988). Spatial, tactile presentation of voice fundamental frequency as a supplement to lipreading: Results of extended training with a single subject. *Journal of Rehabilitation Research and Development*, 25(3), 51–56.

Boothroyd, A., Yeung, E., Hanin, L., Hnath-Chisolm, T., Kishon-Rabin, L., Medwetsky, K., Broecker, B., Eran, O., & Plant, N. (1988). Application of interactive video laserdisc technology to speech perception testing and training. Scientific Exhibit at the annual meeting of the American Speech-Language-Hearing Association, Boston.

Bortman, H. (October, 1993). The Newton generation. *MacUser*, 102–108.

Bowen, K. M. (1985). *Computerized Language Sample Analysis* [Review of computer program]. *Asha*, 27(7), 77–78.

Boyd, D., Rolland, M. B., Lyngaas, K., Zutter-Brose, R., Daggett, B., Gill, M., Kellman, M., Lodholz, C., Pierce, K., Reeves, M. A., Ruchti, L. L., Larson, J., Frieberg, C., Molaska, J. M., Freeman, M. C., Bertolino, K., Miller, J. F., Wyhuske, C., & Odell, B. (1990). Implementing computerized language sample analysis in the public schools. Presentation at the annual meeting of the American Speech-Language-Hearing Association, Seattle, WA. [Abstract in *Asha*, 32(10), 51.]

Boyd, J. M., & Denenberg, M. E. (1992). Innovative uses for Apple II educational software in speech-language programs. Presentation at the annual meeting of the American Speech-Language-Hearing Association, San Antonio, TX. [Abstract in *Asha*, 34(10), 133–134.]

Bracy, O. L. (1983). Computer based cognitive rehabilitation. *Cognitive Rehabilitation*, 1, 7–8.

Bradley, S. (1994). HyperCard applications in occupational hearing conservation. Presentation at the annual meeting of the American Speech-Language-Hearing Association, New Orleans, LA. [Abstract in *Asha*, 36(10), 106.]

Bradley, S., & Krumm, S. (1995). HyperCard applications in recording clinical practicum hours. Presentation at the annual meeting of the American Speech-Language-Hearing Association, Orlando, FL. [Abstract in *Asha*, 37(10), 108.]

Brady, M. E., & Dickson, W. P. (1983). A microcomputer communication game for hearing-impaired students. *American Annals for the Deaf*, 128(6), 835–841.

Brandenburg, S. A., & Vanderheiden, G. C. (Eds.) (1987). *Communication, Control and Computer Access for Disabled & Elderly Individuals: Resource Books 1, 2, 3*. Boston, MA: College-Hill Press/Little, Brown & Company.

Brawley, R., & Peterson, B. (1983). Interactive videodisc: An innovative instructional system. *American Annals of the Deaf*, 128, 685–700.

Brightman, A. J. (1988). *Apple Computer Resources in Special Education and Rehabilitation*. Cupertino, CA: Office of Special Education Programs, Apple Computer.

Brinton, B., Fujiki, M., Ranck, R. L., & Ranck, D. P. (1985). Computer assisted analysis of conversational sequences. Presentation at the annual meeting of the American Speech-Language-Hearing Association, Washington, DC. [Abstract in *Asha*, 27(10), 166.]

Brooks, S., Fallside, F., Gulian, W., & Hinds, P. (1981). Teaching vowel articulation with the computer vowel trainer: Methodology and results. *British Journal of Audiology*, 15(3), 151–163.

Brorson, K., Chlopan, L., Grimmett, J., Humphries, G., Murphy, G., & Kneil, T. (1995). Syndromes in speech and hearing: A hypermedia resource. Presentation at the annual meeting of the American Speech-Language-Hearing Association, Orlando, FL. [Abstract in *Asha*, 37(10), 92.]

Brown, C., Cavalier, A., Sauer, M., & Wyatt, C. (1992). The sound-to-speech translation system using photographic-quality graphic symbols. *The Johns Hopkins APL Technical Digest*, 13(4), 482–489.

Brown, C. J., Osberger, M. J., Hurtig, R. R., & Zimmermann, G. N. (1991). Auditory skills and perceptual learning strategies of hearing-impaired listeners. Presentation at the annual meeting of the American Speech-Language-Hearing Association, Atlanta, GA. [Abstract in *Asha*, 33(10), 193.]

Brown, J. E. (1987a). Aphasia VII: Picture Naming [Review of computer program]. *Asha*, 29(11), 67–68.

Brown, J. E. (1987b). Language Stimulation Software #1, Sentence Completion: Semantics [Review of computer program]. *Asha*, 29(5), 75.

Brown, J. E. (1989). *ASHA* Project IMPACT: #2 Microcomputer Assisted Intervention for Speech and Language Professionals [Review of computer program]. *Asha*, 31(12), 72–73.

Brown, M. J. (1982). Hearing aid selection: A data base approach. *Medical Information* (London), 7(4), 321–330.

Brown, V. L. (1989a). Talking Verbs [Review of computer program]. *Journal for Computer Users in Speech and Hearing*, 5(1), 33–35.

Brown, V. L. (1989b). Twenty Categories [Review of computer program]. *Journal for Computer Users in Speech and Hearing*, 5(1), 36–39.

Brown, V. L. (1989c). Words & Concepts II [Review of computer program]. *Journal for Computer Users in Speech and Hearing*, 5(2), 140–142.

Brubaker, S. H., & Rolnick, M. I. (1985). *Compilation of Clinical Software for Aphasia Rehabilitation and Cognitive Retraining*. Birmingham, MI: Clinical Software Resources.

Bruno, J. (1994). Organizing an advanced pediatric vocabulary for a microcomputer-based AAC system. Presentation at the annual meeting of the American Speech-Language-Hearing Association, New Orleans, LA. [Abstract in *Asha*, 36(10), 173.]

Bruno, J., & Stoughton, A. M. (1984). Computer-aided communication device for a child with cerebral palsy. *Archives of Physical Medicine and Rehabilitation*, 65, 603–605.

Bryant, M. L., Tonkovich, J. D., Horowitz, D. M., & Tan, H. (1992). Voice recognition reporting system for dysphagia documentation. Presentation at the annual meeting of the American Speech-Language-Hearing Association, San Antonio, TX. [Abstract in *Asha*, 34(10), 121.]

Buchanan, L. H., & Jones, G. H. (1987). A computerized audiology database for training in developmental disabilities. Presentation at the annual meeting of the American Speech-Language-Hearing Association, New Orleans, LA. [Abstract in *Asha*, 29(10), 141.]

Buder, E. H., & Kent, R. D. (1995). Survey of microcomputer-based speech acoustic analysis systems. Presentation at the annual meeting of the American Speech-Language-Hearing Association, Orlando, FL. [Abstract in *Asha*, 37(10), 69.]

Bull, G. (1983). Special training for special technology: A curriculum for use of microcomputer-based tools in speech-language pathology. *The Computer Teacher*, 10, 52–56.

Bull, G. L. (1989). Computer applications in speech and hearing: Perspectives for the 1990s. *Journal for Computer Users in Speech and Hearing*, 5(2), 105–109.

Bull, G. L., Chial, M. K., Mahaffey, R. B., & Watkin, K. L. (1986). Teaching computers at the university: Ways and means. Presentation at the annual meeting of the American Speech-Language-Hearing Association, Detroit, MI. [Abstract in *Asha*, 28(10), 157].

Bull, G. L., & Cochran, P. S. (1984). Listful thinking [A monthly column]. *The National Logo Exchange*, 3.

Bull, G. L., & Cochran, P. S. (1985a). Creating tools for clinicians and teachers. *Journal for Computer Users in Speech and Hearing*, 1(1), 45–49.

Bull, G. L., & Cochran, P. S. (1985b). A Logo Tutorial: Tools for clinicians. Presentation at he American Speech and Hearing Foundation conference on microcomputers, New Orleans, LA. [Abstract in the *Journal for Computer Users in Speech and Hearing*, 1(2), 72.]

Bull, G. L., & Cochran, P. S. (1988). Use of BITNET by communication disorders programs. Presentation at the annual meeting of the American Speech-Language-Hearing Association, Boston. [Abstract in *Asha*, 30(10), 166.]

Bull, G. L., & Cochran, P. S. (1992). Hypermedia and traditional clinical materials: A convergence of media. *Journal for Computer Users in Speech and Hearing*, 8(1, 2), 68–74.

Bull, G. L., Cochran, P. S., & Snell, M. E. (1988). Beyond CAI: Computers, language, and persons with mental retardation. *Topics in Language Disorders*, 8, 55–76.

Bull, G., Stoudt, Jr., R. J., & Calderon-Rogers, E. G. (1983). An introduction to some clinical applications of computers using Logo. Presentation at the annual meeting of the American Speech-Language-Hearing Association, Cincinnati. [Abstract in *Asha*, 25(10), 62.]

Burdea, G., & Coiffet, P. (1994). *Virtual Reality Technology*. New York: John Wiley.

Burk, R. W., & Bryant, D. M. (1993). Using interactive videotext in adolescent language intervention. Presentation at the annual meeting of the American Speech-Language-Hearing Association, Anaheim, CA. [Abstract in *Asha*, 35(10), 114.]

Burns, E. (1985). *The Apple Math and Reading Development Kit*. Reston, VA: Reston.

Butterfield, R. (1991). A scope and sequence way to use single switch software. *Journal for Computer Users in Speech and Hearing*, 7(1), 79–82.

Byerly, M. A. (1992). Breakthrough to Language, Volume 1: Multi-sensory Curriculum [Review of computer program]. *Asha*, 34(2), 79.

Calpin, T. C. & Froke, R. A. (1991). A computer program facilitating communication development in hearing-impaired preschoolers. Presentation at the annual meeting of the American Speech-Language-Hearing Association, Atlanta, GA. [Abstract in *Asha*, 33(10), 90.]

Campbell, R. A. (1974). Computer audiometry. *Journal of Speech and Hearing Research*, 17, 134–140.

Carlson, G. S., & Bernstein, J. (1987). Speech recognition of impaired speech. *Proceedings of the 10th Annual Conference on Rehabilitation Engineering*, pp. 103–105.

Carr, K., & England, R. (1995). *Simulated and Virtual Realities*. Bristol, PA: Taylor & Francis.

Carter, J. E. (1991). CELF-R Scoring Assistant [Review of computer program]. *Asha*, 33(5), 89.

Carterette, E. C. (1985). A computer program for estimating thresholds by means of Wetherill's up-down transformed response rule (UDTR). *Journal of Auditory Research*, 24, 191–204.

Cascella, P. W., & Laurent, D. L. (1989). Clinical applications with adult mentally retarded individuals. Presentation at the annual meeting of the American Speech-Language-Hearing Association, St. Louis, MO. [Abstract in *Asha*, 31(10), 83.]

Cassidy, K., & Wynne, M. (1990). Hearing Aid Client Management System [Review of computer program]. *Journal for Computer Users in Speech and Hearing*, 6(1), 63–67.

Cassidy, R., Koller, D., & Schwartz, A. (1984). The uses of word processing for clinical report writing. Part I: Applications, characteristics, and requirements. *Journal of Childhood Communication Disorders*, 8, 7–21.

Catlett, C., Curl, B. A., & Bruskin, D. (1988). Projects of national significance: New developments in *ASHA*'s sponsored program division. Presentation at the annual meeting of the American Speech-Language-Hearing Association, Boston, MA. [Abstract in *Asha*, 30(10), 203.]

Cevette, M. J., Battani, L. R., Smith, G., & Heidlauf, K. (1993). Postural sway differences in vestibular dysfunction by computerized dynamic posturography. Presentation at the annual meeting of the American Speech-Language-Hearing Association, Anaheim, CA. [Abstract in *Asha*, 35(10), 167.]

Cevette, M. J., Wiley, B., & Marion, M. S. (1993). Non-organic patterns of dysfunction in computerized dynamic posturography. Presentation at the annual meeting of the American Speech-Language-Hearing Association, Anaheim, CA. [Abstract in *Asha*, 35(10), 167.]

Chadwell, D. L. (1991a). Computerized Masking Procedure Analysis (COMPASS) [Review of computer program]. *Asha*, 33(2), 82–83.

Chadwell, D. L. (1991b). Sine Wave Introduction Program (SWIP) Version 1.0 and Sine Wave Analysis Practice (SWAP) Version 1.4 [Review of computer programs]. *Asha*, 33(2), 84.

Chan, F. H., Poon, P. W., Cheng, K. H., Li, H. F., & Hwang, J. C. (1984). A microcomputer-based binaural measurement system. *Journal of Biomedical Engineering*, 6(3), 212–218.

Chaney, R. W. (1992). My Macintosh is my speech science classroom instructional aide. Presentation at the annual meeting of the American Speech-Language-Hearing Association, San Antonio, TX. [Abstract in *Asha*, 34(10), 121.]

Channell, R. W. (1983). Development of a microcomputer program for client specific searches of the empirical literature in language training in autism. Unpublished Ph.D. dissertation, University of Utah.

Channell, R. W. (1990). A decision-tree simulator for application of statistical techniques in speech-language pathology and audiology. *Journal for Computer Users in Speech and Hearing*, 6(1), 22–28.

Channell, R. W. (1991). Automated grammatical tagging of children's language samples. Presentation at the annual meeting of the American Speech-Language-Hearing Association, Atlanta, GA. [Abstract in *Asha*, 33(10), 193.]

Channell, R. W., & Berrett, L. G. (1993). Probabilistic grammatical tagging of children's language samples. Presentation at the annual meeting of the American Speech-Language-Hearing Association, Anaheim, CA. [Abstract in *Asha*, 35(10), 183.]

Channell, R. W., Grenfell, S. P., & Hilton, L. M. (1993). Accuracy of automated developmental sentence scoring. Presentation at the annual meeting of the American Speech-Language-Hearing Association, Anaheim, CA. [Abstract in *Asha*, 35(10), 178.]

Channell, R. W., & Liu, T. A. (1994). Software for pitch perception assessment and training. Presentation at the annual meeting of the American Speech-Language-Hearing Association, New Orleans, LA. [Abstract in *Asha*, 36(10), 106.]

Chapman, W. D. (1991). Performance of college level subjects on a software evaluation tutorial. Presentation at the annual meeting of the American Speech-Language-Hearing Association, Atlanta, GA. [Abstract in *Asha*, 33(10), 188.]

Charpied, G. L. (1993). Lights, camera, action: Making the perfect presentation. Presentation at the annual meeting of the American Speech-Language-Hearing Association, Anaheim, CA. [Abstract in *Asha*, 35(10), 145.]

Charpied, G. L. (1994a). *The Clinical Management of the Geriatric Voice in the Nursing Home Environment*. Quincy, MA: Author, 423 Furnace Brook Parkway.

Charpied, G. L. (1994b). Go multimedia, young voice clinician! Presentation at the annual meeting of the American Speech-Language-Hearing Association, New Orleans, LA. [Abstract in *Asha*, 36(10), 175.]

Charpied, G. L. (1995). Voice clinic database: Those exciting GUIs and RDBs. Presentation at the annual meeting of the American Speech-Language-Hearing Association, Orlando, FL. [Abstract in *Asha*, 37(10), 70.]

Charpied, G. L., & Swindell, C. A. (1991). Updating skills in dysphagia diagnosis and treatment: A computerized tutorial. Presentation at the annual meeting of the American Speech-Language-Hearing Association, Atlanta, GA. [Abstract in *Asha*, 33(10), 123.]

Cherney, L. R., Halper, A. S., & Miller, T. K. (1986). Computerized patient progress notes. Presentation at the annual meeting of the American Speech-Language-Hearing Association, Detroit, MI. [Abstract in *Asha*, 28(10), 82.]

Cherow, E., Larkins, P. G., & Kamara, C. A. (1987). *ASHA*'s Program Evaluation System (PES): An automated approach to quality assurance. Presentation at the annual meeting of the American Speech-Language-Hearing Association, New Orleans, LA. [Abstract in *Asha*, 29(10), 138.]

Chial, M. R. (1984a). Evaluating microcomputer hardware. In A. H. Schwartz (Editor), *Handbook of Microcomputer Applications in Communication Disorders*, San Diego: College-Hill, pp. 79–125.

Chial, M. R. (1984b). Glossary of microcomputer terms. In A. H. Schwartz (Editor), *Handbook of Microcomputer Applications in Communication Disorders*, San Diego: College-Hill, pp. 275–309.

Chial, M. R. (1985). Tutorial on speech synthesis. Presentation at the American Speech and Hearing Foundation conference on microcomputers, New Orleans, LA. [Abstract in *Journal for Computer Users in Speech and Hearing*, 1(2), 73.]

Chial, M. R. (1986a). Preliminaries to professional evaluation of software. *Journal for Computer Users in Speech and Hearing*, 2(2), 102–123.

Chial, M. R. (1986b). Student computer facilities: A guide to strategic planning. *Asha*, 28(8), 37–40.

Chial, M. R. (1986c). Tutorial: Program design and troubleshooting. *Journal for Computer Users in Speech and Hearing*, 2(2), 124–146.

Chial, M. R. (1989). Notions, lotions, and potions. *Journal for Computer Users in Speech and Hearing*, 5(2), 125–133.

Chial, M. R., & Kelly, L. J. (1987). Graphical computer tools for instruction and clinical practice. *Journal for Computer Users in Speech and Hearing*, 3(1), 86–93.

Childhood Stuttering: A Second Opinion [Expert system computer program] (no date). Tucson, AZ: Bahill Intelligent Computer Systems, 1622 W. Montenegro.

Clark, H. M., Wilson, A. R., Hass, L., & Olson, I. (1995). Electronic mail: Facilitating multidisciplinary interactions of the dysphagia team. Presentation at the annual meeting of the American Speech-Language-Hearing Association, Orlando, FL. [Abstract in *Asha*, 37(10), 45.]

Clark, M. C. (1993). Computer applications for assessment/training in AAC, LD, and neuropathologies. Presentation at the annual meeting of the American Speech-Language-Hearing Association, Anaheim, CA. [Abstract in *Asha*, 35(10), 109–110.]

Clarke, S. M., & Aagaard, A. A. (1990). *Cue-Write* [Review of computer program]. *Journal for Computer Users in Speech and Hearing*, 6(2), 168–171.

Clarke, S. M., & Kneil, T. (1990). A simple application of HyperCard in speech-language pathology. *Journal for Computer Users in Speech and Hearing*, 6(1), 29–32.

Clymer, E. W. (1985). Using microcomputer authoring languages. Presentation at the American Speech and Hearing Foundation conference on microcomputers, New Orleans, LA. [Abstract in the *Journal for Computer Users in Speech and Hearing*, 1(2), 73–74.]

Clymer, E. W. (1989). *ASHA Project IMPACT. #5 Administrative Applications of Microcomputers for Speech, Language, and Hearing Professionals* [Computer program]. Rockville, MD: American Speech-Language-Hearing Association.

Cochran, P. S. (1989). Clinical computing in the 1990s: There's more to it than which key to press. *Journal for Computer Users in Speech and Hearing*, 5(2), 110–113.

Cochran, P. S., & Applegate, J. A. (1991). Managing information in communication sciences and disorders with AppleWorks Software [Review of computer program]. *Asha*, 33(8), 69.

Cochran, P. S., & Bull, G. L. (1985). Creating a shared context: Using a computer in language therapy. Presentation at the annual meeting of the American Speech-Language-Hearing Association, Washington, DC. [Abstract in *Asha*, 27(10), 60.]

Cochran, P. S., Bull, G. L., & Allen, B. (1988). Creating a shared context: Using videodiscs in language therapy. Presentation at the annual meeting of the American Speech-Language-Hearing Association, Boston, MA. [Abstract in *Asha*, 30(10), 81–82.]

Cochran, P. S., Masterson, J. J., Long, S. H., Katz, R., Seaton, W. H., Wynne, M., Lieberth, A., & Martin, D. (1993). Computing competencies for clinicians. *Asha*, 35(8), 48–49.

Cochran, P. S., & Passe, M. S. (1994). Software sampler: Language therapy with young children. Presentation at the annual meeting of the American Speech-Language-Hearing Association, New Orleans, LA. [Abstract in *Asha*, 36(10), 108.]

Cochran, P. S., Passe, M. S., & Carson, J. A. (1994). Software sampler: Language therapy and classroom curriculum. Presentation at the annual meeting of the American Speech-Language-Hearing Association, New Orleans, LA. [Abstract in *Asha*, 36(10), 108.]

Code, C. (1990). The computerized Boston: Clinical and research applications. Presentation at the annual meeting of the American Speech-Language-Hearing Association, Seattle, WA. [Abstract in *Asha*, 32(10), 121.]

Cohen, C. G. (1984). Implementing microcomputer applications. In A. H. Schwartz (Ed.), *Handbook of Microcomputer Applications in Communication Disorders*, San Diego: College-Hill, pp. 17–33.

Cohen, C. G. (1987). Keytalk [Review of computer program]. *Journal for Computer Users in Speech and Hearing*, 3(1), 95–96.

Cohen, C. G. (1988). Communication, Control, and Computer Access for Disabled and Elderly Individuals: Resource Books 1, 2, 3 (1987) [Review of books]. *Journal for Computer Users in Speech and Hearing*, 4(1), 42–43.

Cohen, C. G., & DeRuyter, F. (1982). Technology for the communicatively impaired: A perspective for future clinicians. *Journal of the National Student Speech and Hearing Association*, 10(1), 67–76.

Cohen, C. G., Frumkin, J. R., & Geiger, C. E. (1987). Interfacing video and computer to augment and teach language skills. Presentation at the annual meeting of the American Speech-Language-Hearing Association, New Orleans, LA. [Abstract in *Asha*, 29(10), 72.]

Cohen, C. G., & Palin, M. W. (1985). Clinical application of speech I/O systems: Synthesis and recognition. Presentation at the annual meeting of the American Speech-Language-Hearing Association, Washington, DC. [Abstract in *Asha*, 27(10), 109.]

Cohen, C. G., & Palin, M. W. (1986). Speech syntheses and speech recognition devices. In M. L. Grossfeld and C. A. Grossfeld (Editors), *Microcomputer Applications in Rehabilitation of Communication Disorders*. Rockville, MD: Aspen, pp. 183–209.

Colan, B. J. (1994). Virtual reality in augmentative communication and rehab. *ADVANCE for Speech-Language Pathologists & Audiologists*, 4(20), 19.

Colby, K. M. (1973). The rationale for computer-based treatment of language difficulties in non-speaking autistic children. *Journal of Autism and Childhood Schizophrenia*, 3, 254–260.

Colby, K. M., Christinaz, D., Parkinson, R. C., Graham, S., & Karpf, C. (1981). A word-finding computer programwith a dynamic lexical-semantic memory for patients with anomia using an intelligent speech prosthesis. *Brain and Language*, 14(2), 272–281.

Coleman, C. L., & Meyers, L. S. (1991). Computer recognition of the speech of adults with cerebral palsy and dysarthria. *Augmentative and Alternative Communication*, 7, 34–42.

Collins, M. (1986). *Multiple Meanings* [Computer program]. Dimondale, MI: Hartley Courseware.

Collins, M. J., Odell, K., Best, S. L., & Dirk, T. (1985). Computer-assisted assessment of visual problem-solving ability in aphasia. Presentation at the annual meeting of the American Speech-Language-Hearing Association, Washington, DC. [Abstract in *Asha*, 27(10), 84.]

Colton, R. H., Casper, J. K., Brewer, D. W., & Conture, E. G. (1989). Digital processing of laryngeal images: A preliminary report. *Journal of Voice*, 3, 132–142.

Comer, D. E. (1995). *The Internet Book*. Englewood Cliffs, NJ: Prentice Hall.

Communication Skill Builders (1984). *Ship Ahoy/Word Scramble* [Computer program]. Tucson, AZ: Communication Skill Builders.

Computerized Speech Research Environment [Computer program] (1994?). London, Ontario, Canada: AVAAZ Innovations. [Advertisement in *Asha*, 36(10), 116.]

Condon, M. (1985). Efficacy of microcomputer scoring of the Staggered Spondaic Word Test. Presentation at the annual meeting of the American Speech-Language-Hearing Association, Washington, D.C. [Abstract in *Asha*, 27(10), 89.]

Condon, M. T. (1983). Micro-computer assisted consumer education: Language/speech problems of aging. Presentation at the annual meeting of the American Speech-Language-Hearing Association, Cincinnati. [Abstract in *Asha*, 25(10), 117.]

Condon, M. T. (1983). Microcomputer assisted consumer education: Hearing loss in aging. Presentation at the annual meeting of the American Speech-Language-Hearing Association, Cincinnati. [Abstract in *Asha*, 25(10), 117.]

Condon, M. T. (1985a). Hearing Aid Manager [Review of computer program]. *Asha*, 27(12), 73–74.

Condon, M. T. (1985b). Selecting a Hearing Aid [Review of computer program]. *Asha*, 27(12), 73.

Condon, M. T., & Blodgett, E. G. (1984). Microcomputer assisted instruction in phonological process identification. Presentation at the annual meeting of the American Speech-Language-Hearing Association, San Francisco, CA. [Abstract in *Asha*, 26(10), 186.]

Connare, L. (1990). Practice Speech for the Laryngectomee [Review of computer program]. *Asha*, 32(8), 71–72.

Connor, N. P. (1992). Clini-base Computer Software for Clinical Supervision in Speech Pathology and Audiology, Release 2 [Review of computer program]. *Asha*, 34(8), 100.

Continuing Education Board (1994). Beyond workshops: Non-traditional types of continuing education. Presentation at the annual meeting of the American Speech-Language-Hearing Association, New Orleans, LA. [Abstract in *Asha*, 36(10), 166.]

Conway, R. J., & Niederjohn, R. J. (1988). Generation of sound spectrograms using a general-purpose digital computer and a dot-matrix printer. *Journal for Computer Users in Speech and Hearing*, 4(1), 14–22.

Cook, G., & Creech, H. B. (1983). Reliability and validity of computer hearing tests. *Hearing Instruments*, 34, 10–13, 39.

Cook, N. (1988). Spide Attack [Review of computer program]. *Asha*, 30(5), 78–79.

Cook, N. (1991). Words & Concepts II/Words & Concepts III [Review of computer programs]. *Asha*, 33(2), 83–84.

Cook, R. (August 1984). Operating system. *Popular Computing*, 3, 111–114, 135–148.

Cooper, J. (1985). Technology infusion: A resource guide. *Journal for Computer Users in Speech and Hearing*, 1(2), 96–116.

Cooper, R., & Neilson, H. (1986). *Computer-aided Speech Production* [Computer program]. Los Angeles, CA: Voice Learning Systems.

Corell, I., Ludvissen, C., & Birk-Nielsen, H. (1983). Experiences with computer-aided hearing aid fitting. *Scandanavian Audiology*, 12(3), 147–150.

Costello, J. M., & Sauer, M. (1990). Computer technology as a tool to develop augmentative communication competence. Presentation at the annual meeting of the American Speech-Language-Hearing Association, Seattle, WA. [Abstract in *Asha*, 32(10), 139.]

Coupland, S. G. (1988). EARS: An expert system approach to ABR interpretation. Presentation at the annual meeting of the American Speech-Language-Hearing Association, Boston, MA. [Abstract in *Asha*, 30(10), 98.]

Cox, D. R. (1993). Computer-assisted cognitive rehabilitation: Designing the THINKable system. Presentation at the annual meeting of the American Speech-Language-Hearing Association, Anaheim, CA. [Abstract in *Asha*, 35(10), 145.]

Cox, N. B., & Morrison, M. D. (1983). Acoustic analysis of voice for computerized laryngeal pathology assessment. *Journal of Otolaryngology*, 12(5), 295–301.

Cox, R. M., Alexander, G., & Gilmore, C. (1987). Development of the Connected Speech Test (CST). *Ear and Hearing*, 8, 1195–1265.

Craig, C. H., & Siegenthaler, B. M. (1981). Preliminary hearing aid selection by computer. *Hearing Aid Journal*, 34, 2.

Craig, H. K., & Hickey, J. J. (1992). Computer use for group and independent practice of sequencing skills. *Journal for Computer Users in Speech and Hearing*, 8(1, 2), 161–164.

Cranley, J. (1985). Aphasia I [Review of computer program]. *Asha*, 27(6), 75.

Creative Learning, Inc. (1991a). *Breakthrough to Language, Volume 1: Multi-sensory Curriculum* [Computer program]. North San Juan, CA: Creative Learning, Inc., P.O. Box 829.

Creative Learning, Inc. (1991b). *Breakthrough to Language, Volume 2: Multi-sensory Curriculum* [Computer program]. North San Juan, CA: Creative Learning, Inc., P.O. Box 829.

Critical Thinking Press and Software (1990) *What's My Logic. Figural and Figural/Verbal* [Computer program]. Pacific Grove, CA: Critical Thinking Press and Software, P. O. Box 448.

Cronk, C. (1986). A clinical application of microcomputer technology in the treatment of stuttering. Presentation at the American Speech and Hearing Foundation Computer Conference, Orlando, FL.

Crump, J. M. (1991). High technology instrumentation and the speech-language pathologist. *Journal for Computer Users in Speech and Hearing*, 7(1), 83–87.

Cuda, R. A. (1990). Managing information in communication sciences and disorders with AppleWorks Software [Review of computer program]. *Journal for Computer Users in Speech and Hearing*, 6(2), 164–167.

Cuda, R. A., & Wynne, M. K. (1991). Preassessment using HyperCard stacks. Presentation at the annual meeting of the American Speech-Language-Hearing Association, Atlanta, GA. [Abstract in *Asha*, 33(10), 187.]

Cuda, R. A., Wynne, M. K., & Sawyer, J. L. (1992). Teaching referral of communicative disorders using HyperCard stacks. *Journal for Computer Users in Speech and Hearing*, 8(1, 2), 105–110.

Curran, J., & Preves, D. (1986). Microcomputers and hearing aids. In J. L. Northern (Ed.), *The Personal Computer for Speech, Language, and Hearing Professionals*, Boston, MA: Little, Brown, pp. 209–228.

Curtis, J. F. (1986). *An Introduction to Microcomputers in Speech, Language, and Hearing*. Boston, MA: College Hill Press/Little, Brown & Company.

Dale, D. A. (1984). Computerized records and information system for speech pathology (CRISSP). Presentation at the annual meeting of the American Speech-Language-Hearing Association, San Francisco, CA. [Abstract in *Asha*, 26(10), 185.]

Dale, P. S., & Cole, K. N. (1988). An empirical comparison of three commercial language analysis programs. *Journal for Computer Users in Speech and Hearing*, 4(2), 100–112.

Dale, P. S., & Marriner, N. (1985). Computerized language analysis: A consumer's guide. Presentation at the annual meeting of the American Speech-Language-Hearing Association, Washington, DC. [Abstract in *Asha*, 27(10), 167–168.]

Dalston, R. M. (1983). Computer-generated reports of speech and language evaluations. *Cleft Palate Journal*, 20, 227–237.

Dalston, R. M., & Keefe, M. J. (1987). The use of a microcomputer in monitoring and modifying velopharyngeal movements. *Journal for Computer Users in Speech and Hearing*, 3(2), 159–169.

Daniels, J., & Mara, M. J. (1988). *Applied HyperCard: Developing and Marketing Superior Stackware*. New York: Simon & Schuster.

Danzer, V. (1986). Computer Managed Articulation Treatment [Review of computer program]. *Asha*, 28(1), 69.

Dashiell, S. E. (1985). Natural Language Processing Program [Review of computer program]. *Asha*, 27(3), 71–72.

Davidson, J., & Eckert, Jr., R. (1986). *Word Attack!* [Computer program]. Torrance, CA: Davidson & Associates, Inc., 3135 Kashiwa Street.

Davis, J. (1990a). Action/Music Play [Review of computer program]. *Journal for Computer Users in Speech and Hearing*, 6(1), 68–70.

Davis, J. (1990b). Words & Concepts II [Review of computer program]. *Journal for Computer Users in Speech and Hearing*, 6(1), 73–75.

Davis, M. L., & Stach, B. A. (1990). The efficiency of computer-based speech audiometry. Presentation at the annual meeting of the American Speech-Language-Hearing Association, Seattle, WA. [Abstract in *Asha*, 32(10), 90.]

Davis, R., & Sammis, B. (1985). Clinical applications for microcomputers. Presentation at the American Speech and Hearing Foundation conference on microcomputers, New Orleans, LA. [Abstract in the *Journal for Computer Users in Speech and Hearing*, 1(2), 74–75.]

Dean, C. R., & Pickering, J. E. (1989). Accessibility to BITNET for communication disorders institutions. Presentation at the annual meeting of the American Speech-Language-Hearing Association, St. Louis, MO. [Abstract in *Asha*, 31(10), 162.]

Dean, C. R., & Pickering, J. E. (1991a). Networking microcomputers for professional and personal benefit. Presentation at the annual meeting of the American Speech-Language-Hearing Association, Atlanta, GA. [Abstract in *Asha*, 33(10), 135.]

Dean, C. R., & Pickering, J. E. (1991b). Telecomputing in communication disorders. *Journal for Computer Users in Speech and Hearing*, 7(1), 35–43.

Dean, R. (1993). Serial Recall Assessment: Michigan Memory Series Software [Review of computer program]. *Asha*, 35(5), 69.

Decker, T. N., & Tice, R. L. (1985). Signal averaging program. Presentation at the American Speech and Hearing Foundation Conference on Microcomputers, New Orleans, LA. [Abstract in the *Journal for Computer Users in Speech and Hearing*,1(2), 75.]

Deem, J. F., Miller, V. P., & Stoner, D. L. (1991). Rural service delivery problems and personnel shortages: One university's answer. Presentation at the annual meeting of the American Speech-Language-Hearing Association, Atlanta, GA. [Abstract in *Asha*, 33(10), 188.]

de Jonge, R. R. (1983). Computer simulation of hearing aid frequency responses. *Hearing Aid Journal*, 36, 27–31.

de Jonge, R. R. (1984). Selecting an aid for maximum intelligibility. Presentation at the annual meeting of the American Speech-Language-Hearing Association, San Francisco, CA. [Abstract in *Asha*, 26(10), 119.]

de Jonge, R. R. (1985). A microcomputer-based hearing aid selection strategy. *Journal for Computer Users in Speech and Hearing*, 1(2), 117–138.

de Jonge, R. R. (1992). HyperCard: A tool for computer-aided instruction in audiology. *Journal for Computer Users in Speech and Hearing*, 137–147

DelCalzo, P. (1988). Practice Speech for the Laryngectomee [Review of computer program]. *Journal for Computer Users in Speech and Hearing*, 4(1), 59–61.

Delgado, R. E., & Miskiel, E. (1991). Innovative computer software and hardware design solutions: Applications in the field of speech and hearing. *Journal for Computer Users in Speech and Hearing*, 7(1), 88–93.

Delgado, R. E., & Ozdamar, O. (1990). Automated ABR peak labelling using matched filters. *Annual International Conference of IEEE EMBS*, 12, 870–871.

Delgado, R. E., Ozdamar, O., & Miskiel, E. (1987). Computer determination of hearing thresholds using evoked potentials. In D. Larnard (Ed.), *Proceedings Miami Technicon '87*. New York: IEEE.

Delgado, R. E., Ozdamar, O., & Miskiel, E. (1988). On-line system for automated auditory evoked response threshold determination. *Annual International Conference of IEEE EMBS*, 10, 1471–1473.

Deliyski, D. D., & Orlikoff, R. F. (1991). Computer system for multidimensional analysis of voice and electroglottographic signals. Presentation at the annual meeting of the American Speech-Language-Hearing Association, Atlanta, GA. [Abstract in *Asha*, 33(10), 188.]

Deller, J. R., Hsu, D., & Ferrier, L. J. (1988). Encouraging results in the automated recognition of cerebral palsy speech. *IEEE Transactions on Biomedical Engineering*, 35, 218–220.

Deller, J. R., Hsu, D., & Ferrier, L. J. (in press). On the use of hidden Markov models for the recognition of dysarthric speech. *Journal of Biomedical Measurement, Information, and Control.*

Dengel, G. A., Robbins, J., & Rosenbek, J. C. (1990). Computerized image processing in videoflouroscopic analysis of oropharyngeal motor functioning. *Journal for Computer Users in Speech and Hearing*, 6(2), 130–133.

Diaz, J. M., Hillman, R. E., Gress, C. D., Bunting, G. W., & Doyle, P.B. (1993). VoiceBase: A clinical and research database for voice disorders. Presentation at the annual meeting of the American Speech-Language-Hearing Association, Anaheim, CA. [Abstract in *Asha*, 35(10), 183.]

Dikeman, K. J., & Kerman-Lerner, P. (1989). Efficacy of microcomputer treatment for reading disorders in adult aphasia. Presentation at the annual meeting of the American Speech-Language-Hearing Association, St. Louis, MO. [Abstract in *Asha*, 31(10), 61.]

Dillingham, L., Roe, J., & Roe, M. (1982). Selected applications of computer assisted video instruction in the education of hearing-impaired students. *American Annals of the Deaf*, 127, 652–658.

Dillon, L. H., & Weiner, F. F. (1995a). *Category Discrimination and Reasoning* [Computer program]. West Bloomfield, MI: Parrot Software.

Dillon, L. H., & Weiner, F. F. (1995b). *Category Naming and Completion* [Computer program]. West Bloomfield, MI: Parrot Software.

Dillon, L. H., & Weiner, F. F. (1995c). *Cognitive Disorders 1: Category Naming and Completion* [Computer program]. West Bloomfield, MI: Parrot Software.

Dillon, L. H., & Weiner, F. F. (1995d). *Cognitive Disorders 2: Category Discrimination and Reasoning* [Computer program]. West Bloomfield, MI: Parrot Software.

Dillon, L. H., & Weiner, F. F. (1995e). *Cognitive Disorders 3: Attention/Perception* [Computer program]. West Bloomfield, MI: Parrot Software.

Dillon, L. H., & Weiner, F. F. (1995f). *Cognitive Disorders 8: Inferential Naming* [Computer program]. West Bloomfield, MI: Parrot Software.

Dillon, L. H., & Weiner, F. F. (1995g). *Cognitive Disorders 12: Antonyms and Synonyms* [Computer program]. West Bloomfield, MI: Parrot Software.

Dillon, L. H., & Weiner, F. F. (1995h). *Cognitive Disorders 13: Homophones* [Computer program]. West Bloomfield, MI: Parrot Software.

Dillon, L. H., & Weiner, F. F. (1995i). *Cognitive Disorders 14: Hierarchical Attention Training* [Computer program]. West Bloomfield, MI: Parrot Software.

Dillon, L. H., & Weiner, F. F. (1995j). *Cognitive Disorders 15: Homographs* [Computer program]. West Bloomfield, MI: Parrot Software.

Dillon, L. H., & Weiner, F. F. (1995k). *Hierarchical Attention Training* [Computer program]. West Bloomfield, MI: Parrot Software.

Dillon, L. H., & Weiner, F. F. (1995l). *Multiple Meaning Words 1* [Computer program]. West Bloomfield, MI: Parrot Software.

Dillon, L. H., & Weiner, F. F. (1995m). *Multiple Meaning Words 2* [Computer program]. West Bloomfield, MI: Parrot Software.

Dillon, L. H., & Weiner, F. F. (1995n). *Visual Confrontation Naming* [Computer program]. West Bloomfield, MI: Parrot Software.

Dinon, D. A., & Parsons, J. M. (1989). *The Computer Assisted Speechreading Training (CAST) Program: An Assessment of Speechreading Training*. Unpublished master's research project, University of Western Ontario, London, Ontario.

Dodson, S. L. (1991). A computer system for auditory evoked potential recording and analysis. Presentation at the annual meeting of the American Speech-Language-Hearing Association, Atlanta, GA. [Abstract in *Asha*, 33(10), 192.]

Domico, W. D. (1985). Audio-Pro [Review of computer program]. *Journal for Computer Users in Speech and Hearing*, 1(1), 51.

Domico, W. D. (1986). Pure-Tone Audiometry Simulation [Review of computer program]. *Journal for Computer Users in Speech and Hearing*, 2(1), 1986.

Don Johnson Developmental Equipment (1990). *Ke:nx* [Computer hardware and program]. Wauconda, IL.

Donnelly, K. G. (1982). Computer assisted hearing aid fitting. *Hearing Instruments*, 33, 7.

Doyle, P. C., Leeper, H. A., Katler, A. L., & Thomas-Stonell, N. (1993). Comparative perceptual and computerized voice recognition functions for dysarthric speakers. Presentation at the annual meeting of the American Speech-Language-Hearing Association, Anaheim, CA. [Abstract in *Asha*, 35(10), 120.]

Doyle, P. C., & Wallace, W. J. B. (1990). Application and clinical use of the Kay Elemetrics Waveform Display System for Photoglottographic (PGG) assessment of vocal function. *Journal for Computer Users in Speech and Hearing*, 6(2), 122–129.

Dr. Speech Science for Windows [Computer program] (1994). Seattle, WA: Tiger Electronics, Box 85126, Seattle, WA 98145.

Dressler, R. A. (1991). Beyond workbooks: The computer as a treatment supplement. Presentation at the annual meeting of the American Speech-Language-Hearing Association, Atlanta, GA. [Abstract in *Asha*, 33(10), 192.]

Dressler, R. A. (1992). Computerized language activity resource kit: A hypercard stack. *Journal for Computer Users in Speech and Hearing*, 8(1, 2), 125–129.

Driscoll, M. S. (1986). Appleworks: For the speech-language pathologist. Presentation at the annual meeting of the American Speech-Language-Hearing Association, Detroit, MI. [Abstract in *Asha*, 28(10), 114.]

Driscoll, M. S. (1987). A computerized articulation training program. Presentation at the annual meeting of the American Speech-Language-Hearing Association, New Orleans, LA. [Abstract in *Asha*, 29(10), 98.]

Driscoll, M. S. (1991). Computerized Continuous Performance Tests. Presentation at the annual meeting of the American Speech-Language-Hearing Association, Atlanta, GA. [Abstract in *Asha*, 33(10), 192.]

Driscoll, M. S., & Driscoll, S. T. (1984). Distinctive feature analysis on an Apple computer. Presentation at the annual meeting of the American Speech-Language-Hearing Association, San Francisco, CA. [Abstract in *Asha*, 26(10), 158.]

Drumright, D. G., Seikel, J. A., & Wilcox, K. A. (1988). Acoustic analysis software for an IBM PC. *Journal for Computer Users in Speech and Hearing*, 4(1), 23–32.

Duncan, B. J., Skarakis-Doyle, E., & Haff, R. (1993). An assessment of young children's semantic/pragmatic comprehension. Presentation at the annual meeting of the American Speech-Language-Hearing Association, Anaheim, CA. [Abstract in *Asha*, 35(10), 183.]

Durham, J. A., Thelin, J. W., & Muenchen, R. A. (1993). Behavioral audiometric simulator (BAS) for teaching visual reinforcement audiometry (VRA). Presentation at the annual meeting of the American Speech-Language-Hearing Association, Anaheim, CA. [Abstract in *Asha*, 35(10), 194.]

Durnford, S. E., Frey, H. J., Hazan, J. H., & Hoffman, A. P. (1994). A diagnostic tutorial and test referencing system for student clinicians. Presentation at the annual meeting of the American Speech-Language-Hearing Association, New Orleans, LA. [Abstract in *Asha*, 36(10), 174.]

Dustrude, S. R. (1990). Thoughts of a speech-language pathologist: An inside perspective. *Journal for Computer Users in Speech and Hearing*, 6(1), 46–49.

Egolf, D. (1978). Computer predictions of hearing aid sound spectra. *Hearing Aid Journal*, 31, 6–8.

Egolf, D. B. (1982). Computer analysis of linguistic protocols. Presentation at the annual meeting of the American Speech-Language-Hearing Association, Toronto, Canada. [Abstract in *Asha*, 24(10), 798.]

Egolf, D. B. (1983). The analysis and synthesis of discourse by computer. Presentation at the annual meeting of the American Speech-Language-Hearing Association, Cincinnati, OH. [Abstract in *Asha*, 25(10), 130.]

Egolf, D. B., & Kikuchi, M. (1985). LISP: Not a speech disorder. Presentation at the annual meeting of the American Speech-Language-Hearing Association, Washington, DC. [Abstract in *Asha*, 27(10), 166.]

Ehren, T. C. (1986). Understanding Questions [Review of computer program]. *Asha*, 28(7), 77–78.

Ehren, T. C. (1989). *ASHA* Project IMPACT: #3 Microcomputer Applications in Assessment for Speech and Language Professionals [Review of computer program]. *Asha*, 31(12), 73.

Eilers, R. E., Miskiel, E., Ozdamar, O., Urbano, R., & Widen, J. E. (1991). Optimization of automated hearing test algorithms: Simulations using an infant response model. *Ear and Hearing*, 12(3), 191–198.

Eilers, R. E., Ozdamar, O., & Steffens, M. L. (1991). CAST—Evaluation of automated behavioral hearing screening of infants. Presentation at the annual meeting of the American Speech-Language-Hearing Association, Atlanta, GA. [Abstract in *Asha*, 33(10), 158.]

Eilers, R. E., Widen, J. E., Urbano, R., Hudson, T., & Gonzalez, L (1991). Optimization of automated hearing test algorithms: A comparison of data from simulations and young children. *Ear and Hearing*, 12(3), 199–204.

Elbert, M., Young, L. L., & Bruce, K. (1981). A computer program for distinctive feature analysis. *Journal of Communication Disorders*, 14(6), 519–523.

Elliot, L., Vegely, A., & Falvey, N. (1971). Description of a computer-oriented record-keeping system. *Asha*, 13, 435–443.

Emanuele, D. D. (1994). On to the 21st century: Computerized documentation. Presentation at the annual meeting of the American Speech-Language-Hearing Association, New Orleans, LA. [Abstract in *Asha*, 36(10), 166.]

Enderby, P. M., & Roworth, M. (1985). *Frenchay Dysarthria Assessment Computer Differential Analysis* [Computer program]. San Diego, CA: College-Hill Press.

Engebretson, A., & Miller, J. (1982). A computer program for fitting a master hearing aid to the residual hearing characteristics of individual patients. *Journal of the Acoustical Society of America*, 72, 426–430.

Epp, M. (1987). *VCR CONTROLLER* [Computer program]. Madison, WI: University of Wisconsin, Waisman Center Research Computing Facility.

Erickson, F. N., Yeung, E., & Boothroyd, A. (1993). Automated assessment of hearing aid effect on phonemic spectral distribution. Presentation at the annual meeting of the American Speech-Language-Hearing Association, Anaheim, CA. [Abstract in *Asha*, 35(10), 216.]

Ernst, M. M., & Wallace, H. M. (1984). *Natural Language Processing Program* [Computer program]. Denver, CO: Educational Audiology Programs, 1077 South Gilpin Street.

Espinoza-Varas, B. (1992). Speech and hearing applications of LabVIEW. Presentation at the annual meeting of the American Speech-Language-Hearing Association, San Antonio, TX. [Abstract in *Asha*, 34(10), 109.]

Esterreicher, C. A. (1985). CAI—Designing and developing your own BASIC microcomputer software programs. Presentation at the annual meeting of the American Speech-Language-Hearing Association, Washington, DC. [Abstract in *Asha*, 27(10), 89.]

Esterreicher, C. A. (1986). *Idioms in America* [Computer program]. Tucson, AZ: Communication Skill Builders, 3130 North Dodge.

Esterreicher, C. A. (1993). *ASHA* session choices? Use your computer to arrange schedule options! Presentation at the annual meeting of the American Speech-Language-Hearing Association, Anaheim, CA. [Abstract in *Asha*, 35(10), 138.]

Esterreicher, C. A., and Shively, P. (1986). Word processing and data base management applications in public schools. Presentation at the annual meeting of the American Speech-Language-Hearing Association, Detroit, MI. [Abstract in *Asha*, 28(10), 114.]

Etter, R. R., & Simmons, S. J. (1993). Computer literacy instruction for individuals with severe developmental disabilities. Presentation at the annual meeting of the American Speech-Language-Hearing Association, Anaheim, CA. [Abstract in *Asha*, 35(10), 220.]

Falla, A. P., & Fausti, S. A. (1990). Managing a multisite ototoxicity study with microcomputer-based communications. Presentation at the annual meeting of the American Speech-Language-Hearing Association, Seattle, WA. [Abstract in *Asha*, 32(10), 64.]

Fausti, S. A., Frey, R. H., Henry, J. A., Knutsen, J. L., & Olson, D. J. (1990). Reliability and validity of high-frequency (8–20 kHz) thresholds obtained on a computer-based audiometer as compared to a documented laboratory system. *Journal of the American Academy of Audiology*, 1, 162–170.

Fausti, S. A., Olson, D. J., Frey, R. H., & Schaffer, H. I. (1991). Managing a multisite research program with microcomputer-based communications. *Journal for Computer Users in Speech and Hearing*, 7(1), 11–21.

Feh, L. L., Gerratt, B. R., Kewley-Port, D., Studebaker, G. A., & Raz, I. (1985). Hardware and software issues in the speech and hearing laboratory. Presentation at the annual meeting of the American Speech-Language-Hearing Association, Washington, DC. [Abstract in *Asha*, 27(10), 146.]

Fein, D. J. (March 1983). Survey report: 1982 *ASHA* Omnibus. *Asha*, 24, 53–57.

Fein, D. J. (1984). Findings from the 1983 *ASHA* omnibus survey. *Asha*, 26, 45–48.

Fell, H. J., Ferrier, L. J., Hariklia, D., & Peterson, R. (1994). Measuring infant communicative precursors: The babble blanket. Presentation at the annual meeting of the American Speech-Language-Hearing Association, New Orleans, LA. [Abstract in *Asha*, 36(10), 106–107.]

Fell, H. J., Ferrier, L. J., & Vogt, C. (1993). An early vocalization analyzer (EVA). Presentation at the annual meeting of the American Speech-Language-Hearing Association, Anaheim, CA. [Abstract in *Asha*, 35(10), 126.]

Ferguson, M. L. (1993). Computer technology: Use in public schools. *Asha*, 35(8), 46–47.

Ferrero, F., Menin, S., Noventa, A., & Rosetti, M. C. (1993). Lo SpeechViewer II: Prime valutazioni. *Acta Phoniatrica Latina*, 15(2), 223–229.

Ferrier, L. J., & Blackmer, E. R. (1992). Computer-assisted accent reduction for non-native speakers of English. Presentation at the annual meeting of the American Speech-Language-Hearing Association, San Antonio, TX. [Abstract in *Asha*, 34(10), 221.]

Ferrier, L. J., Blackmer, E. R., DiGiacomo, J., & Walsh, D. (1993). ESL computer-assisted accent reduction: Does it work? Presentation at the annual meeting of the American Speech-Language-Hearing Association, Anaheim, CA. [Abstract in *Asha*, 35(10), 234.]

Ferrier, L. J., Clough, F. W., & Reid, L. N. (1995). Campus survival guide for ESL speakers: Computer-assisted accent reduction. Presentation at the annual meeting of the American Speech-Language-Hearing Association, Orlando, FL. [Abstract in *Asha*, 37(10), 92.]

Ferrier, L. J., Clough, F. W., Reid, L. N., & Walsh, D. (1994). Computer-assisted accent reduction for non-native speaker. Presentation at the annual meeting of the American Speech-Language-Hearing Association, New Orleans, LA. [Abstract in *Asha*, 36(10), 108.]

Ferrier, L. J., & Fell, H. J. (1992). The Baby-Babble-Blanket providing communication for severely impaired infants. Presentation at the annual meeting of the American Speech-Language-Hearing Association, San Antonio, TX. [Abstract in *Asha*, 34(10), 116.]

Ferrier, L. J., Frazier, H., Carpenter, T., & Shane, H. C. (1993). Intelligibility and computer voice recognition by dysarthric speakers. Presentation at the annual meeting of the American Speech-Language-Hearing Association, Anaheim, CA. [Abstract in *Asha*, 35(10), 207, 241–242.]

Ferrier, L. J., Jarrell, N., Carpenter, T., & Shane, H. C. (1991). Voice recognition by dysarthric speakers. Presentation at the annual meeting of the American Speech-Language-Hearing Association, Atlanta, GA. [Abstract in *Asha*, 33(10), 192.]

Ferrier, L. J., Jarrell, N., Carpenter, T., & Shane, H. C. (1992). A case study of a dysarthric speaker using the DragonDictate voice recognition system. *Journal for Computer Users in Speech and Hearing*, 8(1, 2), 33–52.

Fersting, F. (1984). Word processing for report writing: Skill acquisition and attitudinal change. Presentation at the annual meeting of the American Speech-Language-Hearing Association, San Francisco, CA.. [Abstract in *Asha*, 26(10), 185.]

Fields, T., & Renshaw, S. (1978). Use of the computer in the diagnosis of language of disorders. Presentation at the annual meeting of the American Speech-Language-Hearing Association, San Francisco, CA.

Filter, M. D., Brandell, M. E., Smith, J. E., & Kopin, M. (1990). A CAI method for improving the reliability of supervision. Presentation at the annual meeting of the American Speech-Language-Hearing Association, Seattle, WA. [Abstract in *Asha*, 32(10), 62.]

Filter, M. D., & Hirsh, T. (1987). The Reinforcer [Computer program]. Harrisonburg, VA: CTS Software.

Filter, M. D., Powell, W. L., & Campbell, J. L. (1994). Teaching phonetics with the help of an e-mail system. Presentation at the annual meeting of the American Speech-Language-Hearing Association, New Orleans, LA. [Abstract in *Asha*, 36(10), 107.]

Filter, M. D., & Smith J. E. (1986). Computer assisted instruction in training students to rate voice disorders. Presentation at the annual meeting of the American Speech-Language-Hearing Association, Detroit, MI. [Abstract in *Asha*, 28(10), 148.]

Finley, D. A. (1984). Computer simulation testing: A supplemental mode for assessing clinical competence. Presentation at the annual meeting of the American Speech-Language-Hearing Association, San Francisco, CA. [Abstract in *Asha*, 26(10), 183.]

Fire, K. M., Fox, R. A., & Fligner, M. (1990). Recognition of computer-generated syllables by young and elderly listeners. Presentation at the annual meeting of the American Speech-Language-Hearing Association, Seattle, WA. [Abstract in *Asha*, 32(10), 117.]

Fischer, M. A. (1991a). Hypermedia and the child with language-learning disabilities. Presentation at the annual meeting of the American Speech-Language-Hearing Association, Atlanta, GA. [Abstract in *Asha*, 33(10), 171.]

Fischer, M. A. (1991b). Interactive multimedia: A virtual reality for the LLD child. Presentation at the annual meeting of the American Speech-Language-Hearing Association, Atlanta, GA. [Abstract in *Asha*, 33(10), 81.]

Fischer, M. A. (1992a). Advanced HyperCard applications in speech-language-hearing. Presentation at the annual meeting of the American Speech-Language-Hearing Association, San Antonio, TX. [Abstract in *Asha*, 34(10), 134.]

Fischer, M. A. (1992b). HyperCard: A clinical perspective. *Journal for Computer Users in Speech and Hearing*, 8(1, 2), 111–116.

Fischer, M. A. (1993). HyperCard: The high-tech flannel board. *Asha*, 35(8), 42.

Fisher, J. V., & Pondugula, K. (1993). Mac-based, 6–channel data acquisition system for speech and voice. Presentation at the annual meeting of the American Speech-Language-Hearing Association, Anaheim, CA. [Abstract in *Asha*, 35(10), 116.]

Fishman, I. (1987). *Electronic Communication Aids: Selection and Use*. Boston, MA: College-Hill Press/Little, Brown & Company.

Fitch, J. L. (1982). The computer and speech and hearing services. Presentation at the annual meeting of the American Speech-Language-Hearing Association, Toronto, Canada.

Fitch, J. L. (May 1983a). Computer-based services for the hearing health professional. *Hearing Journal*, 31–34.

Fitch, J. L. (1983b). Telecomputer treatment for aphasia. *Journal of Speech and Hearing Disorders*, 48(3), 335–336.

Fitch, J. L. (1985a). *Computer Managed Articulation Treatment* [Computer program]. Tucson, AZ: Communication Skill Builders.

Fitch, J. L. (1985b). *Computer Managed Articulation Diagnosis* [Computer program]. Tucson, AZ: Communication Skill Builders.

Fitch, J. L. (1985c). *Computer Managed Language Treatment* [Computer program]. Tucson, AZ: Communication Skill Builders.

Fitch, J. L. (1985d). *Computer Managed Screening Test* [Computer program]. Tucson, AZ: Communication Skill Builders.

Fitch, J. L. (1985e). Developing clinical software. Presentation at the American Speech and Hearing Foundation Conference on Microcomputers, New Orleans, LA. [Abstract in the *Journal for Computer Users in Speech and Hearing*, 1(2), 76.]

Fitch, J. L. (1985f). Perspectives on computers in communication disorders. *Journal for Computer Users in Speech and Hearing*, 1(1), 15–16.

Fitch, J. L. (1986a). *Computer Managed Visual Descrimination* [Computer program]. Mobile, AL: Communicology Associates.

Fitch, J. L. (1986b). *Computer Managed Maze Tracking* [Computer program]. Mobile, AL: Communicology Associates.

Fitch, J. L. (1989a). Computer recognition of correct sound production in articulation treatment. *Journal for Computer Users in Speech and Hearing*, 5(1), 8–18.

Fitch, J. L. (1989b). Computers and communication disorders: A perspective. *Journal for Computer Users in Speech and Hearing*, 5(2), 80–83.

Fitch, J. L. (1989c). Computers and the consultive model: Improving efficiency and productivity. Presentation at the annual meeting of the American Speech-Language-Hearing Association, St. Louis, MO. [Abstract in *Asha*, 31(10), 132.]

Fitch, J. L. (1993). Computer technology: History and overview. *Asha*, 35(8), 36–37.

Fitch, J. L., & Cross, S. T. (1983). Telecomputer treatment for aphasia. *Journal of Speech and Hearing Disorders*, 48, 335–336.

Fitch, J. L., Davis, D. A., Evans, W. B., & Sellers, D. E. (1982). Computer managed screening for articulation/language. Presentation at the annual meeting of the American Speech-Language-Hearing Association, Toronto, Canada. [Abstract in *Asha*, 24(10), 770.]

Fitch, J. L., Davis, L. A., Evans, W. B., & Sellers, D. E. (1984). Computer managed screening for communication disorders. *Language, Speech, and Hearing Services in Schools*, 15, 66–69.

Fitch, J. L., Deputy, D., & Dykes, S. (1985). *Goldilocks and the Three Bears* [Review of computer program]. *Journal for Computer Users in Speech and Hearing*, 1(1), 53–54.

Fitch, J. L., Dykes, S., & Deputy, D. (1985). Computer Courseware for the Exceptional Student: Keyboard Training Program [Review of computer program]. *Journal for Computer Users in Speech and Hearing*, 1(1), 52–53.

Fitch, J. L., & Strand, V. (1985). Video voice. *Journal for Computer Users in Speech and Hearing*, 1, 55–56.

Fitch, J. L., & Terrio, L. (1974). Computer assisted articulation therapy. Presentation at the annual meeting of the American Speech-Language-Hearing Association, Las Vagas.

Fitch, J. L., & Wold, J. H. (October 1984). Hearing conservation programs for microcomputers. *Sound and Vibration*, 26–29.

FitzSimons, R. M., & Wright, J. A. (1983). Microcomputers and educational software: Speech-language pathology's new dimensions. Presentation at the annual meeting of the American Speech-Language-Hearing Association, Cincinnati. [Abstract in *Asha*, 25(10), 117.]

Flaherty, C. (1984). Cost-benefit analysis of computer-based instruction of school speech services. Presentation at the annual meeting of the American Speech-Language-Hearing Association, San Francisco, CA. [Abstract in *Asha*, 26(10), 79.]

Flahive, L. K., Nasir, M., & Watson, J. B. (1995). Computer use by speech-language pathologists in public schools. Presentation at the annual meeting of the American Speech-Language-Hearing Association, Orlando, FL. [Abstract in *Asha*, 37(10), 64.]

Flannigan, W. J. (1985). Computerized data base for school speech-language programs. Presentation at the annual meeting of the American Speech-Language-Hearing Association, Washington, DC. [Abstract in *Asha*, 27(10), 128.]

Fletcher, E. C. (1986). Keyboarder [Review of computer program]. *Asha*, 28(4), 85.

Flowers, D. A., Fulks, L. N., Ott-Rose, M. M., Pickering, Jr., J. E., Page, J. L., & Walker, J. W. (1991). Videodisc technology in language assessment and intervention. Presentation at the annual meeting of the American Speech-Language-Hearing Association, Atlanta, GA. [Abstract in *Asha*, 33(10), 85.]

Fox, B. (1980). A study comparing live and computer-assisted receptive syntax items testing the prepositions in, on, and under. Master's thesis, University of Vermont.

Fox, J. P. (1986). Developing computer treatment programs using synthetic speech. Presentation at the ASHF Computer Conference, Orlando, FL.

Fox, J. P. (1990). Computer use by speech-language pathologists. *Journal for Computer Users in Speech and Hearing*, 6(2), 111–117.

Fox, S. (December 20, 1993). EMG biofeedback accelerates dysphagia treatment. *ADVANCE for Speech-Language Pathologists and Audiologists*, 12.

Franzwa, A. (1990). Concentrate! on Words and Concepts Series [Review of computer program]. *Asha*, 32(8), 73.

Franzwa, A. (1991a). Augmentative Communication Series: Scan and Speak [Review of computer program]. *Asha*, 33(5), 90.

Franzwa, A. (1991b). Breakthrough to Writing. Volume 3, Multisensory Curriculum [Review of computer program]. *Asha*, 33(8), 71.

Freeman, A. W., & Hagey, C. M. (1980). A computerized procedure for storing and retrieving comprehensive data on aphasics. Presentation at the annual meeting of the American Speech-Language-Hearing Association, Detroit, MI. [Abstract in *Asha*, 22(9), 789.]

Friedman, S. B. (1989). SpeechViewer [Review of computer program]. *Asha*, 31(8), 45–46.

Fried-Oken, M. (1984). The voice recognition device for computer control by motorically and speech-impaired individuals. *Proceedings of the 2nd International Conference on Rehabilitation Engineering*, 454–455.

Fried-Oken, M. (1985a). DECtalk voice synthesizer for speech input and output: A personal communication system. Presentation at the American Speech and Hearing Foundation Conference on Microcomputers, New Orleans, LA. [Abstract in the *Journal for Computer Users in Speech and Hearing*, 1(2), 77.]

Fried-Oken, M. (1985b). Voice recognition devices as a computer interface for motor and speech impaired people. *Archives of Physical Medicine and Rehabilitation*, 66, 678–681.

Fried-Oken, M. (1988). BOSTON [Review of computer program]. *Journal for Computer Users in Speech and Hearing*, 4(1), 45–48.

Fried-Oken, M. (1989). Future perspectives in augmentative and alternative communication. *Journal for Computer Users in Speech and Hearing*, 5(2), 97–100.

Friedrich, B. W., LaRue, B. L., & Smyke, A. T. (1981). Use of a word processing system for clinical reports. Presentation at the annual meeting of the American Speech-Language-Hearing Association, Los Angeles, CA. [Abstract in *Asha*, 23(10), 722.]

Fritze, W. (1978). A computer-controlled binaural balance test. *Acta Otolaryngologica*, 86, 89–92.

Frydenberg, H., & Wheeler, D. G. (1986). Microcomputer-assisted intervention for the speech and language impaired adult. In M. L. Grossfeld & C. A. Grossfeld (Eds.), *Microcomputer Applications in Rehabilitation of Communication Disorders*. Rockville, MD: Aspen, pp. 97–130.

Fujiu, M. (1989). Design of a Computer-Assisted Speechreading Training System for Japanese. Master's thesis, University of British Columbia.

Fulton, R., Larson, A., & Worthy, R. (1983). The use of microcomputer technology in assessing and training communication skills of young hearing impaired children. *American Annals of the Deaf*, 128, 570–576.

Gagné J.-P., Dinon, D. A., & Parsons, J. M. (1989). Assessment of an interactive video system to train speechreading. Presentation at the annual conference of the Canadian Association of Speech-Language Pathologists and Audiologists, Toronto, Ontario.

Gagné, J.-P., Dinon, D. A., & Parsons, J. M. (1991). An evaluation of CAST: A Computer-Aided Speechreading Training Program. *Journal of Speech and Hearing Research*, 34, 213–221.

Gaines, B. H., & Coupland, S. G. (1984). SMAP: A microcomputer application for assessment of sequential memory. Presentation at the annual meeting of the American Speech-Language-Hearing Association, San Francisco, CA. [Abstract in *Asha*, 26(10), 155.]

Gallaher, A., & Weiner, F. F. (1995a). *Aphasia 9: Initial Phoneme Cueing for Aphasics* [Computer program]. West Bloomfield, MI: Parrot Software.

Gallaher, A., & Weiner, F. F. (1995b). *Aphasia 10: Orientation for Aphasia and Cognitive Disorders: Mastering Personal Information* [Computer program]. West Bloomfield, MI: Parrot Software.

Galsky, A. G. (1984). Funding sources for microcomputers. In A. H. Schwartz (Ed.), *Handbook of Microcomputer Applications in Communication Disorders*. San Diego: College-Hill, pp. 35–52.

Gans, D. P., VerHoef, N., & Berger, K. W. (1983). Hearing aid selection by computer. *Hearing Instruments*, 34, 5.

Gardner, H. J. (1985). *Occupational Hearing Conservation Management on the Kaypro 10 and IBM-PC/XT* [Computer program]. Huntington, NY: Huntington Hearing and Speech Center, 44 Elm Street.

Gardner, H. J. (1991). Occupational hearing conservation data base management software. *Journal for Computer Users in Speech and Hearing*, 7(1), 94–97.

Garrett, E. R. (1989). High tech/high touch: Our challenge for the coming decade. *Journal for Computer Users in Speech and Hearing*, 5(2), 84–88.

Gatehouse, S. (1986). A microcomputer-based trainer for pure-tone audiometry. *British Journal of Audiology*, 20, 141–145.

Gavin, W. (1987). Interactive data management software for language sample analysis. *Child Language Teaching and Therapy*, 3, 183–199.

Gavin, W., & Dismuke, R. P. (1983). CALARSP: The computer assisted LARSP program. Presentation at the annual meeting of the American Speech-Language-Hearing Association, Cincinnati, OH. [Abstract in *Asha*, 25(10), 128.]

Geers, A., Miller, J., Coaker, F., & Rapp, J. (1977). Inexpensive system for computer storage of clinical data. Presentation at the annual meeting of the American Speech-Language-Hearing Association, Chicago, IL.

Gelatt, J. P. (1986). *Needs Assessment Conference: A Final Report.* Rockville, MD: American Speech-Language-Hearing Association.

Gelatt, J. P. (1987). ASHF needs assessment conference: Where next? *Journal for Computer Users in Speech and Hearing*, 3(2), 132–139.

Gelatt, J. P., & Minghetti, N. (1989). Technology: Are we ready to take the lead? *Journal for Computer Users in Speech and Hearing*, 5(2), 75–79.

Gelatt, J. P., Schwartz, A. H., Deily, A. B. S., & Schetz, K. F. (1989). Integrating computer applications in school settings. Presentation at the annual meeting of the American Speech-Language-Hearing Association, St. Louis, MO. [Abstract in *Asha*, 31(10), 51.]

Gibbs, D. P. (1988). Computer applications in augmentative communication. Presentation at the annual meeting of the American Speech-Language-Hearing Association, Boston, MA. [Abstract in *Asha*, 30(10), 121.]

Gibbs, L. K., & Nash, K. (1983). SpecialNet: Instant information/communication. *American Annals of the Deaf*, 128, 631–635.

Gillman, M. G., Feth, L. L., & Barin, K. (1994). A LabView companion for signals and systems. Presentation at the annual meeting of the American Speech-Language-Hearing Association, New Orleans, LA. [Abstract in *Asha*, 36(10), 173.]

Glascoe, G. J. (1984a). *Audiometer Simulator* [Computer program]. State College, PA: Parrot Software.

Glascoe, G. J. (1984b). *Hearing Aid Manager* [Computer program]. State College, PA: Parrot Software.

Glascoe, G. J. (1984c). *Selecting a Hearing Aid* [Computer program]. State College, PA: Parrot Software.

Glasofer, J. T. (1986). Visual/Reading Drills [Review of computer program]. *Asha*, 28(4), 85–86.

Glasofer, J. T. (1992). Tailor Story [Review of computer program]. *Asha*, 34(5), 93–94.

Glassman, D. M. (1986). Computer Managed Screening Test [Review of computer program]. *Asha*, 28(1), 69–70.

Glassman, D. M. (1988). Kidwriter [Review of computer program]. *Asha*, 30(2), 70.

Glassmann, D. M., & Quinoa, J. (1991). The computer, client, and you: An interactive approach. Presentation at the annual meeting of the American Speech-Language-Hearing Association, Atlanta, GA. [Abstract in *Asha*, 33(10), 81.]

Glassman, J. R., & Fickes, R. C. (1991). Stop! look! listen & learn—Computer uses for MR settings. Presentation at the annual meeting of the American Speech-Language-Hearing Association, Atlanta, GA. [Abstract in *Asha*, 33(10), 192.]

Glisky, E. L., Schacter, D. L., & Tulving, E. (1986a). Computer learning by memory-impaired patients: Acquisition and retention of complex knowledge. *Neuropsychologica*, 24, 313–328.

Glisky, E. L., Schacter, D. L., & Tulving, E. (1986b). Learning and retention of computer-related vocabulary in memory-impaired patients: Method of vanishing cues. *Journal of Clinical and Experimental Neuropsychology*, 8, 292–312.

Goalquest: IEP Writer (no date) [Computer program]. Napa, California: Lingquest Software.

Goebel, M. D. (1984). A computer-piloted fluency treatment program using visual biofeeback. Presentation at the annual meeting of the American Speech-Language-Hearing Association, San Francisco, CA. [Abstract in *Asha*, 26(10), 62.]

Goldenberg, E. P., Russell, S. J., and Carter, C. J. (1984). *Computers, Education and Special Needs*. Reading, Massachusetts: Addison Wesley.

Goldman, R., & Dahle, A. J. (1985). Current and emerging applications of microcomputer technology in communication disorders. *Topics in Language Disorders*, 6, 11–25.

Goldojarb, M. F. (1985). A system for organizing computer software. Presentation at the annual meeting of the American Speech-Language-Hearing Association, Washington, DC. [Abstract in *Asha*, 27(10), 89.]

Goldojarb, M. F. (198•). *Goldojarb Software Classification System (GSCS)* [Computer program]. Los Angeles, CA: Sunset Software, 11750 Sunset Blvd.

Goldojarb, M. F., & Secor, J. (1987). *Slow Speech-Rate Drill for Dysarthric Speakers* [Computer program]. Los Angeles, CA: Sunset Software, 11750 Sunset Blvd.

Goldojarb, M. F., & Secor, J. (1989). *Practice Speech for the Laryngectomee* [Computer program]. Los Angeles, CA: Sunset Software, 11750 Sunset Blvd.

Golub, H. L., & Corwin, M. J. (1982). Infant cry: A clue to diagnosis. *Pediatrics*, 69(2), 197–201.

Goodman, D. (1988). *Danny Goodman's HyperCard Developer's Guide*. New York: Bantam Books.

Goodman, D. (1990). *The Complete HyperCard 2.0 Handbook* (3rd Ed.). New York: Bantam Books.

Gould, H. J., & Matesich, J. (1991). A program for obtaining the ABR using an FSP technique. Presentation at the annual meeting of the American Speech-Language-Hearing Association, Atlanta, GA. [Abstract in *Asha*, 33(10), 192.]

Graetz, P. A. M. (1994). The Dutch Speech Pathology Information System for quality improvement. Presentation at the annual meeting of the American Speech-Language-Hearing Association, New Orleans, LA. [Abstract in *Asha*, 36(10), 247.]

Greentree Group (1986). *Parables Plus* [Computer program]. Mohnton, PA: The Greentree Group, P.O. Box 28.

Gregg, E. M., Egan, D. A., & Hanks, J. M. (1991). Evaluating the clinical uses of SALT and Computerized Profiling. Presentation at the annual meeting of the American Speech-Language-Hearing Association, Atlanta, GA. [Abstract in *Asha*, 33(10), 151.]

Gregg, E. M., & Gregg, J. G. (1994). ToolBook: An authoring environment for developing instructional software. Presentation at the annual meeting of the American Speech-Language-Hearing Association, New Orleans, LA. [Abstract in *Asha*, 36(10), 175.]

Greyerbiehl, D., Chial, M. Schwartz, A. Owens, A., & Blackstone, S. (1986). *User System for Evaluating and Reviewing Software: Indepth Review*. Rockville, MD: American Speech-Language-Hearing Association.

Greyerbiehl, D., Schwartz, A., Clymer, W., Owens, A., & Blackstone, S. (1986). *User System for Evaluating and Reviewing Software: Screening and Evaluation*. Rockville, MD: American Speech-Language-Hearing Association.

Grimm, L. (1986a). *Moptown Hotel* [Computer program]. Menlo Park, CA: The Learning Company, 545 Middlefield Road.

Grimm, L. (1986b). *Moptown Parade* [Computer program]. Menlo Park, CA: The Learning Company, 545 Middlefield Road.

Grimm, L., Caswell, D., Genoar, G., Weber, S., Gordon, S., Rowe, P., Suid, M., & Suid, A. (1987). *Writer Rabbit* [Computer program]. Menlo Park, CA: The Learning Company, 545 Middlefield Road.

Grossfeld, M. L., & Grossfeld, C. A. (Eds.) (1986). *Microcomputer Applications in Rehabilitation of Communication Disorders*. Rockville, MD: Aspen.

Grossman, K., Siders, J., & Garraway, H. (1983). Sign Teacher: A microcomputer application for the teaching of sign language. *American Annals of the Deaf*, 128, 577–584.

Gsell, J. (1990). Building a foundation of success within a shared context. *Journal for Computer Users in Speech and Hearing*, 6(1), 44–45.

Guillemin, B. J., & Nguyen, D. T. (1984). Microprocessor based speech processing system. *Journal of Speech and Hearing Research*, 27, 311–317.

Gulian, E., Hinds, P., Fallside, F., & Brooks, S. (1983). Vowel learning and the vowel system of deaf children: Age and feedback-related differences. *Journal of Communication Disorders*, 16(6), 449–469.

Gulian, E., Hinds, P., & Nimmo-Smith, I. (1986). Modifications of deaf children's vowel production: Perceptual evidence. *British Journal of Audiology*, 20, 181–194.

Guss, M. B. (1980). Computer application to literature review in speech, language, and hearing. Presentation at the annual meeting of the American Speech-Language-Hearing Association, Detroit, MI. [Abstract in *Asha*, 23(9), 686.]

GW Instruments (1986). *MacADIOS 411 Instruction Manual, Version 2.0.* Cambridge, MA: GW Instruments.

Hadjian, S., Drumm, M. J., & Haynes-Drumm, M. (1994). Development of an /s/ listener-training program. Presentation at the annual meeting of the American Speech-Language-Hearing Association, New Orleans, LA. [Abstract in *Asha*, 36(10), 107.]

Hadjian, S., Drumm, M. J., & Haynes-Drumm, M. (1995). A computerized /s/ listener-training program. Presentation at the annual meeting of the American Speech-Language-Hearing Association, Orlando, FL. [Abstract in *Asha*, 37(10), 52.]

Hallett, T. L. (1995). Introducing multimedia software: Tools and technology for clinicians and professors. Presentation at the annual meeting of the American Speech-Language-Hearing Association, Orlando, FL. [Abstract in *Asha*, 37(10), 100.]

Hallett, T. L., Pezzaro, D. B., & Pounds, J. L. (1986). Computer-assisted articulation therapy and our changing role. Presentation at the annual meeting of the American Speech-Language-Hearing Association, Detroit, MI. [Abstract in *Asha*, 28(10), 158.]

Hallett, T. L., & Hallett, J. B. (1987). Applying computerized artifical intelligence to language assessment: A new frontier. Presentation at the annual meeting of the American Speech-Language-Hearing Association, New Orleans, LA. [Abstract in *Asha*, 29(10), 102.]

Hallis, J. W. (1992). Perceptual scaling of speech attributes: A clinical assessment procedure. Presentation at the annual meeting of the American Speech-Language-Hearing Association, San Antonio, TX. [Abstract in *Asha*, 34(10), 134.]

Halpin, C., Wynne, M., Wilson, W., & Gravel, J. (1992). A detailed look at VRA using video disc. Presentation at the annual meeting of the American Speech-Language-Hearing Association, San Antonio, TX. [Abstract in *Asha*, 34(10), 141.]

Han, Y., Hou, Z., & Thornton, A. R. (1993). Expert system audiometry report generator. Presentation at the annual meeting of the American Speech-Language-Hearing Association, Anaheim, CA. [Abstract in *Asha*, 35(10), 216.]

Han, Y., Thornton, A. R., & Halpin, C. F. (1994). Expert-system decision support for clinical pure tone masking. Presentation at the annual meeting of the American Speech-Language-Hearing Association, New Orleans, LA. [Abstract in *Asha*, 36(10), 106.]

Hanavan, P. C. (1992). Delta Hearing Handicap and Presbycusis Software [Review of computer program]. *Asha*, 34(12), 90.

Hancock, R. S. (1986). *MacSpeech Lab Manual Version 2.0.* Cambridge, MA: GW Instruments.

Hanin, L., Boothroyd, A., & Hnath-Chisolm, T. (1988). The presentation of voice fundamental frequency as an aid to the speechreading of sentences. *Ear and Hearing*, 9, 335–341.

Hanson, J. K., & Hooper, C. R. (1988). A computerized treatment program for alexia without agraphia. Presentation at the annual meeting of the American Speech-Language-Hearing Association, Boston, MA. [Abstract in *Asha*, 30(10), 93.]

Harden, J. R., & Harden, R. W. (1983). Interactive computer collation of clinical practicum. Presentation at the annual meeting of the American Speech-Language-Hearing Association, Cincinnati, OH. [Abstract in *Asha*, 25(10), 118.]

Harden, J. C., & Harden, R. W. (1984). Microcomputer collation of clinical practice. Presentation at the annual meeting of the American Speech-Language-Hearing Association, San Francisco, CA. [Abstract in *Asha*, 26(10), 187.]

Harden, J. R., & Harden, R. W. (1985). Microcomputer collation of clinical practicum. Presentation at the annual meeting of the American Speech-Language-Hearing Association, Washington, DC. [Abstract in *Asha*, 27(10), 132.]

Harden, J. R., & Harden, R. W. (1986). Microcomputer program for the analysis of student's practicum performance. Presentation at the annual meeting of the American Speech-Language-Hearing Association, Detroit, MI. [Abstract in *Asha*, 28(10), 84.]

Harden, J. R., Harden, R. W., & Norris, M. (1977). Computer program for the analysis of clinical enrollment. *Asha*, 19, 472–474.

Harding, R., & Tidball, L. (1982). A national microcomputer software survey of current microcomputer usage in schools for the hearing impaired. *American Annals of the Deaf*, 127, 673–683.

Harlan, C. L. (1986). Telecommunication boards in speech-language pathology and audiology. Presentation at the annual meeting of the American Speech-Language-Hearing Association, Detroit, MI. [Abstract in *Asha*, 28(10), 168.]

Harlan, C. L. (1988). Customized computer augmentative communication via HyperCard. Presentation at the annual meeting of the American Speech-Language-Hearing Association, Boston, MA. [Abstract in *Asha*, 30(10), 113.]

Harlan, D. (1983). Computer-assisted procedures for processing communication disorders data. Unpublished thesis, Colorado State University.

Harlan, D. E., Larimore, H. W., & Smith, M. A. (1984). Computer processing of SICD data. *Asha*, 26(5), 23–25.

Harlan, N., & Hasegawa, A. (1976). Computer processing of graduate students' clinical clock hours as needed for *ASHA* certification. *Asha*, 18, 295–300.

Harley Courseware (1987). *Language Arts Series II: Antonyms/Synonyms* [Computer program]. Dimondale, MI: Harley Courseware.

Harn, W. E. (1986). Facilitating acquisition of subject-verb utterances in children: Actions, Animation and pictures. *Journal for Computer Users in Speech and Hearing*, 2(2), 95–101.

Harn, W. E. (1992). Computerized Language Error Analysis Report (CLEAR) [Review of computer program]. *Journal for Computer Users in Speech and Hearing*, 8(1, 2), 154–156.

Harn, W. E., & Ruder, K. F. (1987). Microcomputer animation: Clinical and research applications. Presentation at the annual meeting of the American Speech-Language-Hearing Association, New Orleans, LA. [Abstract in *Asha*, 29(10), 163.]

Harnadek, A., & Boeing, B. (1991). *Mind Benders: Sets A1, A2, and B1* [Computer programs]. Pacific Grove, PA: Critical Thinking Press & Software, P. O. Box 448.

Harris, D. A. (1979). Microprocessor, self-recording and manual audiometry. *Journal of Auditory Research*, 19(3), 159–166.

Harris, D. A. (1979). Microprocessor versus self-recording audiometry in industry. *Journal of Auditory Research*, 19(2), 137–149.

Harris, J. D. (1980). A comparison of computerized audiometry by ANSI, Bekesy fixed-frequency, and modified ISO procedures in an industrial hearing conservation program. *Journal of Auditory Research*, 20, 143–167.

Harris, L. M., Skarakis-Doyle, E., Haaf, R., & Doyle, P. (1993). Language intervention for children with severe speech and physical impairments. Presentation at the annual meeting of the American Speech-Language-Hearing Association, Anaheim, CA. [Abstract in *Asha*, 35(10), 126.]

Harris, R. W., & Channell, R. W. (1993). Automated presentation of speech audiometry material on compact disc. Presentation at the annual meeting of the American Speech-Language-Hearing Association, Anaheim, CA. [Abstract in *Asha*, 35(10), 222.]

Harris, R. W., Hilton, L. M., McPherson, D. M., & Hanks, W. D. (1993). Digital audio editing, sample editing, and compact disc mastering. Presentation at the annual meeting of the American Speech-Language-Hearing Association, Anaheim, CA. [Abstract in *Asha*, 35(10), 173.]

Harrison, J. E., & Engelman, D. A. (1992). Teaching basic concepts: Does commercial software help? Presentation at the annual meeting of the American Speech-Language-Hearing Association, San Antonio, TX. [Abstract in *Asha*, 34(10), 161.]

Hart, T. L. (1983). Computer assisted teaching of basic concepts and sight words. Presentation at the annual meeting of the American Speech-Language-Hearing Association, Cincinnati, OH. [Abstract in *Asha*, 25(10), 80.]

Hartley Software (1987). *Opposites* [Computer program]. Dimondale, MI: Hartley Software.

Hartman, K. M. (1989). Microcomputer use in supervision: Current practices. Presentation at the annual meeting of the American Speech-Language-Hearing Association, St. Louis, MO. [Abstract in *Asha*, 31(10), 132.]

Hasegawa, A., and Mahshie, J. J. (1984). Computerized approach to improvement of deaf speakers' voice production. Presentation at the annual meeting of the American Speech-Language-Hearing Association, San Francisco, CA. [Abstract in *Asha*, 26(10), 100.]

Hashimoto, T., Murata, K., Minami, S., Taniguchi, I., & Katayama, Y. (1977). Computer-aided group audiometry. *Journal of Auditory Research*, 17, 59–76.

Haux, S., & Shewan, C. M. (December, 1991). Computers and professional use. *Asha*, 33, 47.

Hazan, P. (Ed.) (1981). *Proceedings of the Johns Hopkins First National Search for Applications of Personal Computing to Aid the Handicapped.* Los Angeles, CA: IEEE Society Press.

Healey, E. C., & Tice, R. L. (1986). Vocal fundamental frequency and intensity analysis program. Presentation at the American Speech-Language-Hearing Foundation Conference, Orlando, FL.

Healey, E. C., & Tice, R. L. (1991). A fundamental frequency and intensity analysis program for the Apple IIe/gs. *Journal for Computer Users in Speech and Hearing*, 7(1), 29–34.

Healey, E. C., & Beukelman, D. R. (1988). Computerized cueing therapy. Presentation at the annual meeting of the American Speech-Language-Hearing Association, Boston, MA. [Abstract in *Asha*, 30(10), 179.]

Healey, E. C., Beukelman, D., Turton, L., & Cronk, C. (1987). A comparison of microcomputer software for the acoustical analysis of the voice. Presentation at the American Speech-Language-Hearing Foundation Conference, Houston.

Heinbaugh, C., Evans, T., & Weiner, F. F. (1995). *Minimal Contrast Stories* [Computer program]. West Bloomfield, MI: Parrot Software.

Heob, W. G., Carter, R. G., Jochum, J. A., & Dutcher, L. (1984). Computer application in a school hearing screening program. Presentation at the annual meeting of the American Speech-Language-Hearing Association, San Francisco, CA. [Abstract in *Asha*, 26(10), 78.]

Herman, G. (1989). MacADIOS and MacSpeech Lab as instructional tools. *Journal for Computer Users in Speech and Hearing*, 5(2), 62–72.

Hetzroni, O. E., Lloyd, L. L., & Quist, R. W. (1994). Computer versus teacher effectiveness on Blissymbol learning by AAC students. Presentation at the annual meeting of the American Speech-Language-Hearing Association, New Orleans, LA. [Abstract in *Asha*, 36(10), 174.]

Higgins, J. M., Baker, B. R., Nyberg 3rd, E. H., & Kushler, C. A. (1989). The future of artifical intelligence in augmentative and alternative communication. Presentation at the annual meeting of the American Speech-Language-Hearing Association, St. Louis, MO. [Abstract in *Asha*, 31(10), 56.]

Hight, R. L. (1981). Lip-reader trainer: A computer program for the hearing impaired. In *Proceedings of the John Hopkins First National Search for Applications of Personal Computing to Aid the Handicapped.* Los Angeles, CA: IEEE Computer Society Press.

Hillard, S. W., & Gilbertson, M. L. (1987). Computer-assisted intervention with the school-age child who stutters. Presentation at the annual meeting of the American Speech-Language-Hearing Association, New Orleans, LA. [Abstract in *Asha*, 29(10), 99.]

Hillinger, M., Fox, B., & Wilson, M. (1981). Computer-enhanced communication systems for the Apple II. In *Proceedings of the Johns Hopkins First National Search for Applications of Personal Computing to Aid the Handicapped.* Los Angeles, CA: IEEE Computer Society Press.

Hillis, J. W. (1991a). Computer-assisted supervision in the management of speech fluency disorders. Presentation at the annual meeting of the American Speech-Language-Hearing Association, Atlanta, GA. [Abstract in *Asha*, 33(10), 188.]

Hillis, J. W. (1991b). A method for improving perceptual identification of speech characteristics. Presentation at the annual meeting of the American Speech-Language-Hearing Association, Atlanta, GA. [Abstract in *Asha*, 33(10), 123.]

Hillis, J. W. (1994). Perceptual managment of "speechflow obstructions": A treatment approach for stuttering. Presentation at the annual meeting of the American Speech-Language-Hearing Association, New Orleans, LA. [Abstract in *Asha*, 36(10), 107–108.]

Hinckley, J. J., Packard, M. W., & Bardach, L. (1995). Computers as tools to achieve functional outcomes in language rehabilitation. Presentation at the annual meeting of the American Speech-Language-Hearing Association, Orlando, FL. [Abstract in *Asha*, 37(10), 94.]

Hixon, T. J., Bayles, K. A., Tomoeda, C. K., & Lynch, II, D. J. (1992). CENTER-NET and TELEROUNDS: Linking scientists and practitioners. Presentation at the annual meeting of the American Speech-Language-Hearing Association, San Antonio, TX. [Abstract in *Asha*, 34(10), 126.]

Hmelo, C. (1990). Computer-assisted instruction in health professions education: A review of the published literature. *Journal of Educational Technology Systems*, 18(2), 83–101.

Hnath-Chisolm, T., & Kishon-Rabin, L. (1988). Tactile presentation of voice fundamental frequency as an aid to the perception of speech pattern contrasts. *Ear and Hearing*, 9, 329–334.

Hodson, B. W. (1985). *Computer Analysis of Phonological Processes* [Computer program]. Stonington, IL: Phono Comp, Box 46.

Hodson, B. W., & Oller, D. K. (1992). Clinician-friendly computer analysis of phonological deviations: English and Spanish. Presentation at the annual meeting of the American Speech-Language-Hearing Association, San Antonio, TX. [Abstract in *Asha*, 34(10), 141–142.]

Holcombe, M. W., & Stein, J. K. (1983). *Presentations for Decision Makers* New York: Van Nostrand Reinhold.

Hood, J. R. (1984). *Articulation Error Analysis (AEA) Software* [Computer program]. Burlington, NC: Southern MicroSystems.

Hood, R. B., & Zimmerman, H. R. (1980). Computerized audiometric programmable simulator (CAPS). Scientific exhibit presented at the annual meeting of the American Speech-Language-Hearing Association, Detroit, MI.

Hood, R. B., & Zimmerman, H. R. (1981). Computerized audiometric programmable simulator. *Hearing Aid Journal*, 34, 6, 20.

Hood, S. B. (1986). The Clock Hours Program [Review of computer program]. *Journal for Computer Users in Speech and Hearing*, 2(1), 38–39.

Hood, S. B., & Miller, L. R. (1982). Computer assisted management of client, clinician, and clinic records. Presentation at the annual meeting of the American Speech-Language-Hearing Association, Toronto, Canada. [Abstract in *Asha*, 24(10), 746.]

Hood, S. B., & Miller, L. R. (1984). Administrative applications for microcomputers. In A. H. Schwartz (Ed.), *Handbook of Microcomputer Applications in Communication Disorders.* San Diego, CA: College-Hill, 219–245.

Horii, Y. (1986). Finger-tapping tasks in studying hemispheric specialization for language processing. *Journal for Computer Users in Speech and Hearing*, 2(1), 18–24.

Horn, D. (1986). Computer-Managed Articulation Diagnosis [Review of computer program]. *Journal for Computer Users in Speech and Hearing*, 2(1), 43.

Horton, W. K. (1990). *Designing and Writing Online Documentation: Help Files to Hypertext.* New York: John Wiley & Sons.

Houle, G. R. (1988). Computer usage by speech-language pathologists in public schools. Presentation at the annual meeting of the American Speech-Language-Hearing Association, Boston, MA. [Abstract in *Asha*, 30(10), 166–167.]

House, L. I., & House, T. D. (1994). Using touch window programs with severe/profound individuals. Presentation at the annual meeting of the American Speech-Language-Hearing Association, New Orleans, LA. [Abstract in *Asha*, 36(10), 76.]

Howard, R. A. (1986). Microcomputer applications in speech pathology. In J. L. Northern (Ed.), *The Personal Computer for Speech, Language, and Hearing Professionals*, Boston: Little, Brown, 75–84.

Huang, D., Minifie, F. D., & Lin, S. (1992). An integrated clinical program for voice evaluation and therapy. Presentation at the annual meeting of the American Speech-Language-Hearing Association, San Antonio, TX. [Abstract in *Asha*, 34(10), 109.]

Huckabee, M. L., Kelly-Arsenault, J., & Goldsmith, T. (1993). An accelerated dysphagia treatment program: Utilization of EMG biofeedback. Presentation at the annual meeting of the American Speech-Language-Hearing Association, Anaheim, CA. [Abstract in *Asha*, 35(10), 222.]

Huckle, N., Haaf, R. G., & Doyle, P. C. (1995). Computerized recognition of consonants produced by a severely dysarthric speaker. Presentation at the annual meeting of the American Speech-Language-Hearing Association, Orlando, FL. [Abstract in *Asha*, 37(10), 77.]

Huer, M. K. (1986). The Clock Hour Program [Review of computer program]. *Asha*, 28(4), 86–87.

Huer, M. K. (1991). Boardmaker: The PCS Libraries on Disk [Review of computer program]. *Asha*, 33(2), 83.

Hugghins, M. (1987). Using the Radio Shack Color Computer. *Journal for Computer Users in Speech and Hearing*, 3(2), 131.

Hughes, D. L., Fey, M. E., Kertoy, M. K., & Nelson, N. W. (1994). Computer-assisted instruction for learning developmental sentence scoring: An experimental comparison. *American Journal of Speech-Language Pathology*, 3(3), 89–95.

Hughes, D. L., Lehman, M. E., Soukanec, G. P., & Tatchell, R. H. (1993). Computer technology: Use in training programs. *Asha*, 35(8), 38–39.

Hughes, D. L., & Low, W. C. (1989). Computer-assisted tutorial for learning DDS. Presentation at the annual meeting of the American Speech-Language-Hearing Association, St. Louis, MO. [Abstract in *Asha*, 31(10), 86.]

Hughes, D. L., & Low, W. C. (1990). Learning Developmental Sentence Scoring: A computerized tutorial. *Journal for Computer Users in Speech and Hearing*, 6(2), 149–157.

Hughes, D. L., Low, W., Fey, M., & Alsop, W. (1990). *Computer-Assisted Tutorial for Learning Developmental Sentence Scoring* [Computer program]. Mt. Pleasant, MI: Central Michigan University, Department of Communication Disorders.

Humanities Software (1991). *Story Tailor* [Computer program]. Hood River, OR: Humanities Software, 408 Columbia, Suite 222.

Humes, L. E. (1990). *Shape (Selecting Hearing Aids for Patients Effectively)* [Computer program]. Bloomington, IN: Venture 4th, 2003 Montclair Avenue.

Huntley, R. A., Williams, A. L., & Gonzalez-Rothi, L. J. (1985). Computerized treatment of surface dyslexia. Presentation at the annual meeting of the American Speech-Language-Hearing Association, Washington, DC. [Abstract in *Asha*, 27(10), 123.]

Hurvitz, J. A., Goldojarb, M. F., Walcek, A. M., & Levin, K. L. M. (1987). Comparison of two aural rehabilitation methods in a nursing home. Presentation at the annual meeting of the

American Speech-Language-Hearing Association, New Orleans, LA. [Abstract in *Asha*, 29(10), 129.]

Hyman, C. S. (1985). Computer usage in the speech-language pathology and audiology profession. Presentation at the annual meeting of the American Speech-Language-Hearing Association, Washington, DC. [Abstract in *Asha*, 27(10), 89.]

Hyman, C. S. (1985). Computer usage in the speech-language-hearing profession. *Asha*, 27(11), 25.

Ifft, L. M. (1991). CAFET with functional and organic voice disorders. Presentation at the annual meeting of the American Speech-Language-Hearing Association, Atlanta, GA. [Abstract in *Asha*, 33(10), 135.]

Ilecki, H. J. (1985). Computer-controlled diagnostic audiology: Validity and reliability. Presentation at the American Speech and Hearing Conference on Microcomputers, New Orleans, LA. [Abstract in the *Journal for Computer Users in Speech and Hearing*, 1(2), 78–79.]

Ilecki, H. J., & Picard, M. (1991). The use of computerized audiometry in different clinical groups. Presentation at the annual meeting of the American Speech-Language-Hearing Association, Atlanta, GA. [Abstract in *Asha*, 33(10), 161.]

Imhoff, T. E. (1986). Computer print shop: Entrepreneurship, a vehicle for head injury rehabilitation. Presentation at the annual meeting of the American Speech-Language-Hearing Association, Detroit, MI. [Abstract in *Asha*, 28(10), 116.]

Ingram, D., & Pye, C. (1992). The use of computer adventure games as a research tool. Presentation at the annual meeting of the American Speech-Language-Hearing Association, San Antonio, TX. [Abstract in *Asha*, 34(10), 187.]

Internet (1995). *Asha*, 37(5), 28.

Iverson, A. M. (1990). *SunTool Speech/Language IEP Writer+* [Computer program]. Bedford, IA: Ivy Sun, Rt. 2 Box 66.

Iverson, A. M., & Iverson, S. J. (1991). Confessions of a small software developer: How to get rich in a short time with very little effort. *Journal for Computer Users in Speech and Hearing*, 7(1), 98–103.

Jackson, C. O. (1983). Use of microcomputers for school hearing screening and evaluation records. Presentation at the annual meeting of the American Speech-Language-Hearing Association, Cincinnati, OH. [Abstract in *Asha*, 25(10), 117.]

Jackson, C. O. (1986a). Hearing aid software selection. *Asha*, 28(7), 25–28.

Jackson, C. O. (1986b).Microcomputers in assessment and rehabilitation of the hearing-impaired. In M. L. Grossfeld & C. A. Grossfeld (Eds.), *Microcomputer Applications in Rehabilitation of Communication Disorders*. Rockville, MD: Aspen, pp. 43–66.

Jay, R. E., & Kifer, L. M. (1981). Computer assisted selection of hearing aids. Presentation at the annual meeting of the American Speech-Language-Hearing Association, Los Angeles, CA. [Abstract in *Asha*, 23(10), 808.]

Jay, R. E., & Mahaffey, R. B. (1984). Adaptation of a microcomputer to pseudohypoacusis detection. Presentation at the annual meeting of the American Speech-Language-Hearing Association, San Francisco, CA. [Abstract in *Asha*, 26(10), 148.]

Jenkins, M. (1987). Effect of a computerized individual education program (IEP) writer on time savings and quality. *Journal of Special Education Technology*, 3, 55–66.

Jerivall, L., Dryselius, H., & Arlinger, S. (1983). Comparison of manual and computer-controlled audiometry using identical procedures. *Scandinavian Audiology*, 12(3), 209–213.

Jinks, A. F. (1985). Using the home computer for language treatment. Presentation at the American Speech and Hearing Foundation Conference on Microcomputers, New Orleans, LA. [Abstract in the *Journal for Computer Users in Speech and Hearing*, 1(2), 79–80.]

Johnson, B., & Johnson, R. (1984). *Computer Software for the Exceptional Student* [Computer program]. Tucson, AZ: Communication Skill Builders.

Johnson, B. W., & Channell, R. W. (1992). Automated grammatical tagging of spoken and written language samples. Presentation at the annual meeting of the American Speech-Language-Hearing Association, San Antonio, TX. [Abstract in *Asha*, 34(10), 166.]

Johnson, C. L., & Kasica, A. (1984). Computer system programmed for use by adult aphasics. Presentation at the annual meeting of the American Speech-Language-Hearing Association, San Francisco, CA. [Abstract in *Asha*, 26(10), 188.]

Johnson, W. (1946). *People in Quandaries*. New York: Harper & Row.

Jones, B. W., & Grygar, J. (1982). The test of syntactic abilities and microcomputers. *American Annals of the Deaf*, 127, 5–7, 638–644.

Jones, R. S., Beukelman, D. R., & Ulrich, P. A. (1993). Comparison of keystroke savings for Macintosh computers. Presentation at the annual meeting of the American Speech-Language-Hearing Association, Anaheim, CA. [Abstract in *Asha*, 35(10), 171.]

Jordahl, N., Harris, M. D., & Hayden, P. A. (1981). A computerized tracking center for developmentally delayed children: Rural model. Presentation at the annual meeting of the American Speech-Language-Hearing Association, Los Angeles, CA. [Abstract in *Asha*, 23(10), 723.]

Kaasgaard, K., & Lauritsen, P. (1995). The use of computers in cognitive rehabilitation in Denmark. *American Journal of Speech-Language Pathology*, 4(2), 5–8.

Kamara, C., & Kamara, A. (1976). Computer billing, service analysis, and financial reporting in a hearing and speech agency. *Asha*, 18, 229–236.

Kamin, A., Joblin, M., & Weiner, F. F. (1995a). *Cognitive Disorders* 4: Memory for Pictures [Computer program]. West Bloomfield, MI: Parrot Software.

Kamin, A., Joblin, M., & Weiner, F. F. (1995b). *Preposition Fill-ins* [Computer program]. West Bloomfield, MI: Parrot Software.

Kamin, A., Joblin, M., & Weiner, F. F. (1995c). *Verb Fill-ins* [Computer program]. West Bloomfield, MI: Parrot Software.

Kapur, R. (1989). Words and Concepts [Review of computer program]. *Asha*, 31(12), 71.

Karnell, M. P. (1992a). Data base storage, retrieval, and reporting of videoendoscopic velopharyngeal evaluations. Presentation at the annual meeting of the American Speech-Language-Hearing Association, San Antonio, TX. [Abstract in *Asha*, 34(10), 115].

Karnell, M. P. (1992b). Data base storage, retrieval, and reporting of videostroboscopic voice data. Presentation at the annual meeting of the American Speech-Language-Hearing Association, San Antonio, TX. [Abstract in *Asha*, 34(10), 156.]

Karnell, M. P., & MacCracken, E. (1992). Data base storage, retrieval, and reporting of videofluorographic swallowing evaluations. Presentation at the annual meeting of the American Speech-Language-Hearing Association, San Antonio, TX. [Abstract in *Asha*, 34(10), 121.]

Karnell, M. P., & MacCracken, E. (1993). Data base storage, retrieval, and reporting of videofluorographic swallowing. Presentation at the annual meeting of the American Speech-Language-Hearing Association, Anaheim, CA. [Abstract in *Asha*, 35(10), 105.]

Karnell, M. P., & MacCracken, E. (1994). A database information storage and reporting system for videofluorographic oropharyngeal motility (OPM) swallowing evaluations. *American Journal of Speech-Language Pathology*, 3(2), 54–60.

Kataoka, R., Mayo, R., Zajac, D., Kataoka, T., & Warren, D. W. (1995). A microcomputer-based system for assessing hypernasality in cleft palate speakers. Presentation at the annual meeting of the American Speech-Language-Hearing Association, Orlando, FL. [Abstract in *Asha*, 37(10), 49.]

Katz, J., Yeung, E., & Medwetsky, L. (1990). *SSW C*I*R* [Computer program]. Amherst, NY: JIMM Company, 113 Kaymar Drive.

Katz, K. (1983). Computers . . . every office needs one! *Hearing Instruments*, 34, 7.

Katz, R. C. (1983a). *Keyboarder* [Computer program]. Los Angeles, CA: Sunset Software.

Katz, R. C. (1983b). *PICAPAD* [Computer program]. Los Angeles, CA: Sunset Software.

Katz, R. C. (1983c). *Understanding Questions* [Computer program]. Los Angeles, CA: Sunset Software.

Katz, R. C. (1983d). *Understanding Stories* [Computer program]. Los Angeles, CA: Sunset Software.

Katz, R. C. (1984). Using microcomputers in the diagnosis and treatment of chronic aphasic adults. *Seminars in Speech and Language*, 5, 11–22.

Katz, R. C. (1985a). Coding treatment in BASIC. Presentation at the annual meeting of the American Speech-Language-Hearing Association, Washington, DC. [Abstract in *Asha*, 27(10), 59.]

Katz, R. C. (1985b). *Holiday* [Computer program]. Los Angeles, CA: Sunset Software, 11750 Sunset Boulevard.

Katz, R. C. (1985c). *Understanding Questions* [Computer program]. Los Angeles, CA: Sunset Software, 11750 Sunset Boulevard.

Katz, R. C. (1985d). *Visual/Reading Drills* [Computer program]. Los Angeles, CA: Sunset Software, 11750 Sunset Boulevard.

Katz, R. C. (1986). *Aphasia Treatment and Microcomputers*. San Diego: College-Hill Press/Little, Brown & Company.

Katz, R. C. (1991). *Cognitive Drills Set 1: Visual Tasks* [Computer program]. Scottsdale, AZ: Sunset Software, 9277 East Corrine Drive.

Katz, R. C., & Nagy, V. T. (1982). A computerized treatment system for chronic aphasic adults. In R. H. Brookshire (Ed.), *Clinical Aphasiology: Conference Proceedings 1982*. Minneapolis, MN: BRK Publishers.

Katz, R. C., & Porch, B. E. (1987). *PICApad II: PICA Report Generating Program* [Computer program]. Los Angeles, CA: Sunset Software.

Katz, R. C., Wertz, R. T., Davidoff, M., Shubitowski, Y. D., & Devitt, E. W. (1988). Improving written confrontation naming in aphasia using a computer program. Presentation at the annual meeting of the American Speech-Language-Hearing Association, Boston, MA. [Abstract in *Asha*, 30(10), 93.]

Katz, R. C., Wertz, R. T., Lewis, S. M., Esparza, C., & Goldojarb, M. (1989). Computerized reading treatment versus stimulation and no treatment for aphasia. Presentation at the annual meeting of the American Speech-Language-Hearing Association, St. Louis, MO. [Abstract in *Asha*, 31(10), 61.]

Kavanaugh, K. T. (1991). *Delta Hearing Handicap and Presbycusis Software* [Computer program]. Bartlett, TN: Delta Medical Shareware, Inc., 9170 Ellen Davies Drive.

Keating, D. L., Evans, A. L., Wyper, D. J., & Cunningham, E. (1986). A comparison of the intelligibility of some low cost speech synthesis devices. *British Journal of Disorders of Communication*, 21, 167–172.

Kehr, K., & Gumbiner-Roeder, T. (1993). Computer use for expanding preschool language for children with disabilities. Presentation at the annual meeting of the American Speech-Language-Hearing Association, Anaheim, CA. [Abstract in *Asha*, 35(10), 178.]

Kellum, G. D., Robinson, Jr., T. L., & Cole, P. A. (1990). Computerized library/information systems as a clinical tool. Presentation at the annual meeting of the American Speech-Language-Hearing Association, Seattle, WA. [Abstract in *Asha*, 32(10), 89.]

Kelly, B. R., Hegde, G., Hegde, P., Azevado, D., Roberts, S. D., & Bryant, J. (1992). You too can program interactive instructional modules. Presentation at the annual meeting of the American Speech-Language-Hearing Association, San Antonio, TX. [Abstract in *Asha*, 34(10), 177–178.]

Kelly, P. A., Richmond, D. M., Wesolowski, B. D., & Heuer, B. (1987). Computer based speech-language phase II IEPs using Appleworks. Presentation at the annual meeting of the American Speech-Language-Hearing Association, New Orleans, LA. [Abstract in *Asha*, 29(10), 99.]

Kennedy, K. A. (1986). Computer Analysis of Phonological Processes [Review of computer program]. *Asha*, 28(8), 71.

Kennedy, K. A. (1989). *ASHA* Project Impact: #1 Overview of Microcomputer Applications for Speech, Language, and Hearing Professionals [Review of computer program]. *Asha*, 31(12), 72.

Kennedy, M. D., Radlinski, S. S., & Sheridan, M. K. (1991). Using the IBM SpeechViewer with severely delayed young children. Presentation at the annual meeting of the American Speech-Language-Hearing Association, Atlanta, GA. [Abstract in *Asha*, 33(10), 188.]

Kennedy, S., & Yonovitz, A. (1991). A computer-enabled 32–channel FM auditory trainer. Presentation at the annual meeting of the American Speech-Language-Hearing Association, Atlanta, GA. [Abstract in *Asha*, 33(10), 93.]

Kerr, M., Healey, E. C., & Votipka, J. (1990). Comparisons of fundamental frequency measures across three microprocessor systems. Presentation at the annual meeting of the American Speech-Language-Hearing Association, Seattle, WA. [Abstract in *Asha*, 32(10), 76.]

Kersting, F. M. (1983). Clinic management information systems using a microcomputer. Presentation at the annual meeting of the American Speech-Language-Hearing Association, Cincinnati, OH. [Abstract in *Asha*, 25(10), 117.]

Kersting, F. M., & Beckner, C. L. (1979). Data system for retrieving and storing pertinent clinical information. Presentation at the annual meeting of the American Speech-Language-Hearing Association, Atlanta, GA. [Abstract in *Asha*, 21(9), 748.]

Kewley-Port, D., Watson, C. S., & Maki, D. P. (1991). Evaluation of speech recognizers for speech training applications. Presentation at the annual meeting of the American Speech-Language-Hearing Association, Atlanta, GA. [Abstract in *Asha*, 33(10), 161.]

Khoo, K. I., & Allington, T. B. (1993). Three modes of learning in an undergraduate hearing science course. Presentation at the annual meeting of the American Speech-Language-Hearing Association, Anaheim, CA. [Abstract in *Asha*, 35(10), 132.]

Kihneman, K. C., & Salathiel, R. M. (1981). Computer fingerspelling. In *Proceedings of the John Hopkins First National Search for Applications of Personal Computing to Aid the Handicapped*. Los Angeles, CA: IEEE Computer Society Press.

Killorin, V. S., & King, J. V. (1992). Using interactive video to train preservice personnel in communicative disorders. Presentation at the annual meeting of the American Speech-Language-Hearing Association, San Antonio, TX. [Abstract in *Asha*, 34(10), 156.]

Kimmerly, S. L. (1983). Using microcomputers for language intervention in public schools. Presentation at the annual meeting of the American Speech-Language-Hearing Association, Cincinnati, OH. [Abstract in *Asha*, 25(10), 100.]

Kimmerly, S. L., Fox, B. J., & Wilson, M. S. (1982). Developing microcomputer based augmentative communication systems: Pragmatic and linguistic considerations. Presentation at the annual meeting of the American Speech-Language-Hearing Association, Toronto, Canada. [Abstract in *Asha*, 24(10), 714.]

King, D. (1990). *Talking Symbols* [Computer program]. Solana Beach, CA: Mayer-Johnson.

King, J. M., & Hux, H. (1995). Intervention using talking word processing software: An aphasia case study. Presentation at the annual meeting of the American Speech-Language-Hearing Association, Orlando, FL. [Abstract in *Asha*, 37(10), 44.]

King, T. W. (1990). Morse code: Your next language. *Closing the Gap*, 9(3), 14.

King, T. W., Noel, E. M., Rounds, L. A., & Bergo, T. J. (1991). A comparison of visual and auditory methods of teaching Morse code in rehabilitation applications. *Closing the Gap*, 11, 12–13 & 31.

Klatt, D. H. (1985). Speech synthesis and recognition: Present and future. Presentation at the American Speech and Hearing Foundation Conference on Microcomputers, New

Orleans, LA. [Abstract in the *Journal for Computer Users in Speech and Hearing*, 1(2), 80.]

Klatt, D. H., Tetschner, W., Tiao, J., & Pisoni, D. (1984). Using DECtalk as an aid for the handicapped. Presentation at the annual meeting of the American Speech-Language-Hearing Association, San Francisco, CA. [Abstract in *Asha*, 26(10), 103.]

Kleczewska, M. K., Shapiro, L. P., Steele, R. D., & Weinrich, M. (1987). Design considerations for a Computer-Based Visual Communication System. Presentation at the annual meeting of the American Speech-Language-Hearing Association, New Orleans, LA. [Abstract in *Asha*, 29(10), 117.]

Klee, T. (1991). Transcribing children's language in real time. Presentation at the annual meeting of the American Speech-Language-Hearing Association, Atlanta, GA. [Abstract in *Asha*, 33(10), 151.]

Klee, T., Gavin, W. J., & Dismuke, R. P. (1985). Computer data base management for language sample analyses. Presentation at the annual meeting of the American Speech-Language-Hearing Association, Washington, DC. [Abstract in *Asha*, 27(10), 180.]

Klodd, D. A., & Hoyt, H. R. (1991). Managing your practice: The untapped resources of the microcomputer. Presentation at the annual meeting of the American Speech-Language-Hearing Association, Atlanta, GA. [Abstract in *Asha*, 33(10), 88.]

Kneil, T. R. (1991). Introduction to the decibel scale—A HyperCard stack. Presentation at the annual meeting of the American Speech-Language-Hearing Association, Atlanta, GA. [Abstract in *Asha*, 33(10), 187.]

Kneil, T. R. (1992a). Bringing sound and animation to HyperCard stacks. Presentation at the annual meeting of the American Speech-Language-Hearing Association, San Antonio, TX. [Abstract in *Asha*, 34(10), 134.]

Kneil, T. R. (1992b). Why HyperCard? *Journal for Computer Users in Speech and Hearing*, 8(1, 2), 75–78.

Kneil, T. R., Gordon, M. E., & Hodson, B. W. (1991). HyperCard instructional program for phonological processes. Presentation at the annual meeting of the American Speech-Language-Hearing Association, Atlanta, GA. [Abstract in *Asha*, 33(10), 187.]

Knox, J. A. (1986). Language Stimulation Software Series #2, Rebuilding Sentences: Syntax [Review of computer program]. *Asha*, 28(9), 77–78.

Knox, J. A. (1988a). Language Arts Series II: Antonyms/Synonyms [Review of computer program]. *Asha*, 30(2), 71.

Knox, J. A. (1988b). Opposites [Review of computer program]. *Asha*, 30(5), 79–80.

Knox, J. A. (1989). 40,000 Selected Words [Review of computer program]. *Asha*, 31(12), 71–72.

Knox, J. A. (1991). *What's My Logic. Figural and Figural/Verbal* [Review of computer program]. *Asha*, 33(8), 69.

Kojima, H., Gould, W. J., Lambiase, A., & Isshiki, N. (1980). Computer analysis of hoarseness. *Acta Otolaryngologica*, 89(5–6), 547–554.

Kopra, L. L., Dunlop, R. J., Kopra, M. A., & Abrahamson, J. E. (1985). Computer-assisted instruction in lipreading with a laser videodisc interactive system. Presentation at the American Speech and Hearing Foundation conference on microcomputers, New Orleans, LA. [Abstract in the *Journal for Computer Users in Speech and Hearing*, 1(2), 81.]

Kopra, L. L., Kopra, M. A., Abrahamson, J. E., & Dunlop, R. J. (1987). Lipreading drill and practice software for an auditory-visual laser videodisc interactive system (ALVIS). *Journal for Computer Users in Speech and Hearing*, 3(1), 58–68.

Korabic, E. W. (1993). Easy as 1–2–3: Using an electronic spreadsheet to calculate AIs. *Hearing Instruments*, 44(1), 28–29.

Korabic, E. W., Kuo, S. C., & Linville, S. E. (1986). Analysis of pitch perturbation (jitter) using a Visi-pitch and a microcomputer. *Journal for Computer Users in Speech and Hearing*, 2(2), 86–93.

Korabic, E. W., & Silverman, F. H. (1983). Low cost microcomputer-based augmentative communication system. Scientific exhibit at the annual meeting of the American Speech-Language-Hearing Association, Cincinnati, OH.

Korabic, E. W., Silverman, F. H., & Rosera, M. (1987). An inexpensive single-switch scanning communication aid. *Journal for Computer Users in Speech and Hearing*, 3(1), 34–38.

Kotler, A.-L., & Thomas-Stonell, N. L. (1993). Improving voice recognition of dysarthric speech through speech training. Presentation at the annual meeting of the American Speech-Language-Hearing Association, Anaheim, CA. [Abstract in *Asha*, 35(10), 120.]

Kouri, T. A., & Savage, M. L. (1993). Multimedia applications in clinical research: Desktop. Presentation at the annual meeting of the American Speech-Language-Hearing Association, Anaheim, CA. [Abstract in *Asha*, 35(10), 107.]

Kozma-Spytek, L., Bakke, M. H., & Chute, P. M. (1995). Computer-assisted notetaking: Providing access to classroom information. Presentation at the annual meeting of the American Speech-Language-Hearing Association, Orlando, FL. [Abstract in *Asha*, 37(10), 86.]

Krogulski, P. (1988). Aphasia VII: Picture Identification [Review of computer program]. *Asha*, 30(5), 78.

Krol, E. (1992). *The Whole Internet: User's Guide and Catalog*. Sebastopol, CA: O'Reilly & Associates.

Krueger, B. (1985). Computerized reporting in a public school program. *Language, Speech, and Hearing Services in Schools*, 16, 135–139.

Krueger, B. M., & Barker, K. D. (1983). Implementing use of computerized reporting in a public school program. Presentation at the annual meeting of the American Speech-Language-Hearing Association, Cincinnati, OH. [Abstract in *Asha*, 25(10), 129.]

Krupke, D. L. (1990). Making connections-networking: An Iowa effort. *Journal for Computer Users in Speech and Hearing*, 6(1), 54–56.

Kunicki, E. (1989). Words & Concepts III [Review of computer program]. *Journal for Computer Users in Speech and Hearing*, 5(2), 143–147.

Kurtis, J. (1990). PICAPAD II. Report Generator for the Porch Index of Communicative Ability [Review of computer program]. *Asha*, 32(12), 96–97.

Kuster, J. M. (1995a). The Internet—Providing important links for practicing professionals. *Asha*, 37(4), 29–30.

Kuster, J. M. (1995b). Internet in the news. *Asha*, 37(6/7), 34–35.

Kuster, J. M., & Kuster, T. A. (1995). Finding treasures on the Internet. *Asha*, 37(2), 43–47.

Lancker, D. V., Hall, E., Goldojarb, M., & Treiman, S. (1993). An interactive computer workstation for testing and training nonliteral expressions. Presentation at the annual meeting of the American Speech-Language-Hearing Association, Anaheim, CA. [Abstract in *Asha*, 35(10), 114.]

Langford, D. (1995). *Practical Computer Ethics*. London, England: McGraw-Hill Book Company Europe.

LaPine, P. R. (1990). Utilizing laptop technology in clinical practice. *Journal for Computer Users in Speech and Hearing*, 6(2), 158–162.

Larijani, L. C. (1993). *The Virtual Reality Primer*. New York: McGraw-Hill.

LaRiviere, C., & Sherblom, J. (1986). Speech synthesis and speech recognition by microcomputer. In J. L. Northern (Ed.), *The Personal Computer for Speech, Language, and Hearing Professionals*. San Diego, CA: College-Hill, pp. 177–208.

Larkins, P. G., & Tishman, A. (1984). Computer assisted instruction in establishing diagnostic competencies. Presentation at the annual meeting of the American Speech-Language-Hearing Association, San Francisco, CA. [Abstract in *Asha*, 26(10), 84.]

Larkins, P. G., Boykin, P. T., & Tishman, A. (1983). Computer technology utilized in a university training program. Presentation at the annual meeting of the American Speech-Language-Hearing Association, Cincinnati, OH. [Abstract in *Asha*, 25(10), 58.]

Larrick, W. R. (1992). Using multimedia in the treatment of bilingual speech/language disorders. Presentation at the annual meeting of the American Speech-Language-Hearing Association, San Antonio, TX. [Abstract in *Asha*, 34(10), 109.]

Larson, L. C., & Thornton, N. E. (1991). Use of a phonetic word finder program in clinical settings. Presentation at the annual meeting of the American Speech-Language-Hearing Association, Atlanta, GA. [Abstract in *Asha*, 33(10), 188.]

Larson, L. C., & Whiteside, J. D. (1986). Assessing students' concerns about microcomputer applications. *Journal for Computer Users in Speech and Hearing*, 2(1), 8–17.

Larson, V. L., & Steiner, S. (1985). Language intervention using microcomputers. *Topics in Language Disorders*, 6(1), 41–55.

Laughton, J., Jones, G., & Hasenstab, M. S. (1986). Microcomputers for learning discourse repair strategies. Presentation at the annual meeting of the American Speech-Language-Hearing Association, Detroit, MI. [Abstract in *Asha*, 28(10), 118.]

Lauridsen, O., & Nielsen, H. B. (1981). A new computerized method of hearing aid fitting based on measurement at the ear drum. *Scandinavian Audiology*, 10, 109–113.

Lauter, J. L. (1991). MacCAD: Central auditory diagnostics for the Macintosh. Presentation at the annual meeting of the American Speech-Language-Hearing Association, Atlanta, GA. [Abstract in *Asha*, 33(10), 187.]

Lawler, S. (1990). Communication systems for special populations. *Journal for Computer Users in Speech and Hearing*, 6(1), 42–43.

Layte, D. L., & Lefkowitz, N. (1985). Instituting a computer assisted treatment program in a rehabilitation hospital. Presentation at the annual meeting of the American Speech-Language-Hearing Association, Washington, DC. [Abstract in *Asha*, 27(10), 90.]

Layton, T. L. (1990). *ASHA* Project IMPACT. #5 Administrative Applications of Microcomputers for Speech, Language, and Hearing Professionals [Review of computer program]. *Asha*, 32(5), 74.

Layton, T. L. (1991). Augmentative Communication Series: Touch & Speak [Review of computer program]. *Asha*, 33(12), 105.

Layton, T. L. (1992). Words & Concepts, Words & Concepts II, and Words & Concepts III [Review of computer programs]. *Asha*, 34(12), 92.

Lea, W. (1986). *Trends in Speech Recognition*. Apple Valley, MN: Speech Science Publications.

Lee, K. S., & Thomas, D. J. (1990). *Control of Computer-Based Technology for People with Physical Disabilities: An Assessment Manual*. Buffalo, NY: University of Toronto Press. [Review in *Asha*, 32(8), 70.]

Lee, L. (1986). *Verbal Reasoning* [Computer program]. Mohnton, PA: The Greentree Group, P.O. Box 28.

Lee, W. C., Blackstone, S. W., & Poock, G. K. (1987). Dysarthric speech input to expert systems, electronic mail, and daily job activities. *Proceedings of the Voice I/O Systems Applications Conference*, 33–43.

Leeper, L. H. (1991a). Hypermedia applications in speech-language pathology. Presentation at the annual meeting of the American Speech-Language-Hearing Association, Atlanta, GA. [Abstract in *Asha*, 33(10), 86.]

Leeper, L. H. (1991b). Teaching basic clinical computing skills using self-paced instructional modules. Presentation at the annual meeting of the American Speech-Language-Hearing Association, Atlanta, GA. [Abstract in *Asha*, 33(10), 187.]

Leeper, L. H. (1992a). Developing clinical treatment materials in hypermedia environments. Presentation at the annual meeting of the American Speech-Language-Hearing Association, San Antonio, TX. [Abstract in *Asha*, 34(10), 185.]

Leeper, L. H. 1992b). First Words and First Words II [Review of computer programs]. *Asha*, 34(12), 92–93.

Leeper, L. H. (1992c). Hypermedia development: Simultaneous use of HyperCard IIGS and HyperStudio for stack-building efficiency. *Journal for Computer Users in Speech and Hearing*, 8(1, 2), 148–152.

Leeper, L. H. (1994). Using Hyper-stackware to create individualized service delivery materials. Presentation at the annual meeting of the American Speech-Language-Hearing Association, New Orleans, LA. [Abstract in *Asha*, 36(10), 175.]

Leeper, L. H., & Stuart, S. (1993). HyperCard how-to: Using efficient design and learning strategies in stack-building. Presentation at the annual meeting of the American Speech-Language-Hearing Association, Anaheim, CA. [Abstract in *Asha*, 35(10), 145.]

Lefkowitz, N. G., & Layte, D. L. (1988). Update the data! Modernizing through computing. Presentation at the annual meeting of the American Speech-Language-Hearing Association, Boston, MA. [Abstract in *Asha*, 30(10), 203.]

Lehnhardt, E., Battmer, R. D., & Becker, D. (1980). Storage of audiometric data—online—with a small computer. *Archives of Otorhinolaryngology*, 226, 199–206.

Leonard, R. J. (1994). Clinical instrumentation for Macintosh computers: Novel designs, unique applications. Presentation at the annual meeting of the American Speech-Language-Hearing Association, New Orleans, LA. [Abstract in *Asha*, 36(10), 173.]

Levey, S. K., Dietrich, J. M., Dickerson, M., & Lieman, B. (1993). Voice-input computer control by a dysarthric speaker. Presentation at the annual meeting of the American Speech-Language-Hearing Association, Anaheim, CA. [Abstract in *Asha*, 35(10), 171.]

Levitt, H. (1980). Computer applications in audiology and rehabilitation of the hearing impaired. *Journal of Communication Disorders*, 13, 471–481.

Levitt, H., & Boothroyd, A. (1982). Computers and audiology. Presentation at the annual meeting of the American Speech-Language-Hearing Association, Toronto, Canada. [Abstract in *Asha*, 24(10), 760.]

Levitt, H., Slosberg, R., Hawie, D., Mazor, R., & Rosenstein, M. (1978). Computer-based techniques for enhancement of clinical techniques. *Asha*, 20, 398–402.

Lieberth, A. K. (1991). Computerized speech training aids and hearing impaired children. Presentation at the annual meeting of the American Speech-Language-Hearing Association, Seattle, WA. [Abstract in *Asha*, 32(10), 64.]

Lieberth, A. K. (1992). Multimedia HyperCard applications for children's aural rehabilitation. Presentation at the annual meeting of the American Speech-Language-Hearing Association, San Antonio, TX. [Abstract in *Asha*, 34(10), 156.]

Lieberth, A. K., & Martin, D. R. (1992). HyperSign: A HyperCard-driven sign language dictionary. Presentation at the annual meeting of the American Speech-Language-Hearing Association, San Antonio, TX. [Abstract in *Asha*, 34(10), 156.]

Lieberth, A. K., & Martin, D. R. (1993). Our favorite Macintosh shareware. Presentation at the annual meeting of the American Speech-Language-Hearing Association, Anaheim, CA. [Abstract in *Asha*, 35(10), 227.]

Lieberth, A. K., Martin, D. R., & Kitchens, L. (1994). Hands-on introduction to HyperCard authoring for NSSLHA members. Presentation at the annual meeting of the American Speech-Language-Hearing Association, New Orleans, LA. [Abstract in *Asha*, 36(10), 218.]

Lieberth, A. K., Martin, D. R., & Scherz, J. W. (1994). Our favorite shareware and freeware for the Macintosh. Presentation at the annual meeting of the American Speech-Language-Hearing Association, New Orleans, LA. [Abstract in *Asha*, 36(10), 175–176.]

Lillie, K. D., Kneil, T. R., & Wynne, M. K. (1993). Educational strategies for hearing-impaired students. Presentation at the annual meeting of the American Speech-Language-Hearing Association, Anaheim, CA. [Abstract in *Asha*, 35(10), 222.]

Linebaugh, C., & Mills, R. H. (1985). Computer applications in clinical management of neurogenic communicative disorders. In J. Darby (Ed.), *Speech and Language Evaluation in Neurology* (Volume 3).

Lipscomb, D. M., & Fankhouser, R. J. (1986). Computer technology in hearing conservation programs: Schools & industry. In J. L. Northern (Ed.), *The Personal Computer for Speech, Language, and Hearing Professionals*. Boston, MA: Little, Brown, pp. 135–156.

Litke, R. E. (1991). Keep it simple. *Journal for Computer Users in Speech and Hearing*, 7(1), 104–105.

Logemann, J. A., Kahrilas, P. J., Begelman, J., Dodds, W. J., & Pauloski, B. R. (1989). Interactive computer program for biomechanical analysis of videoradiographic studies of swallowing. *American Journal of Radiology*, 153, 277–280.

Long, S. H. (1991) Integrating microcomputer applications into speech and language assessment. *Topics in Language Disorders*, 11(2), 1–17.

Long, S. H. (1992). An extension to Computerized Profiling: The Index of Productive Syntax. Presentation at the annual meeting of the American Speech-Language-Hearing Association, San Antonio, TX. [Abstract in *Asha*, 34(10), 126.]

Long, S. H. (1993). WordPerfect macros to facilitate the coding of SALT transcripts. Presentation at the annual meeting of the American Speech-Language-Hearing Association, Anaheim, CA. [Abstract in *Asha*, 35(10), 183.]

Long, S. H., & Clezy, G. (1994). The Lincoln Interactive Profile: Computerized version. Presentation at the annual meeting of the American Speech-Language-Hearing Association, New Orleans, LA. [Abstract in *Asha*, 36(10), 106.]

Long, S. H., & Dale, P. S. (1994). Productivity analysis using PANEL and Computerized Profiling. Presentation at the annual meeting of the American Speech-Language-Hearing Association, New Orleans, LA. [Abstract in *Asha*, 36(10), 174.]

Long, S. H., & Fey, M. E., (1987). Computerized profiling of grammatical performance and social-interactional participation. Presentation at the annual meeting of the American Speech-Language-Hearing Association, New Orleans, LA. [Abstract in *Asha*, 29(10), 103.]

Long, S. H., & Fey, M. E. (1988). A computerized system for multilevel analysis of language samples. Presentation at the annual meeting of the American Speech-Language-Hearing Association, Boston, MA. [Abstract in *Asha*, 30(10), 129.]

Long, S. H., & Fey, M. E. (1990a). Language sample analysis with the Macintosh. Presentation at the annual meeting of the American Speech-Language-Hearing Association, Seattle, WA. [Abstract in *Asha*, 32(10), 88.]

Long, S. H., & Fey, M. E. (1990b). Reciprocal use of SALT and Computerized Profiling. Presentation at the annual meeting of the American Speech-Language-Hearing Association, Seattle, WA. [Abstract in *Asha*, 32(10), 88.]

Long, S. H., & Fey, M. E. (1993a). *Computerized Profiling* [Computer program]. San Antonio, TX: The Psychological Corporation.

Long, S. H., & Fey, M. E. (1993b). Syntactic analysis techniques with Computerized Profiling. Presentation at the annual meeting of the American Speech-Language-Hearing Association, Anaheim, CA. [Abstract in *Asha*, 35(10), 227.]

Long, S. H., & Fey, M. E. (1995). Computer-assisted instruction in linguistics and language analysis. Presentation at the annual meeting of the American Speech-Language-Hearing Association, Orlando, FL. [Abstract in *Asha*, 37(10), 82.]

Long, S. H., & Long, S. T. (1990). Computer-assisted instruction (CAI) for LARSP profiling. Presentation at the annual meeting of the American Speech-Language-Hearing Association, Seattle, WA. [Abstract in *Asha*, 32(10), 88.]

Long, S. H., & Masterson, J. J. (1993). Computer technology: Use in language analysis. *Asha*, 35(8), 40–41, 51.

Lorendo, L. C. (1988a). *Computer Implementation in Communication Sciences and Disorders*. Unpublished Ph.D. dissertation, University of Mississippi.

Lorendo, L. C. (1988b). Computer implementation in communication sciences and disorders education programs. Presentation at the annual meeting of the American Speech-Language-Hearing Association, Boston, MA. [Abstract in *Asha*, 30(10), 123.]

Lotterman, S. H. (1983). Computer assisted instruction in audiology. Presentation at the annual meeting of the American Speech-Language-Hearing Association, Cincinnati, OH. [Abstract in *Asha*, 25(10), 58.]

Lotterman, S. H. (1984a). Computer assisted introduction to audiology. Presentation at the annual meeting of the American Speech-Language-Hearing Association, San Francisco, CA. [Abstract in *Asha*, 26(10), 187.]

Lotterman, S. H. (1984b). Computer generated audiologic reports. Presentation at the annual meeting of the American Speech-Language-Hearing Association, San Francisco, CA. [Abstract in *Asha*, 26(10), 185.]

Lotterman, S. H. (1985). Audiologic report generator. Presentation at the American Speech and Hearing Foundation Conference on Microcomputers, New Orleans, LA. [Abstract in the *Journal for Computer Users in Speech and Hearing*, 1(2), 82–83.]

Lotterman, S. H. (1985). Introduction to audiology. Presentation at the American Speech and Hearing Foundation Conference on Microcomputers, New Orleans, LA. [Abstract in the *Journal for Computer Users in Speech and Hearing*, 1(2), 83–84.]

Lotterman, S. H. (1988). INSTANT Hearing Performance Inventory [Review of computer program]. *Asha*, 30(2), 68–69.

Lotterman, S. H., & Barry, M. (1985). Instruction in audiological case history technique through computer simulation. Presentation at the annual meeting of the American Speech-Language-Hearing Association, Washington, DC. [Abstract in *Asha*, 27(10), 92.]

Lotterman, S. H., & Cox, B. P. (1987). Artifical intelligence and expert systems in audiologic training. Presentation at the annual meeting of the American Speech-Language-Hearing Association, New Orleans, LA. [Abstract in *Asha*, 29(10), 141.]

Loverso, F. L., & Prescott, T. M. (1986). Data versus intuition in using microcomputers for aphasia rehabilitation. Presentation at the annual meeting of the American Speech-Language-Hearing Association, Detroit, MI. [Abstract in *Asha*, 28(10), 157.]

Loverso, F. L., Prescott, T. E., Selinger, M., & Riley, L. (1989). Comparison of two modes of aphasia treatment: Clinician and computer-clinical assisted therapy. In T. E. Prescott (Ed.), *Clinical Aphasiology*. Boston, MA: College-Hill Press.

Lu, C. (September, 1993). A small revelation: Newton has arrived at long last. *McWorld*, 102–106.

Luschei, E. S., & Robin, D. A. (1991). Taking the fear out of instrumentation: Suggestions for speech-language clinicians. Presentation at the annual meeting of the American Speech-Language-Hearing Association, Atlanta, GA. [Abstract in *Asha*, 33(10), 81.]

Lutman, M. E. (1983). Microcomputer-controlled psychoacoustics in clinical audiology. *British Journal of Audiology*, 17(2), 109–114.

Lynch, W. J. (1983). Cognitive retraining using microcomputer games and commercially available software. *Cognitive Rehabilitation*, 1, 19–22.

Lynn, C. A. (1991). Telecommunication for the deaf devices. *Journal for Computer Users in Speech and Hearing*, 7(1), 10.

Lynn, J. M. (1986). *Phonemic Symbols* [Computer program]. Alliance, OH: L/M Enterprises, Inc., 1194 West State Street.

Lynn, J. M., & Lesner, S. A. (1987). *INSTANT Hearing Performance Inventory* [Computer program]. Alliance, OH: L/M Enterprises, Inc., 1194 West State Street.

Ma, M. T. L. (March, 1985). The future of educational computing. *High Technology*.

Macurik, K. (1981). A vocalization trainer for the hearing impaired. In *Proceedings of the Johns Hopkins First National Search for Applications of Personal Computing to Aid the Handicapped. Los Angeles*, CA: IEEE Computer Society Press.

MacWhinney, B. (1991). *The CHILDES Project: Tools for Analyzing Talk*. Lawrence Erlbaum Associates.

MacWhinney, B., Rosenthal-Rollins, P., Evans, J., & Alexander-Pan, B. (1991). Introduction to the Child Language Data Exchange System (CHILDES). Presentation at the annual meeting of the American Speech-Language-Hearing Association, Atlanta, GA. [Abstract in *Asha*, 33(10), 123.]

Magilen, G. (1990). *Why Choose a Mac Rather Than an MS-DOS Computer?* Vallejo, CA: MacHear/Hearing Centers' Network, 426 Virginia St.

Magilen, G. (1991). Hearing aid office management and the Macintosh. *Journal for Computer Users in Speech and Hearing*, 7(1), 106–112.

Mahaffey, R. B. (1973). Computerized procedure for keeping student records for *ASHA*-CCC requirements. *Asha*, 15, 590.

Mahaffey, R. B. (1975). The measurement of hearing by computer. In S. Singh (Ed.), *Measurement Procedures in Speech, Hearing, and Language*. Baltimore: University Park Press.

Mahaffey, R. B. (1980). Computer-assisted instruction in speech and hearing sciences. Scientific exhibit presented at the annual meeting of the American Speech-Language-Hearing Association, Detroit, MI.

Mahaffey, R. B. (1981). Strategies for using digital computers in adult education. Short course presented at the annual meeting of the American Speech-Language-Hearing Association, Los Angeles, CA. [Abstract in *Asha*, 23(10), 737.]

Mahaffey, R. B. (1984). Research applications in communication disorders. In A. H. Schwartz (Ed.), *Handbook of Microcomputer Applications in Communication Disorders*. San Diego, CA: College-Hill, pp. 174–192.

Mahaffer, R. B. (1985). An overview of computer applications. *Topics in Language Disorders*, 6, 1–10.

Mahshie, J. J. (1985). Interactive video in the classroom and clinic. Presentation at the American Speech and Hearing Foundation Conference on Microcomputers, New Orleans, LA. [Abstract in the *Journal for Computer Users in Speech and Hearing*, 1(2), 84.]

Mahshie, J. J. (1987). A primer on interactive video. *Journal for Computer Users in Speech and Hearing*, 3(1), 39–57.

Mahshie, J. J. (1992). Using computers to improve the speech of hearing-impaired children. Presentation at the annual meeting of the American Speech-Language-Hearing Association, San Antonio, TX. [Abstract in *Asha*, 34(10), 221.]

Mahshie, J. J., Bernstein, L. E., Goldstein Jr., M. H., Vari-Alquist, D., & Waddy-Smith, B. (1988). Computerized speech training/practice aids for hearing-impaired children. Presentation at the annual meeting of the American Speech-Language-Hearing Association, Boston, MA. [Abstract in *Asha*, 30(10), 103–104.]

Mahshie, J. J., Wilson-Favors, V., Schneider, D., & Brandt, F. D. (1991). Computer-based speech training with deaf children. Presentation at the annual meeting of the American Speech-Language-Hearing Association, Atlanta, GA. [Abstract in *Asha*, 33(10), 211.]

Mahshie, J. J., & Yadav, P. K. (1990). The Gallaudet University speech training and evaluation system for deaf children. Presentation at the annual meeting of the American Speech-Language-Hearing Association, Seattle, WA. [Abstract in *Asha*, 32(10),

Major, B., & Wilson, K. (1985). *Computerized Reading for Aphasics*. San Diego: College-Hill.

Major, R. R. C. (1994). VARBRUL analysis and interlanguage phonology. Presentation at the annual meeting of the American Speech-Language-Hearing Association, New Orleans, LA. [Abstract in *Asha*, 36(10), 175.]

Maki, J. E., Mershon, S., & Silver, G. D. (1993). Development of a computer-based speech training system. Presentation at the annual meeting of the American Speech-Language-Hearing Association, Anaheim, CA. [Abstract in *Asha*, 35(10), 222.]

Mann, V. A. (1987). DSPS Realtime Signal Lab [Review of computer program]. *Asha*, 29(11), 64–65.

Mansour, P. (1987). *Print Your Own Calendar* [Computer program]. Dimondale, MI: Hartley Courseware.

Marchbanks, R. J., & Martin, A. M. (1985). A computer-based test system for implementing pure-tone audiometry, acoustic immittance and tympanic membrane displacement measurements. *British Journal of Audiology*, 19(1), 19–28.

Marriner, N. A. (1985). Computer applications: Review of FIRST WORDS. *Child Language Teaching and Therapy*, 1(1), 105–109.

Marriner, N. A., Dowden, P. A., & Hesketh, L. H. (1985). Adapting microcomputers for the nonreading communicative impaired. Videotape presented at the annual meeting of the American Speech-Language-Hearing Association, Washington, DC. [Abstract in *Asha*, 27(10), 95.]

Martin, C. W., & Lewis, F. C. (1982). Computer implemented frequency/time analysis of vocal pathologies. Presentation at the annual meeting of the American Speech-Language-Hearing Association, Toronto, Canada. [Abstract in *Asha*, 24(10), 746.]

Martin, D. R. (1991). AudioPro 2 [Review of a computer program]. *Journal for Computer Users in Speech and Hearing*, 7(1), 183–188.

Martin, D. R., & Lieberth, A. K. (1991). Introduction to HyperCard authoring: Programming for the nonprogrammer. Presentation at the annual meeting of the American Speech-Language-Hearing Association, Atlanta, GA. [Abstract in *Asha*, 33(10),

Martin, D. R., & Lieberth, A. K. (1992a). A hands-on introduction to HyperCard authoring. Presentation at the annual meeting of the American Speech-Language-Hearing Association, San Antonio, TX. [Abstract in *Asha*, 34(10), 133.]

Martin, D. R., & Lieberth, A. K. (1992b). An introduction to HyperTalk: Programming with HyperCard. *Journal for Computer Users in Speech and Hearing*, 8(1, 2), 53–66.

Martin, D. R., & Lieberth, A. K. (1993a). A hands-on introduction at HyperCard authoring. Presentation at the annual meeting of the American Speech-Language-Hearing Association, Anaheim, CA. [Abstract in *Asha*, 35(10), 145.]

Martin, D. R., & Lieberth, A. K. (1993b). Our favorite Macintosh shareware. Presentation at the annual meeting of the American Speech-Language-Hearing Association, Anaheim, CA.

Mason, S. M., & Adams, W. (1984). An automated microcomputer based electric response audiometry system for machine scoring of auditory evoked potentials. *Clinical Physiology and Physiological Measurement*, 5(3), 219–222.

Massey, H. J. (1988). Language-impaired children's comprehension of synthesized speech. *Language, Speech, and Hearing Services in Schools*, 19, 401–409.

Masterson, J. J. (1994). Capitalizing on microcomputer applications in clinical phonology. Presentation at the annual meeting of the American Speech-Language-Hearing Association, New Orleans, LA. [Abstract in *Asha*, 36(10), 106.]

Masterson, J. J., Channell, R., Fey, M., Hughes, D., Pollock, K., & Matesich, J. (1991). Enhancing linguistic analysis skills with microcomputer software. Presentation at the annual meeting of the American Speech-Language-Hearing Association, Atlanta, GA. [Abstract in *Asha*, 33(10), 122.]

Masterson, J. J., Evans, L. H., & Clayton, J. (1991). An overview of Macintosh applications in speech-language pathology. Presentation at the annual meeting of the American Speech-Language-Hearing Association, Atlanta, GA. [Abstract in *Asha*, 33(10), 170.]

Masterson, J. J., Katz, R., Cochran, P. S., Wynne, M. K., McGuire, R. A., Martin, D., & Lieberth, A. K. (1992). Microcomputer applications: What we can do, what we should do. Presentation at the annual meeting of the American Speech-Language-Hearing Association, San Antonio, TX. [Abstract in *Asha*, 34(10), 101.]

Masterson, J. J., Katz, R., Lieberth, A., & Wynne, M. (1993). Clinical computing competencies: Shooting at a moving target. Presentation at the annual meeting of the American Speech-Language-Hearing Association, Anaheim, CA. [Abstract in *Asha*, 35(10), 161.]

Masterson, J. J., & Long, S. (1990). Issues in the design and use of phonological analysis software. Presentation at the annual meeting of the American Speech-Language-Hearing Association, Seattle, WA. [Abstract in *Asha*, 32(10), 154.]

Masterson, J. J., Long, S., Fey, M., Pye, C., Oller, K., Miller, J., MacWhinney, B., & Evans, J. (1995a). Evaluation and use of language analysis software. Presentation at the annual meeting of the American Speech-Language-Hearing Association, Orlando, FL. [Abstract in *Asha*, 37(10), 82.]

Masterson, J. J., Long, S., Fey, M., Pye, C., Oller, K., Miller, J., MacWhinney, B., & Evans, J. (1995b). Evaluation and use of phonological analysis software. Presentation at the annual meeting of the American Speech-Language-Hearing Association, Orlando, FL. [Abstract in *Asha*, 37(10), 116.]

Masterson, J. J., Martin, D. J., & Lieberth, A. (1992). Introduction to the use of the Macintosh in speech-language pathology. Presentation at the annual meeting of the American Speech-Language-Hearing Association, San Antonio, TX. [Abstract in *Asha*, 34(10), 133.]

Masterson, J. J., Masterson, G. L., & Turner, N. J. (1994). Introduction to Macintosh applications for speech-language pathology. Presentation at the annual meeting of the American Speech-Language-Hearing Association, New Orleans, LA. [Abstract in *Asha*, 36(10), 219.]

Masterson, J. J., Matesich, J. S., & Pagan, F. G. (1988). The speech-language pathologist and the computer scientist: Interdisciplinary "handshaking." Presentation at the annual meeting of the American Speech-Language-Hearing Association, Boston, MA. [Abstract in *Asha*, 30(10), 203.]

Masterson, J. J., McGuire, R., Masterson, G. L., & Turner, N. J. (1993). Introduction to IBM-PC applications for speech-language pathology. Presentation at the annual meeting of the American Speech-Language-Hearing Association, Anaheim, CA. [Abstract in *Asha*, 35(10), 145.]

Masterson, J. J., Mistric, C., & Jordon, D. (1987). Computerized scheduling: An end to the clinical coordinator's nightmare. Presentation at the annual meeting of the American Speech-Language-Hearing Association, New Orleans, LA. [Abstract in *Asha*, 29(10), 141.]

Masterson, J. J., & Pagan, F. G. (1990). Phonological analysis with the Macintosh. Presentation at the annual meeting of the American Speech-Language-Hearing Association, Seattle, WA. [Abstract in *Asha*, 32(10), 154.]

Masterson, J. J., Spiser-Albert, V., Laurent, J., & Waryas, C. (1994). Using microcomputers in phonological assessment and intervention. Presentation at the annual meeting of the American Speech-Language-Hearing Association, New Orleans, LA. [Abstract in *Asha*, 36(10), 175.]

Matesich, J. S. (1992). First Verbs: IBM compatible version [Review of computer program]. *Asha*, 34(12), 93.

Matesich, J. S. (1993). First Categories: IBM compatible version [Review of computer program]. *Asha*, 35(2), 70.

Mauer, D. M., & Sanders-Wann, J. A. (1992). Using technology to enhance language acquisition in young handicapped children. Presentation at the annual meeting of the American Speech-Language-Hearing Association, San Antonio, TX. [Abstract in *Asha*, 34(10), 116.]

Mayer-Johnson Company (1990). *Boardmaker* [Computer program]. Solana Beach, CA: Mayer-Johnson Company.

McCabe, S. J., Lawton, S., & Weinreb, G. S. (1994). Designing acoustic sound editing and analysis tools using SoundScope. Presentation at the annual meeting of the American Speech-Language-Hearing Association, New Orleans, LA. [Abstract in *Asha*, 36(10), 247.]

McCabe, S. J., Lawton, S., & Weinreb, G. S. (1994). The use of SoundScope in the analysis of speech. Presentation at the annual meeting of the American Speech-Language-Hearing Association, New Orleans, LA. [Abstract in *Asha*, 36(10), 219.]

McCabe, S. J., & Weinreb, G. S. (1995). Sound analysis: Measurement through report generation using the SoundScope model. Presentation at the annual meeting of the American Speech-Language-Hearing Association, Orlando, FL. [Abstract in *Asha*, 37(10), 116.]

McCullough, J. A., Birck, J. D., & Wilson, R. H. (1991). Computer application of auditory/visual word identification material. Presentation at the annual meeting of the American Speech-Language-Hearing Association, Atlanta, GA. [Abstract in *Asha*, 33(10), 187.]

McCullough, J. A., Cunningham, L. B., & Wilson, R. H. (1991). Computer application and standardization of auditory/visual word-identification materials. Presentation at the annual meeting of the American Speech-Language-Hearing Association, Atlanta, GA. [Abstract in *Asha*, 33(10), 108.]

McCullough, J. A., Wilson, R. H., & Birck, J. D. (1993). Performance of Spanish speakers on multimedia speech audiometry materials. Presentation at the annual meeting of the American Speech-Language-Hearing Association, Anaheim, CA. [Abstract in *Asha*, 35(10), 173.]

McCullough, J. A., Wilson, R. H., Birck, J. D., & Anderson, L. G. (1994). A multimedia approach for estimating speech recognition of multilingual clients. *American Journal of Audiology*, 3(1), 19–22.

McFarlane, S. C. (1990a). Clinicians and computers: The interaction. *Journal for Computer Users in Speech and Hearing*, 6(2), 118–121.

McFarlane, S. C. (1990b). Videolaryngoendoscopy and voice disorders. *Seminars in Speech and Language*, 11, 1–59.

McGhee, W. G. (1987). Idioms in America [Review of computer program]. *Asha*, 29(5), 76–77.

McGuire, R. A. (1991). Microcomputer assisted speech assessment and treatment: Tips, tricks, and traps. Presentation at the annual meeting of the American Speech-Language-Hearing Association, Atlanta, GA. [Abstract in *Asha*, 33(10), 137.]

McGuire, R. A. (1995). Development of virtual instruments for the clinic and lab. Presentation at the annual meeting of the American Speech-Language-Hearing Association, Orlando, FL. [Abstract in *Asha*, 37(10), 109.]

McGuire, R. A., & Elliot, H. M. (1994). Enhancement of speech science instruction using SoundScope's self-authoring features. Presentation at the annual meeting of the American Speech-Language-Hearing Association, New Orleans, LA. [Abstract in *Asha*, 36(10), 173.]

McGuire, R. A., Kouri, T. A., & Woods, J. D. (1993). Getting the most out of SpeechViewer II. Presentation at the annual meeting of the American Speech-Language-Hearing Association, Anaheim, CA. [Abstract in *Asha*, 35(10), 195.]

McGuire, R. A., Lorang, T. L., McCoy, K. L., & Zillig, L. L. (1994). Maximizing the clinical potential of SpeechViewer II. Presentation at the annual meeting of the American Speech-Language-Hearing Association, New Orleans, LA. [Abstract in *Asha*, 36(10), 219.]

McMillan, W. W., Gardiner, C. J., & McMillan, P. M. (1990). An expert system for audiology. Presentation at the annual meeting of the American Speech-Language-Hearing Association, Seattle, WA. [Abstract in *Asha*, 32(10), 90.]

McRay, L. B., & Fitch, J. L. (1994). Microcomputer applications in the public schools: A survey. Presentation at the annual meeting of the American Speech-Language-Hearing Association, New Orleans, LA. [Abstract in *Asha*, 36(10), 162.]

MDC Software (1991). *Clini-base Computer Software for Clinical Supervision in Speech Pathology and Audiology, Release 2* [Computer program]. Carlsbad, CA: MDC Software, 7926 La Capela Place.

Meng, B. (April, 1988). Get to the Point: Win audiences by mastering the tools and techniques of presentation graphics. *Macworld*, 136–143.

Menosky, J. A. (May, 1984). Computer worship. *Science 84*, 40–46

Merson, R. M., Rolnick, M. I., & Weiner, F. F. (1995a). *The Beaumont Outcome Software System* [Computer program]. West Bloomfield, MI: Parrot Software.

Merson, R. M., Rolnick, M. I., & Weiner, F. F. (1995b). The Beaumont Outcome Software System: An approach to reporting outcome measures. Presentation at the annual meeting of the American Speech-Language-Hearing Association, Orlando, FL. [Abstract in *Asha*, 37(10), 42.]

Mervine, P. L., & Ziegler, B. (1994). *I Can Play Too!* [Computer program]. Solana Beach, CA: Mayer-Johnson Company.

Metz, D. E., Schiavetti, N., & Knight, S. D. (1991). Comparison of computer artificial neural networks used in speech research. Presentation at the annual meeting of the American Speech-Language-Hearing Association, Atlanta, GA. [Abstract in *Asha*, 33(10), 143.]

Meyers, L. (1990). *Keytalk* [Computer program]. Los Angeles, CA: Peal software, 3200 Wilshire Boulevard.

Meyers, L. F. (1984). Using microprocessors to augment language skills in handicapped children. Presentation at the annual meeting of the American Speech-Language-Hearing Association, San Francisco, CA. [Abstract in *Asha*, 26(10), 128.]

Meyers, L. F. (1985). *Programs for Early Acquisition of Language (PEAL)* [Computer program]. Calabasas, CA: PEAL Software, P. O. Box 8188.

Meyers, L. F., & Lansky, P. S. (1990). *Action/Music Play* [Computer program]. Calabasas, CA: PEAL Software, P. O. Box 8188.

Meyers, L. F., & Lansky, P. S. (1988). Computer-enhanced language scaffolding with severely visually impaired preschoolers. Presentation at the annual meeting of the American Speech-Language-Hearing Association, Boston, MA. [Abstract in *Asha*, 30(10), 82.]

Meyers, S. C., & Strang, H. R. (1988). Computer-simulated training on student-clinicians' intervention effectiveness with preschool stutterers. Presentation at the annual meeting of the American Speech-Language-Hearing Association, Boston, MA. [Abstract in *Asha*, 30(10), 170.]

Miles, J. (1987). *Design for Desktop Publishing*. San Francisco, CA: Chronicle Books.

Miller, C. J., & Daniloff, R. G. (1990). ONLINE: Subject-interactive experiment controller for perceptual research. Presentation at the annual meeting of the American Speech-Language-Hearing Association, Seattle, WA. [Abstract in *Asha*, 32(10), 76.]

Miller, G. D., Slike, S. B., Bailey, H. J., & Hobbis, D. H. (1987). Interactive videodisc technology: Audiometric testing and sign language instruction. Presentation at the annual meeting of the American Speech-Language-Hearing Association, New Orleans, LA. [Abstract in *Asha*, 29(10), 158–159.]

Miller, J. F., & Chapman, R. S. (1983). A computer solution to free speech sample analysis. Presentation at the annual meeting of the American Speech-Language-Hearing Association, Cincinnati, OH. [Abstract in *Asha*, 25(10), 59.]

Miller, J. F., & Chapman, R. S. (1991). *Systematic Analysis of Language Transcripts (SALT).* Madison, WI: Language Analysis Laboratory, University of Wisconsin-Madison.

Miller, J. F., & Nockerts, A. (1993). Making language sample analysis decisions using SALT database profiler. Presentation at the annual meeting of the American Speech-Language-Hearing Association, Anaheim, CA. [Abstract in *Asha*, 35(10), 195.]

Miller, J. M., & Page, J. L. (1994). The effectiveness of computer-assisted instruction in language intervention. Presentation at the annual meeting of the American Speech-Language-Hearing Association, New Orleans, LA. [Abstract in *Asha*, 36(10), 67.]

Mills, R. H. (1985). Computers in the communication sciences—Personal notes on a short history. *Journal for Computer Users in Speech and Hearing*, 1(1), 12–14.

Mills, R. H. (1986a). Annotated bibliography of computer literature in the communication sciences: Part I. *Journal for Computer Users in Speech and Hearing*, 2(2), 65–85.

Mills, R. H. (1986b). Computerized management of aphasia. In R. Chapey (Ed.), *Language Intervention Strategies in Adult Aphasia*. Baltimore: Williams & Wilkins, 333–344.

Mills, R. H. (1986c). Funding microcomputers: Dealing with remote decision making. *Cognitive Rehabilitation*, 4, 1–6.

Mills, R. H. (1986d). Microcomputer applications in aphasia and head trauma. In J. L. Northern (Ed.), *The Personal Computer for Speech, Language, and Hearing Professionals*. Boston: Little, Brown, pp. 85–100.

Mills, R. H. (1986e). Peripheral devices and the clinical microcomputer. In M. L. Grossfeld & C. A. Grossfeld (Eds.), *Microcomputer Applications in Rehabilitation of Communication Disorders*. Rockville, MD: Aspen, pp.155–182.

Mills, R. H. (1991). Machine vision technology: Quantification of videofluoroscopic swallowing data. *Journal for Computer Users in Speech and Hearing*, 7(1), 132–142.

Mills, R. H., Burkhead, C., & Shappiro, M. (1986?). *Reading Recognition Programs* [Computer programs]. Ann Arbor, MI: Brain-Link Software, 317 Montgomery.

Mills, R. H., & Langmore, S. E. (1980). A microcomputer system in aphasia rehabilitation. Scientific exhibit presented at the annual meeting of the American Speech-Language-Hearing Association, Detroit, MI.

Mills, R. H., Schatz, K. H., & Langmore, S. E. (1986). Microcomputers as home-based therapy aids for aphasia and congnitive dysfunction. Presentation at the annual meeting of the American Speech-Language-Hearing Association, Detroit, MI. [Abstract in *Asha*, 28(10), 157.]

Mills, R. H., & Stewman, D. Y. (1991). Computerized image analysis of dysphagia in ALS: A case study. Presentation at the annual meeting of the American Speech-Language-Hearing Association, Atlanta, GA. [Abstract in *Asha*, 33(10), 111.]

Mills, R. H., & Thomas, R. P. (1981). Microcomputerized language therapy for the aphasic patient. In *Proceedings of the Johns Hopkins First National Search for Applications of Personal Computing to Aid the Handicapped*. Los Angeles, CA: IEEE Computer Society Press.

Mills, R. H., & Thomas, R. P. (1983a). The talking Apple: Comparisons of three microcomputerized speech production methods. Presentation at the annual meeting of the American Speech-Language-Hearing Association, Cincinnati, OH. [Abstract in *Asha*, 25(10), 117.]

Mills, R. H., & Thomas, R. P. (1983b). *Word Recognition Programs* [Computer programs]. Ann Arbor, MI: Brain-Link Software.

Mills, R. H., & Volin, R. A. (1987). Annotated bibliography of computer literature in the communication sciences: Part II. *Journal for Computer Users in Speech and Hearing*, 3(1), 8–25.

Miltich, S. H., & Miltich, A. J. (1994). Interactive phonetics teaching system. Presentation at the annual meeting of the American Speech-Language-Hearing Association, New Orleans, LA. [Abstract in *Asha*, 36(10), 174.]

Mineo, B. A., Demasco, P. W., & Gray, J. (1993). Systematic assessment of picture-based language performance via computer. Presentation at the annual meeting of the American Speech-Language-Hearing Association, Anaheim, CA. [Abstract in *Asha*, 35(10), 226–227.]

Minghetti, N. J., Stach, B. A., Palmer, C. V., Lauter, J., Beukelman, D. R., Long, S. H., Cochran, P. S., & Fiegel, C. L. (1989). The "Building Bridges" project: Innovative software for communication disorders. Presentation at the annual meeting of the American Speech-Language-Hearing Association, St. Louis, MO. [Abstract in *Asha*, 31(10), 103.]

Minifie, F. D. (1984). The personal computer as a professional tool. *Asha*, 26(6), 23–25.

Mitch, J. L. (1988). Performance of a system for automatic course transcription of spectrograms. Presentation at the annual meeting of the American Speech-Language-Hearing Association, Boston, MA. [Abstract in *Asha*, 30(10), 88.]

Mitchell, A. (1986). Cognitive Rehabilitation [Review of computer program]. *Journal for Computer Users in Speech and Hearing*, 2(1), 41–42.

Mitchell, A., & Owens, B. (1985). Visual Recognition Programs [Review of computer programs]. *Journal for Computer Users in Speech and Hearing*, 1(2), 147–148.

Mitchell, P. R. (1986). BITNET: An international link for universities. *Journal for Computer Users in Speech and Hearing*, 2(1), 35–36.

Mitchell, P. R., Caruso, A. J., & Dean, C. R. (1994). Telecomputing and the Internet: Application to communication disorders. Presentation at the annual meeting of the American Speech-Language-Hearing Association, New Orleans, LA. [Abstract in *Asha*, 36(10), 173.]

Mitchell, P. R., McClowry, M. T., Salmon, C., & Yu, J. H. (1994). Internet gopher resources for speech-language pathologists and audiologists. Presentation at the annual meeting of the American Speech-Language-Hearing Association, New Orleans, LA. [Abstract in *Asha*, 36(10), 106.]

Mitchell, P. R., McComas, K., McClowry, M. T., & Prichard, C. L. (1995). ELSA gopher and Diversity University: Virtual School of Speech Pathology and Audiology. Presentation at the annual meeting of the American Speech-Language-Hearing Association, Orlando, FL. [Abstract in *Asha*, 37(10), 98.]

Mizuko, M. I. (1991). Simulation of a communication device on the Macintosh. Presentation at the annual meeting of the American Speech-Language-Hearing Association, Atlanta, GA. [Abstract in *Asha*, 33(10), 191.]

Mizuko, M. I. (1992). The use of the Macintosh as an augmentative and alternative communication aid. *Journal for Computer Users in Speech and Hearing*, 8(1, 2), 117–124.

Mizuko, M. I. (1993). Personal computers as augmentative and alternative communication aids. *American Journal of Speech-Language Pathology*, 2(3), 8–10.

Mizuko, M. I. (1995). Use of HyperStudio tools to create inexpensive scanning programs. Presentation at the annual meeting of the American Speech-Language-Hearing Association, Orlando, FL. [Abstract in *Asha*, 37(10), 62.]

Mizuko, M. I., & Erickson, A. L. (1994). The use of HyperStudio to create color communication boards. Presentation at the annual meeting of the American Speech-Language-Hearing Association, New Orleans, LA. [Abstract in *Asha*, 36(10), 106.]

Mizuko, M. I., & Hatten, J. T. (1994). Computer-assisted cognitive rehabilitation: Feature analysis guide. Presentation at the annual meeting of the American Speech-Language-Hearing Association, New Orleans, LA. [Abstract in *Asha*, 36(10), 174.]

Mizuko, M. I., & Hornstadt, H. (1992a). The use of alternate input devices with Macintosh computers. Presentation at the annual meeting of the American Speech-Language-Hearing Association, San Antonio, TX. [Abstract in *Asha*, 34(10), 160–161.]

Mizuko, M. I., & Hornstadt, H. (1992b). The use of HyperCard utilities to create communication boards. Presentation at the annual meeting of the American Speech-Language-Hearing Association, San Antonio, TX. [Abstract in *Asha*, 34(10), 115.]

Mizuko, M. I., Hornstadt, H., & Erickson, A. (1993). The use of HyperCard utilities to create color communication boards. Presentation at the annual meeting of the American Speech-Language-Hearing Association, Anaheim, CA. [Abstract in *Asha*, 35(10), 138.]

Modugno, P. A., & Tiegerman, E. (1986). A high-tech lifestyle for the speech and hearing center: Pragmatic considerations and operational issues. In M. L. Grossfeld & C. A. Grossfeld (Ed.), *Microcomputer Applications in Rehabilitation of Communication Disorders*. Rockville, MD: Aspen, pp. 213–238.

Monk, W. H. (1992). The army's hearing evaluation automated registry system. Presentation at the annual meeting of the American Speech-Language-Hearing Association, San Antonio, TX. [Abstract in *Asha*, 34(10), 166.]

Montgomery, A. A., Walden, B. E., & Prosek, R. A. (1986). Demonstration of a computer-based system for generating clinical material. *Journal for Computer Users in Speech and Hearing*, 2(1), 25–34.

Montgomery, J. K. (1985). Development of the software review process used in the *ASHA* Journal. Presentation at the American Speech and Hearing Foundation Conference on Microcomputers, New Orleans, LA. [Abstract in the *Journal for Computer Users in Speech and Hearing*, 1(2), 85.]

Montgomery, J. K. (1989). Computer applications in speech, language, and hearing: An essay on the 1990s. *Journal for Computer Users in Speech and Hearing*, 5(2), 101–104.

Montgomery, J. K., & Dean, C. R. (1988). Reading Recognition [Review of computer program]. *Journal for Computer Users in Speech and Hearing*, 4(1), 64–66.

Mooers, J. E. (1986). Spelltronics [Review of computer program]. *Asha*, 28(8), 71–72.

Mooers, J. E. (1987). *Word Attack!* [Review of computer program]. *Asha*, 29(8), 61–62.

Mooers, J. E. (1988). Wally's Word Works [Review of computer program]. *Asha*, 30(8), 59.

Moomaw, D. E. (No Date). *Systematic Hearing Aid Prescription (SHAP)* [Computer program]. San Diego: College-Hill.

Mordecai, D., Palin, M., & Palmer, C. (1985). *Lingquist I Language Sample Analysis* [Computer program]. Columbus, OH: Charles E. Merrill.

Morgan, B. T., & Webster, R. L. (1984). Computer assisted evaluation of voice onsets in stutterers. Presentation at the annual meeting of the American Speech-Language-Hearing Association, San Francisco, CA. [Abstract in *Asha*, 26(10), 158.]

Morris, M. S., Reggia, J. A., Ahuja, S. B., Hart, J.. & Watson, V. (1984). SLIPS: A data base system for computer storage and analysis of phonological errors. *Journal of Medical Systems*, 8, 197–204.

Morris, N. T., & Ray, S. (1991). Computer use in augmentative communication service provision. *Journal for Computer Users in Speech and Hearing*, 7(1), 113–120.

Morris, R. (1986). *DSPS Realtime Signal Lab* [Computer program]. Ottawa, Canada: DSPS, Inc., P.O. Box 5348, Station F.

Morris, R., Brown, W. S., & Sapienza, C. (1995). Comparison of fundamental frequency extraction software using disordered voices. Presentation at the annual meeting of the American Speech-Language-Hearing Association, Orlando, FL. [Abstract in *Asha*, 37(10), 109.]

Moseley, M. J. (1992). Tests of Syntactic Ability (TSA): Screening Test Form 1 [Review of computer program]. *Asha*, 34(5), 94.

Mower, D. E. (1995). The electronic forum: New ways to maximize student learning. Presentation at the annual meeting of the American Speech-Language-Hearing Association, Orlando, FL. [Abstract in *Asha*, 37(10), 66.]

Mueller, P., & Peters, T. (1976). Clinical Recordkeeping system. *Asha*, 18, pp. 352–353.

Mullendore, J. M. (1984). Microcomputer applications: A perspective in the development of the Profession. In A. H. Schwartz (Ed.), *Handbook of Microcomputer Applications in Communication Disorders*. San Diego, CA: College-Hill, 259–273.

Murray, L. (November, 1983). Computer sex therapists. *Science Digest*.

Murveit, H., & Brodersen, R. W. (1986). An integrated circuit-based speech recognition system. *IEEE Transactions on Acoustics, Speech and Signal Processing*, ASSP-34, 6, 1465–1472.

Navarro, R., Fucci, D., Leach, E., Wilson, K., & Thompson, B. (1995). Computer analysis of hearing aid processed speech. Presentation at the annual meeting of the American Speech-Language-Hearing Association, Orlando, FL. [Abstract in *Asha*, 37(10), 113.]

Naylor, C. (1983). *Build Your Own Expert System*. Cheshire,UK: Sigma Technical Press.
Neely, A., & Aaronson, T. (1984). *Wizard of Words* [Computer program]. Tucson, AZ: Communication Skill Builders.
Neff, S. R. (1992a). W.O.R.D. Benders Complete the Phrase [Review of computer program]. *Asha*, 34(8), 100–101.
Neff, S. R. (1992b). W.O.R.D. Benders Definition [Review of computer program]. *Asha*, 34(8), 100.
Neilson, H. R., & Cooper, R. J. (1984). Computer-aided speech production training (CASPT) for the speech handicapped. Scientific exhibit at the annual meeting of the American Speech-Language-Hearing Association, San Francisco, CA. [Abstract in *Asha*, 26(10), 201.]
Neilson, H. R., Cooper, R. J., & Koike, K. (1986). Use of computer-aided speech production and training (CASPT) in articulation therapy. Presentation at the annual meeting of the American Speech-Language-Hearing Association, Detroit, MI.
Nelson, L. K. (1991). Ten reasons to start using database software. Presentation at the annual meeting of the American Speech-Language-Hearing Association, Atlanta, GA. [Abstract in *Asha*, 33(10), 122.]
Nelson, L. K. (1992). Take control—Video tape logging and analysis with a Macintosh. Presentation at the annual meeting of the American Speech-Language-Hearing Association, San Antonio, TX. [Abstract in *Asha*, 34(10), 189.]
Nelson, L. K. (1993). Microcomputer control of videotape: One multimedia approach for treatment delivery. Presentation at the annual meeting of the American Speech-Language-Hearing Association, Anaheim, CA. [Abstract in *Asha*, 35(10), 108.]
Nelson, N. W. (1991). Generating IEP objectives with computer software. Presentation at the annual meeting of the American Speech-Language-Hearing Association, Atlanta, GA. [Abstract in *Asha*, 33(10), 171.]
Netsell, R. W. (1994). Instrumentation and special procedures for individuals with dysarthria. *American Journal of Speech-Language Pathology*, 3(2), 9–11.
Neu, P. (1985). *Moptown Parade Builds Problem-Solving Skills* [Computer program]. Menlo Park, CA: The Learning Company.
Newell, W. J., ldims, D., & Meyers, T. (1983). Principles and requisites of computer-assisted interactive video instruction: A sign language lesson. *American Annals of the Deaf*, 128, 662–672.
Newell, W. J., Sims, D., & Clymer, E. W. (March 1984). Meet David, our teacher's helper. *Perspectives* [Gallaudet University Press], 14–18.
Newman, C. W., Jacobson, G. P., & Weinstein, B. E. (1993). Developing hearing handicap profiles: Application of macro statements. Presentation at the annual meeting of the American Speech-Language-Hearing Association, Anaheim, CA. [Abstract in *Asha*, 35(10), 216.]
Newton, M. (1986a). Computer applications in private practice: Getting started. In K. G. Butler (Ed.), *Prospering in Private Practice: A Handbook for Speech-Language Pathology and Audiology*. Rockville, MD: Aspen.
Newton, M. (1986b). Standard computer software applications in private practice. In K. G. Butler (Ed.), *Prospering in Private Practice: A Handbook for Speech-Language Pathology and Audiology*. Rockville, MD: Aspen.
Nicholas, M. L., Elliott, S. T., Baker, E., & Weiss, S. (1994). Computerized AAC system for severe aphasia: Person talk using computer. Presentation at the annual meeting of the American Speech-Language-Hearing Association, New Orleans, LA. [Abstract in *Asha*, 36(10), 246.]
Nickerson, R. S., Kalikow, C. D., & Stevens, K. N. (1976). Computer-aided speech training for the deaf. *Journal of Speech and Hearing Disorders*, 41(1), 120–132.

Nickerson, R., Stevens, K., Rollins, A., & Zue, V. (1983). Computers and speech aids. In I. Hocberg, H. Levitt, & M. Osberger (Eds.), *Speech of the Hearing Impaired.* Baltimore, MD: University Park Press.

Nicolaou, E. (1988). The Computer-Assisted Speechreading Training (CAST) Program: The equivalency of pre and post tests. Unpublished master's research project, University of Western Ontario, London, Ontario.

Nippold, M., Schwarz, I., & Lewis, M. (1992). Analyzing the potential benefit of microcomputer use for teaching figurative language. *American Journal of Speech-Language Pathology*, 1(2), 36–53.

Northern, J. L. (1986). The personal computer as a professional tool. In J. L. Northern (Ed.), *The Personal Computer for Speech, Language, and Hearing Professionals*. Boston, MA: Little, Brown, 1–10.

Northern, J. L. (Ed.) (1986). *The Personal Computer for Speech, Language, and Hearing Professionals*. Boston, MA: Little, Brown.

Nye, C., & Pentz, A. (1987). Computer Graphics for the Photo Articulation Test [Review of this computer program]. *Journal for Computer Users in Speech and Hearing*, 3(2), 173–175.

Nye, C., & Weems, L. (1989). Concentrate on Words and Concepts I, II and III [Review of computer program]. *Journal for Computer Users in Speech and Hearing*, 5(1), 44–47.

O'Connor, L. C., & Schery, T. (1986). A comparison of microcomputer-aided and traditional language therapy for developing communication skills in nonoral toddlers. *Journal of Speech and Hearing Disorders*, 51, 356–361.

Odom, C. (1991a). Action Music Play [Review of computer program]. *Asha*, 33(5), 88–89.

Odom, C. (1991b). Keytalk [Review of computer program]. *Asha*, 33(12), 106.

Oliveira, A. (1991). Office automation and its benefits to the hearing health care professional. *Journal for Computer Users in Speech and Hearing*, 7(1), 121–122.

Oller, D. K. (1991). Computational approaches to transcription and analysis in child phonology. *Journal for Computer Users in Speech and Hearing*, 7(1), 44–59.

Oller, D. K., & Delgado, R. E. (1991). Phonetic transcription and phonological analysis using LIPP. Presentation at the annual meeting of the American Speech-Language-Hearing Association, Atlanta, GA. [Abstract in *Asha*, 33(10), 122.]

Oller, D. K., Hodson, B. W., & Delgado, R. E. (1992). Computerized phonological analysis: Tool for the clinician implemented in LIPP. Presentation at the annual meeting of the American Speech-Language-Hearing Association, San Antonio, TX. [Abstract in *Asha*, 34(10), 134.]

O'Malley, H., Barlow, S. M., Harris, D. M., Kahane, J. C., Prosek, R. A., Shannon, R. V., Wier, C. C., & Wightman, F. L. (1987). Computer applications in the laboratory. Presentation at the annual meeting of the American Speech-Language-Hearing Association, New Orleans, LA. [Abstract in *Asha*, 29(10), 65–66.]

O'Neal, L. (1987a). Language Stimulation Software #6, Selecting Modifiers: Semantics [Review of computer program]. *Asha*, 29(8), 61.

O'Neal, L. (1987b). Parables Plus [Review of Computer Program]. *Asha*, 29(11), 68.

O'Neal, L. (1988). Cognitive Disorders 1: Category Naming and Completion [Review of computer program]. *Asha*, 30(5), 77–78.

Optimum Resources (1986). *Stickybear ABC* [Computer program]. Middletown, CT: Weekly Reader Family Software.

Oratio, A. R. (1979). Computer assisted interaction analysis in speech-language pathology and audiology. *Asha*, 21(3), 179–184.

O'Rouke-Jackson, C. (1985). Audiometer Simulator [Review of computer program]. *Asha*, 27(9), 73–74.

Orsten, M. M. (1986). Computerized diagnostic summary for the speech-language pathologist. Presentation at the annual meeting of the American Speech-Language-Hearing Association, Detroit, MI. [Abstract in *Asha*, 28(10), 98.]

Orwig, G. W., & Hodges, W. S. (1982). *The Computer Tutor: Apple Computer Edition.* Boston: Little, Brown.

Osberger, M., Moeller, M., Kroese, J., and Lippmann, R. (1981). Computer-assisted speech training for the hearing impaired. *Journal of the Academy of Rehabilitation Audiology*, 14, 145–158.

Osborne, G. S. (1985). Computer assistance in the management of a speech and hearing center. Presentation at the American Speech and Hearing Foundation Conference on Microcomputers, New Orleans, LA. [Abstract in the *Journal for Computer Users in Speech and Hearing*, 1(2), 86–87.]

Oshrin, S. E. (1985). A first programming language: BASIC or Pascal. *Journal for Computer Users in Speech and Hearing*, 1(2), 139–143.

Oshrin, S. E. (1994). Navigating the information superhighway. Presentation at the annual meeting of the American Speech-Language-Hearing Association, New Orleans, LA. [Abstract in *Asha*, 36(10), 106.]

Oshrin, S. E., & Terrio, L. M. (1990a). *Sine Wave Analysis Practice version 1.4* [Computer program]. Hattiesburg, MS: Diversified Education Management Systems, Inc., Software Products Division, 123 South 25th Avenue.

Oshrin, S. E., & Terrio, L. M. (1990b). *Sine Wave Introduction Program version 1.0* [Computer program]. Hattiesburg, MS: Diversified Education Management Systems, Inc., Software Products Division, 123 South 25th Avenue.

Oshrin, S. E., & Terrio, L. M. (1991). An integration of audiometric data analysis and customized report generation. Presentation at the annual meeting of the American Speech-Language-Hearing Association, Atlanta, GA. [Abstract in *Asha*, 33(10), 192.]

Osredkar, M. M., & Horii, Y. (1991). Accelerometric, videoflurographic and IBM SpeechViewer assessment pre-and post-pharyngeal flap. Presentation at the annual meeting of the American Speech-Language-Hearing Association, Atlanta, GA. [Abstract in *Asha*, 33(10), 147.]

Ostergren, D. E., & Rodel, M. J. (1987). Managing audiological records in an educational setting: Computer applications. Presentation at the annual meeting of the American Speech-Language-Hearing Association, New Orleans, LA. [Abstract in *Asha*, 29(10), 138.]

Ott-Rose, M., & Cochran, P. S. (1992). Teaching action verbs with computer-controlled videodisc vs. traditional picture stimuli. *Journal for Computer Users in Speech and Hearing*, 8(1, 2), 15–32.

Owen, A. S., Hilbert, J. E., & Owen, W. L. (1994). Computer aided instruction for speech and hearing science. Presentation at the annual meeting of the American Speech-Language-Hearing Association, New Orleans, LA. [Abstract in *Asha*, 36(10), 219.]

Owen, A. S., & Owen, W. L. (1989a). Computer assisted computation of supervisory hours. Presentation at the annual meeting of the American Speech-Language-Hearing Association, St. Louis, MO. [Abstract in *Asha*, 31(10), 132.]

Owen, A. S., & Owen, W. L. (1989b). Computer recorded analysis of student hours. Presentation at the annual meeting of the American Speech-Language-Hearing Association, St. Louis, MO. [Abstract in *Asha*, 31(10), 132.]

Owen, A. S., & Owen, W. L. (1995). Charting management progress with spreadsheets. Presentation at the annual meeting of the American Speech-Language-Hearing Association, Orlando, FL. [Abstract in *Asha*, 37(10), 83.]

Owen, A. S., Owen, W. L., & Schicht, M. D. (1991). How to save time and increase accountability. Presentation at the annual meeting of the American Speech-Language-Hearing Association, Atlanta, GA. [Abstract in *Asha*, 33(10), 170.]

Owen, A. S., Owen, W. L., Schicht, M. D., Hilbert, J. E. (1995). Use of computer-aided instruction in communication sciences and disorders. Presentation at the annual meeting of the American Speech-Language-Hearing Association, Orlando, FL. [Abstract in *Asha*, 37(10), 83.]

Ozdamar, O., Delgado, R. E., Eilers, R. E., & Widen, J. E. (1990). Computer methods for on-line hearing testing with auditory brainstem responses. *Ear and Hearing*, 6, 417–422.

Ozdamar, O., Kaplan, R., Miskiel, E., & Delgado, R. E. (1987). Human-machine interface for an interactive evoked potential system. In S. S. Asfour (Ed.), *Trends in Ergonomics/ Human Factors IV*. Amsterdam: Elsevier Science Publishing BV.

Ozdamar, O., Eilers, R. E., Miskiel, E. & Widen, J. E. (199?). Classification of audiograms by sequential testing using a dynamic Bayesian procedure. *Journal of the Acoustical Society of America*.

Palin, M. W., & Cohen, C. G. (1986). Technology in the schools. *Asha*, 28(5), 35.

Palin, M. W., & Mordecai, D. (1982). *Lingquest 2: Phonological Analysis* [Computer program]. Napa, CA: Lingquest Software.

Palmer, C. V. (1990). Shape (Selecting Hearing Aids for Patients Effectively), Version 3.0 [Review of computer program]. *Asha*, 32(8), 70–71.

Palmer, C. V. (1991a). The computer in audiology supervision. Presentation at the annual meeting of the American Speech-Language-Hearing Association, Atlanta, GA. [Abstract in *Asha*, 33(10), 187.]

Palmer, C. V. (1991b). An overview of Macintosh applications in audiology. Presentation at the annual meeting of the American Speech-Language-Hearing Association, Atlanta, GA. [Abstract in *Asha*, 33(10), 122–123.]

Palmer, C. V. (1992). Using the HyperCard/HyperTalk programming environment in the clinical and educational audiology setting. *Journal for Computer Users in Speech and Hearing*, 8(1, 2), 130–136.

Palmer, C. V., Garstecki, D., & Rauterkus, M. (1990). An interactive product locator for the selection of assistive devices. Presentation at the annual meeting of the American Speech-Language-Hearing Association, Seattle.

Parent Reporting (No Date)[Computer program]. Dimondale, MI: Hartley Courseware.

Parish, H. M., Wynne, M. K., & Kneil, T. R. (1993). Hypertext modules and their advantage over traditional student projects. Presentation at the annual meeting of the American Speech-Language-Hearing Association, Anaheim, CA. [Abstract in *Asha*, 35(10), 132.]

Parker, B. S., Arnett, A. A., & Eldred, J. (1993). MacAid: A computer application in aural rehabilitation. *Journal of the Academy of Rehabilitative Audiology*, 26, 13–23.

Parker, B. S., & Eldred, J. (1992). MacAid: An interactive program for new hearing aid users. Presentation at the annual meeting of the American Speech-Language-Hearing Association, San Antonio, TX. [Abstract in *Asha*, 34(10), 126.]

Parker, R. C. (1990). *Looking Good in Print*. Chapel Hill, NC: Vantana Press.

Parkhurst, B. G., & MacEachron, M. P. (1980). Computer-assisted analysis of written language: Assessing the written language of deaf children. *Journal of Communication Disorders*, 13(6), 493–504.

Patterson, J. P., & Punch, J. (1994). Launching multimedia applications: Issues in design and development. Presentation at the annual meeting of the American Speech-Language-Hearing Association, New Orleans, LA. [Abstract in *Asha*, 36(10), 218.]

Pawluk, M. F. (1985). *Creating Audiology and Speech-Language Pathology Programs on Your Apple Computer*. Austin, TX: PRO-ED.

Pawluk, M. F. (1986). Pure Tone Audiometry Simulation [Review of computer program]. *Asha*, 28(5), 85–86.

Pejsa, J., & Pejsa, J. (1987). *Kidwriter* [Computer program]. Tucson, AZ: Communication Skill Builders.

Peletier, C. A., & Weiner, F. F. (1995). *Aphasia 4: Reading Comprehension* [Computer program]. West Bloomfield, MI: Parrot Software.

Pentz, A. L. Jr. (1987a). Professional staff orientation and training in the use of microcomputers. *Journal for Computer Users in Speech and Hearing*, 3(2), 140–147.

Pentz, A. L. Jr. (1987b). The Reinforcer [Review of computer program]. *Journal for Computer Users in Speech and Hearing*, 3(2), 171–172.

Pentz, A. L. Jr. (1991). Computer-generated stimulus materials, *Journal for Computer Users in Speech and Hearing*, 7(1), 143–148.

Perez, W. E. B., Alba, L., Reimer, T., & Oboudi, A. L. (1993). An adult linguistic/pragmatic database report utilizing a 7–point rating scale. Presentation at the annual meeting of the American Speech-Language-Hearing Association, Anaheim, CA. [Abstract in *Asha*, 35(10), 126.]

Perron, J. D., Nichols, M., & Arnstrong, A. (1987?). *Wally's Word Works* [Computer program]. Pleasantville, NY: Sunburst Communications, 39 Washington Avenue.

Peterson, H. A. (1977). More about computer assisted clinical record keeping. *Asha*, 19(9), 617–618.

Petheram, B. (1991). Microcomputers as a supplement to aphasia therapy. *Journal of Neurolinguistics*, 6, 177–195.

Pflaum, M. (1982). The California connection: Interfacing the TDD and the Apple computer. *American Annals of the Deaf*, 127, 573–584.

Phonological Project, Waisman Center on Mental Retardation and Human Development, University of Wisconsin-Madison (1987). *Computer Graphics for the Photo Articulation Test* [Computer program]. Danville, IL: Interstate Printers and Publishers, Inc., P.O. Box 50.

Pichora-Fuller, M. K., & Benguerel, A.-P. (1990). Development of CAST: A Computer-Aided Speechreading Training program. *Journal of Speech and Hearing Research*, 34, 202–212.

Pichora-Fuller, M. K., & Benguerel, A.-P. (1991). The design of CAST (Computer-Aided Speechreading Training). *Journal of Speech and Hearing Research*, 34, 202–212.

Pichora-Fuller, M. K., & Cicchelli, M. (1986). *Computer Aided Speechreading Training (CAST) Owner's Manual*. Mississauga, Ontario: Department of Psychology, University of Toronto, Canada.

Pickering, Jr., J. E. (1992). Pictures, sounds, and button-making: A perspective on the appeal of HyperCard for communication disorders. *Journal for Computer Users in Speech and Hearing*, 8(1, 2), 100–104.

Pickett, J. (1981). Speech technology and communication for the hearing impaired. *Volta Review*, 83, 301–309.

Pimentel, K., & Teixeira, K. (1995). *Virtual Reality: Through the New Looking Glass* (2nd Ed.). New York: McGraw-Hill.

Pitts, W. M. (1991). Personal computers for language retrieval. *Journal for Computer Users in Speech and Hearing*, 7(1), 123–125.

Plakke, B. L. (1987). Audio-PC Version 2.0 [Review of computer program]. *Asha*, 29(2), 75–76.

Plakke, B. L. (1988). The Ear [Review of computer program]. *Asha*, 30(12), 67.

Plakke, B. L. (1994). Utilizing SoundScope applications for teaching measurement of sound. Presentation at the annual meeting of the American Speech-Language-Hearing Association, New Orleans, LA. [Abstract in *Asha*, 36(10), 107.]

Plakke, B. L., & Royster, J. D. (1991). Utilizing N.A.N. computer program for assessment of hearing loss claims. Presentation at the annual meeting of the American Speech-Language-Hearing Association, Atlanta, GA. [Abstract in *Asha*, 33(10), 192.]

Poburka, B. J. (1995). Teaching acoustic phonetics. Presentation at the annual meeting of the American Speech-Language-Hearing Association, Orlando, FL. [Abstract in *Asha*, 37(10), 73.]

Poburka, B. J., & Bless, D. M. (1994). Interpretation of videostroboscopy. Presentation at the annual meeting of the American Speech-Language-Hearing Association, New Orleans, LA. [Abstract in *Asha*, 36(10), 107.]

Pollock, K. E. (1988). PEPPER: Programs to Examine Phonetic and Phonologic Evaluation Records [Review of computer program]. *Asha*, 30(8), 57–58.

Pollock, K. E., & Dana, D. (1989). A comparison of the results of three computerized phonological analyses. Presentation at the annual meeting of the American Speech-Language-Hearing Association, St. Louis, MO. [Abstract in *Asha*, 31(10), 155.]

Pollock, K. E., Matesich, J. S., & Ward, M. F. (1992). Determining the relative effect of various phonological errors on intelligibility. Presentation at the annual meeting of the American Speech-Language-Hearing Association, San Antonio, TX. [Abstract in *Asha*, 34(10), 121.]

Ponsford, J. L. (1990). The use of computers in the rehabilitation of attention disorders. In R. L. Wood & I. Fussey (Eds.), *Cognitive Rehabilitation in Perspective*. London: Taylor & Francis, 48–68.

Popelka, G. R. (1983). Computer assisted hearing aid fitting. Presentation at the American Speech-Language-Hearing Association, Cincinnati, OH. [Abstract in *Asha*, 25(10), 87.]

Popelka, G. R. (1986). Computer-assisted hearing aid fitting. In M. L. Grossfeld & C. A. Grossfeld (Eds.), *Microcomputer Applications in Rehabilitation of Communication Disorders*. Rockville, MD: Aspen, 67–96.

Popelka, G., & Engebretson, A. M. (1983). A computer-based system for hearing aid assessment. *Hearing Instruments*, 34, 6.

Porter, D. (1978). Patient responses to computer counseling. *Proceedings: The Second Annual Symposium on Computer Application* Care, Washington, DC., 104–108.

Portnoy, R. A., & Aronson, A. E. (1982). Diadochokinetic syllable rate and regularity in normal and in spastic and ataxic dysarthric subjects. *Journal of Speech and Hearing Disorders*, 47, 324–328.

Povel, D. J., & Wansink, M. A. (1986). A computer-controlled vowel corrector for the hearing impaired. *Journal of Speech and Hearing Research*, 29, 99–105.

Prater, R. J. (1988). Microcomputer-based program for students' *ASHA* clinical hours and client billing. Presentation at the annual meeting of the American Speech-Language-Hearing Association, Boston, MA. [Abstract in *Asha*, 30(10), 149.]

Pratt, S. R., Heintzelman, A. T., & Deming, S. E. (1993). The efficacy of using the IBM SpeechViewer Vowel Accuracy Module to treat young children with hearing impairment. *Journal of Speech and Hearing Research*, 36, 1063–1074.

Prescott, T. E., & Loverso, F. L. (1985). Computerized aphasia rehabilitation: State of the art. Presentation at the annual meeting of the American Speech-Language-Hearing Association, Washington, DC. [Abstract in *Asha*, 27(10), 84.]

Preves, D. (1982). The potential of computers and signal processing for hearing aids. *Hearing Instruments*, 31, 15–16.

Printz, P. M. (1991). Literacy and language development within microcomputer-videodisc-assisted interactive contexts. *Journal of Childhood Communication Disorders*, 14(1), 67–80.

Printz, P. M., & Nelson, K. E. (1983). Interactive microcomputer system for reading/language development in deaf children. Presentation at the annual meeting of the American Speech-Language-Hearing Association, Cincinnati, OH. [Abstract in *Asha*, 25(10), 99.]

Printz, P. M., & Nelson, K. E. (1984). ALPHA interactive microcomputer system for reading/language development in children. Presentation at the annual meeting of the American Speech-Language-Hearing Association, San Francisco, CA. [Abstract in *Asha*, 26(10), 157.]

Printz, P. M., Nelson, K. E., Arford, L. M., & Mugg, S. E. (1988). "Recasting" during microcomputer-aided language intervention with multihandicapped children. Presentation at the annual meeting of the American Speech-Language-Hearing Association, Boston, MA. [Abstract in *Asha*, 30(10), 173.]

Propp, G., Nugent, G., & Stone, C. (1980). Videodisc update. *American Annals of the Deaf*, 125, 679–684.

Psychological Corporation (1994). *PictureGallery* [Computer program]. San Antonio: The Psychological Corporation.

Punch, J., & Weinstein, B. (1994). Hearing Handicap Inventory for the Elderly: A multimedia version. Presentation at the annual meeting of the American Speech-Language-Hearing Association, New Orleans, LA. [Abstract in *Asha*, 36(10), 218.]

Punch, J. L., Levitt, H., Mahaffey, R. B., & Wilson, M. S. (1983). Computer technology: The revolution has started without us. Presentation at the annual meeting of the American Speech-Language-Hearing Association, Cincinnati, OH. [Abstract in *Asha*, 25(10), 96.]

Pye, C. (1987). *Pye Analysis of Language* (PAL). Lawrence, KS: Author, 200 Arrowhead Drive.

Pye, C. (1988). The Pye analysis of language. *Working Papers in Language Development*. University of Kansas Child Language Program, 1–37.

Quigley, S. M. (1991). Teaching audiogram interpretation through computer aided instruction (CAI). Presentation at the annual meeting of the American Speech-Language-Hearing Association, Atlanta, GA. [Abstract in *Asha*, 33(10), 187.]

Quigley, S. M., & Sanborn, E. S. (1992). Interactive computer software for speechreading training. Presentation at the annual meeting of the American Speech-Language-Hearing Association, San Antonio, TX. [Abstract in *Asha*, 34(10), 109.]

Quigley, S. P., Steinkamp, M. W., Power, D. J., & Jones, B. W. (1991). *Tests of Syntactic Abilities (TSA). Screening Test Form 1* [Computer program]. Austin, TX: ProEd.

Quinoa, J. (1988). Computer Graphics for the Photo Articulation Test [Review of computer program]. *Asha*, 30(2), 69–70.

Raade, A. S., & Reaburn, B. L. A. (1993). Computerized Visual Communication: Response Elaboration Training (RET). Presentation at the annual meeting of the American Speech-Language-Hearing Association, Anaheim, CA. [Abstract in *Asha*, 35(10), 171.]

Rabb, M. Y. (1990). *The Presentation Design Book*. Chapel Hill, NC: Ventana Press.

Randolph, K. J., & Lynch, O. C. (1988). Spreadsheet applications in hearing aid prescription and evaluation. Presentation at the annual meeting of the American Speech-Language-Hearing Association, Boston, MA. [Abstract in *Asha*, 30(10), 146.]

Ratcliff, A., Lehman, M., & Hughes, D. (1994). Diverse applications for HyperCard in a communication disorders training program. Presentation at the annual meeting of the American Speech-Language-Hearing Association, New Orleans, LA. [Abstract in *Asha*, 36(10), 174.]

Regents of the University of Michigan (no date). *Serial Recall Assessment: Michigan Memory Series Software* [Computer program]. Ann Arbor, MI: Intellectual Property Office, University of Michigan.

Reiner, B. J., & Ludlow, C. L. (1979a). *MEDLINE Users Manual and Thesaurus for Specialists in Communicative Disorders*, Volume I (Users Manual NIH 79–1997). Bethesda: U.S. Department of Health Services, Public Health Service, National Institutes of Health.

Reiner, B. J., & Ludlow, C. L. (1979b). *MEDLINE Users Manual and Thesaurus for Specialists in Communicative Disorders*, Volume II (Thesaurus NIH 79–1198). Bethesda: U.S. Department of Health Services, Public Health Service, National Institutes of Health .

Reiner, B. J., & Ludlow, C. L. (1981). Using MEDLINE for literature retieval in the communicative disorders. *Asha*, 23(9), 655–661.

Rentschler, G. J. (1984). Computer literacy: Meeting the needs of the profession. Presentation at the annual meeting of the American Speech-Language-Hearing Association, San Francisco, CA. [Abstract in *Asha*, 26(10), 79.]

Rentschler, G. J. (1985). Computer synthesized speech: Intelligibility and the language-impaired child. Presentation at the annual meeting of the American Speech-Language-Hearing Association, Washington, DC. [Abstract in *Asha*, 27(10), 88.]

Revit, L. J. (1991). Computerized tailoring of hearing aid prescriptions to the individual ear. Presentation at the annual meeting of the American Speech-Language-Hearing Association, Atlanta, GA. [Abstract in *Asha*, 33(10), 193.]

Reynolds, M. E., Fucci, D., Bettagere, R., & Gonzales, M. D. (1995). Factors influencing the intelligibility of DECtalk. Presentation at the annual meeting of the American Speech-Language-Hearing Association, Orlando, FL. [Abstract in *Asha*, 37(10), 46.]

Rickard, J. K., Shuler, J. F., & Jackson, C. A. (1995). Microcomputer applications in aphasia treatment. Presentation at the annual meeting of the American Speech-Language-Hearing Association, Orlando, FL. [Abstract in *Asha*, 37(10), 87.]

Rimac, R. T. (1991). How to make "talking" communication boards on the Macintosh computer. Presentation at the annual meeting of the American Speech-Language-Hearing Association, Atlanta, GA. [Abstract in *Asha*, 33(10), 191.]

Riski, J. E., & Delong, E. R. (1982). Computer-assisted analysis of articulation data. Presentation at the annual meeting of the American Speech-Language-Hearing Association, Toronto, Canada. [Abstract in *Asha*, 24(10), 835.]

Robertson, I. (1990). Does computerized cognitive rehabilitation work? A review. *Aphasiology*, 4(4), 381–405.

Robey, R., & Olsen, B. (1978). Computer-assisted analysis of PICA raw scores. Presentation at the annual meeting of the American Speech-Language-Hearing Association, San Francisco, CA.

Robins, A. (1996). Technology tutorial will open doors. *ASHA Leader*, 1(8), 5.

Rodman, R. D., Moody, T., & Price, J. A. (1984). Speech recognizer performance of the voice handicapped. *Proceedings of the Voice I/O Systems Applications Conference* (Arlington, VA).

Rolnick, M. I. (1985). Clinical use of the Apple microcomputer during language and cognitive rehabilitation. Presentation at the American Speech and Hearing Foundation Conference on Microcomputers, New Orleans, LA. [Abstract in the *Journal for Computer Users in Speech and Hearing*, 1(2), 87–88.]

Rolnick, M. I., Koster, M. H., Brabaker, S. H., Gordon, C., Smith, J.B., & Sell, D. (1983). Microcomputers in language and cognitive rehabilitation. Presentation at the annual meeting of the American Speech-Language-Hearing Association, Cincinnati, OH. [Abstract in *Asha*, 25(10), 126.]

Rose, S., & Waldron, M. (1984). Microcomputer use in programs for hearing-impaired children: A national survey. American Annals for the Deaf, 129(3), 338–342.

Rosen, L. D., & Weil, M. M. (1995). Computer availability, computer experience, and technophobia among public school teachers. *Computers in Human Behavior*, 11(1) 9–31.

Rosenblum, M. (1991). Marketing products for new platforms: A difficult and frustrating task. *Journal for Computer Users in Speech and Hearing*, 7(1), 126–127.

Roske, L. M., McCann, C. A., & Thomas-Stonell, N. L. (1991). Evaluation of a computer-based program for training stop-consonants. Presentation at the annual meeting of the American Speech-Language-Hearing Association, Atlanta, GA. [Abstract in *Asha*, 33(10), 188.]

Ross, L. L., Butt, D. S., & Williams, J. K. (1991). Learning and recalling symbol sequences in augmentative communication using computers. Presentation at the annual meeting of the American Speech-Language-Hearing Association, Atlanta, GA. [Abstract in *Asha*, 33(10), 192.]

Roush, J., & Horii, Y. (1986). Microcomputer applications in the university setting. In J. L. Northern (Ed.), *The Personal Computer for Speech, Language, and Hearing Professionals*. Boston, MA: Little, Brown.

Rubin, C., & Bollinger, R. L. (1983). Aphasia: Treatment considerations, graphic output. *Topics in Language Disorders*, 3(4), 67–75.

Rubin, P. (1987). MacSpeech Lab [Review of computer program]. *Asha*, 29(2), 74–75.

Rubow, R. T., & Swift, E. (1985). Microcomputer-based wearable biofeedback device to improve the transfer of treatment in Parkinson dysarthria. *Journal of Speech and Hearing Disorders*, 50, 178–185.

Ruder, K., Blache, S., & Harn, W. (1988). *ASHA Project IMPACT: #2 Microcomputer Assisted Intervention for Speech and Language Professionals* [Computer program]. Rockville, MD: American Speech-Language-Hearing Association.

Ruff, R., Mahaffey, R., Engel, J., Farrow, C., Cox, D., & Karzmark, P. (1994). Efficacy study of THINKable in the attention and memory retraining of traumatically head-injured patients. *Brain Injury*, 8(1), 3–14.

Ruge, J. P. (1992). Mind Benders: Sets A1, A2, and B1 [Review of computer programs]. *Asha*, 34(12), 91.

Rusch, C. R. (1987). *Multiple Meanings* [Review of computer program]. *Asha*, 29(11), 66.

Rushakoff, G. E. (1982). Design and implementation of a course of instruction in clinical microcomputer applications for speech-language pathologists and audiologists. Unpublished Ph.D. dissertation, University of Florida.

Rushakoff, G. E. (1983). The /s/ meter: A beginning for microcomputer assisted articulation therapy. Presentation at the annual meeting of the American Speech-Language-Hearing Association, Los Angeles, CA.

Rushakoff, G. E. (1984a). Clinical applications in communication disorders. In A. H. Schwartz (Ed.), *Handbook of Microcomputer Applications in Communication Disorders*, San Diego, CA: College-Hill, pp. 147–173.

Rushakoff, G. E. (1984b). A clinician's model for the review of speech, language, and hearing microcomputer software. *Asha*, 26(8), 43–44.

Rushakoff, G. E. (1984c). Microcomputer assisted instruction in communication disorders. *Journal of Childhood Communication Disorders*, 8(1), 51–61.

Rushakoff, G. E. (1984d). The microcomputer as an efficient and versatile speech-output communication aid. In M. Behrmann & L. Lahm (Eds.). *Proceedings of the National Conference on the Use of Microcomputers in Special Education*. Reston, Virginia: Council for Exceptional Children, pp. 201–205.

Rushakoff, G. E. (1985). Evaluating educational software in communication disorders. Presentation at the American Speech and Hearing Foundation Conference on Microcomputers, New Orleans, LA. [Abstract in the *Journal for Computer Users in Speech and Hearing*, 1(2), 88.]

Rushakoff, G. E. (1986). Microcomputer-based client-record management. In J. L. Northern (Ed.), *The Personal Computer for Speech, Language, and Hearing Professionals*. Boston: Little, Brown, pp. 39–52.

Rushakoff, G. E., & Edwards, W. G. (1982). The /s/ meter: A beginning for microcomputer assisted articulation therapy. Presentation at the annual meeting of the American Speech-Language-Hearing Association, Toronto, Canada. [Abstract in *Asha*, 24(10), 839.]

Rushakoff, G. E., & Lombardino, L. J. (1983). Comprehensive microcomputer applications for severely physically handicapped children. *Teaching Exceptional Children*, 16(1), 18–22.

Rushakoff, G. E., & Lombardino, L. J. (1984). Microcomputer applications. *Asha*, 26(6), 27–31.

Rushakoff, G. E., & Schwartz, A. H. (1986). Clinical assessment software. In M. L. Grossfeld & C. A. Grossfeld (Eds.), *Microcomputer Applications in Rehabilitation of Communication Disorders*. Rockville, MD: Aspen, pp. 1–24.

Rushakoff, G. E., Vinson, B. P., & Messal, S. E. (1979). A computer for clinicians: The future . . . is here today. Presentation at the annual meeting of the American Speech-Language-Hearing Association, Atlanta, GA. [Abstract in *Asha*, 21(9), 748.]

Russel, M. (1990). The Messenger (keyboard and scan access versions) [Review of computer program]. *Asha*, 32(5), 73–74.

Russel, M. (1992). Breakthrough to Language, Volume 2: Multisensory curriculum [Review of computer program]. *Asha*, 34(2), 79–80.

Ryalls, J. (1989). Comparison of two computerized speech training systems: SpeechViewer and ISTRA. *Revue d'Orthophonie et d'Audiologie*, 14, 65–70.

Ryalls, J., Cloutier, M., & Cloutier, D. (1991). Two clinical applications of IBM's SpeechViewer: Therapy and its evaluation on the same machine. *Journal for Computer Users in Speech and Hearing*, 7(1), 22–27.

Sakabe, N., Hirai, Y., & Itami, E. (1978). Modification and application of the computerized automatic audiometer. *Scandinavian Audiology*, 7, 105–109.

Sakabe, N., Miyashita, Y., & Itami, E. (1981). A computerized automatic audiometer. *Medical Information* (London), 6(4), 285–291.

Sakabe, N., Ooki, T., Terai, E., Shinozaki, K., & Itami, E. (1975). A computerized automatic audiometer. *Scandinavian Audiology*, 4, 75–81.

Salciccia, C. E. (1986).The microcomputer as an augmentative communication system. In M. L. Grossfeld & C. A. Grossfeld (Eds.), *Microcomputer Applications in Rehabilitation of Communication Disorders*. Rockville, MD: Aspen, pp. 131–154.

Sanders, J. (1986a). *Microcomputer Applications for Speech-Language Services in the Schools*. Boston, MA: College-Hill Press/Little, Brown & Company.

Sanders, J. (1986b). *Microcomputers and Systems Analysis for Speech-Language Clinicians*. Boston, MA: College-Hill/Little, Brown & Company.

Sanders, J. S. (1984). Application of computer science methodology to speech-language delivery systems. Presentation at the annual meeting of the American Speech-Language-Hearing Association, San Francisco, CA. [Abstract in *Asha*, 26(10), 78–79.]

Sandstedt, C. R., Sonnenberg, E. A., Brinton, B., Lyon, J. G., & Fujiki, M. (1984). The use of word processing software for language sample analysis. Presentation at the annual meeting of the American Speech-Language-Hearing Association, San Francisco, CA. [Abstract in *Asha*, 26(10), 88.]

Saniga, R. D., Carlin, M. F., & Weiner, M. J. (1992). *Voice Conservation Index* [Computer program]. State College, PA: Parrot Software, P.O. Box 1139.

Sansone, F. E., & Acker III. J. F. (1993). Computer-assisted academic programming and practicum tracking. Presentation at the annual meeting of the American Speech-Language-Hearing Association, Anaheim, CA. [Abstract in *Asha*, 35(10), 131–132.]

Sarachan-Deily, A. B. (1990). Can microcomputers help the school speech-language pathologist? *Journal for Computer Users in Speech and Hearing*, 6(1), 57–61.

Sarachan-Deily, A. B. (1992). Beyond the one-room schoolhouse. *Asha*, 34(4), 34–37, 42.

Sarachan-Deily, A. B., & Volin, R. A. (1991). An introduction to the use of the Apple II in speech-language pathology. Presentation at the annual meeting of the American Speech-Language-Hearing Association, Atlanta, GA. [Abstract in *Asha*, 33(10), 170.]

Sauer, M., Brown, C., Wyatt, C., & Cavalier, A. (1992). Research findings for a voice-activated communication system with graphics. Presentation at the annual meeting of the American Speech-Language-Hearing Association, San Antonio, TX. [Abstract in *Asha*, 34(10), 126.]

Savage, H. E., & Zukerman, R. A. (1991). Computerized video data acquisition and analysis in social interaction research. Presentation at the annual meeting of the American Speech-Language-Hearing Association, Atlanta, GA. [Abstract in *Asha*, 33(10), 193.]

Sawyer, J. L., & Sawyer, R. (1994). A management system for clinic and student practicum. Presentation at the annual meeting of the American Speech-Language-Hearing Association, New Orleans, LA. [Abstract in *Asha*, 36(10), 173.]

Sawyer, J. L., Sawyer, R., & Wynne, M. K. (1993). Clinic and student practicum management system using Paradox 4.0. Presentation at the annual meeting of the American Speech-Language-Hearing Association, Anaheim, CA. [Abstract in *Asha*, 35(10), 172.]

Sbordone, R. J. (1983). A computerized approach to cognitive rehabilitation for individuals with traumatic head injury. Presentation at the International Conference on the Management of Traumatic Brain Injury, London, England.

Schaker, B. E. (1990). *Breakthrough to Writing. Volume 3, Multisensory Curriculum* [Computer program]. North San Juan, CA: Creative Learning, Inc., P.O. Box 829.

Schatz, K. H., Joyce, P. E., & O'Shaughnessey, M. S. (1988). Computerized patient tracking for audiologists. Presentation at the annual meeting of the American Speech-Language-Hearing Association, Boston, MA. [Abstract in *Asha*, 30(10), 166.]

Schery, T. K., & O'Connor, L. C. (1986). A comparison of microcomputer aided and traditional language therapy for developing communication skills in nonoral toddlers. *Journal of Speech and Hearing Disorders*, 51, 356–361.

Schery, T. K., & O'Connor, L. C. (1989). Assessing effectiveness of computer language intervention with severely handicapped students. Presentation at the annual meeting of the American Speech-Language-Hearing Association, St. Louis, MO. [Abstract in *Asha*, 31(10), 149.]

Scherz, J. W. (1990). We've come a long way . . . or have we? *Journal for Computer Users in Speech and Hearing*, 6(2), 107–110.

Scherz, J. W. (1992a). Auditory Anatomy [Review of computer program]. *Asha*, 34(5), 93.

Scherz, J. W. (1992b). Software evaluation—A method to the madness. Presentation at the annual meeting of the American Speech-Language-Hearing Association, San Antonio, TX. [Abstract in *Asha*, 34(10), 166.]

Scherz, J. W. (1992c). An undergraduate course in microcomputer applications—An example. Presentation at the annual meeting of the American Speech-Language-Hearing Association, San Antonio, TX. [Abstract in *Asha*, 34(10), 109.]

Scherz, J. W. (1993a). The computer's great—How's the software? Introduction to software review. Presentation at the annual meeting of the American Speech-Language-Hearing Association, Anaheim, CA. [Abstract in *Asha*, 35(10), 227.]

Scherz, J. W. (1993b). Undergraduate speech science: "Nightmare on Elm Street" no more. Presentation at the annual meeting of the American Speech-Language-Hearing Association, Anaheim, CA. [Abstract in *Asha*, 35(10), 132.]

Scherz, J. W. (1995). I Can Play Too! [Review of computer program]. *Asha*, 37(6/7), 59.

Scherz, J. W., & Koch, K. F. (1991). Computer animation or line drawings—An advantage for identifying verbs? Presentation at the annual meeting of the American Speech-Language-Hearing Association, Atlanta, GA. [Abstract in *Asha*, 33(10), 193.]

Scherz, J. W., & Kuster, J. M. (1995). Teaching communicative disorders classes by "surfing the 'net'." Presentation at the annual meeting of the American Speech-Language-Hearing Association, Orlando, FL. [Abstract in *Asha*, 37(10), 69.]

Scherz, J. W., & Lieberth, A. (1995). Modifying commercial software and shareware for clinical use. Presentation at the annual meeting of the American Speech-Language-Hearing Association, Orlando, FL. [Abstract in *Asha*, 37(10), 69.]

Schetz, K. F. (1990). Computer technology in schools: Insights on the future. *Journal for Computer Users in Speech and Hearing*, 6(1), 39–41.

Schetz, K. F., Miller, J. M., & Bernier, C. A. (1991). Computerized IEPs: Praises and precautions. Presentation at the annual meeting of the American Speech-Language-Hearing Association, Atlanta, GA. [Abstract in *Asha*, 33(10), 140.]

Schetz, K. F., & Sheese, R. J. (1989). Software that works in school settings. *Asha*, 31(1), 65–68.

Scheurer, R. (1985). Computerizing a hearing aid office. *Audecibel*, 34, 10–12.

Schneider, P., & Holdgrafer, G. (1994). Using SALT for language research. Presentation at the annual meeting of the American Speech-Language-Hearing Association, New Orleans, LA. [Abstract in *Asha*, 36(10), 107.]

Schodorf, J. K. (1988). Print Your Own Calendar [Review of computer program]. *Asha*, 30(5), 80.

Schodorf, J. K. (1993). My House: Language Activities of Daily Living [Review of computer program]. *Asha*, 35(2), 70.

Schoenberg, M. C. (1995). Use of Speech Viewer MLO and ELLIS with Hispanic college students. Presentation at the annual meeting of the American Speech-Language-Hearing Association, Orlando, FL. [Abstract in *Asha*, 37(10), 78.]

Scholl, K. J., Norris, J., Friehe, M. J., & Davis, P. (1979). Computerized evaluation of diagnostic clinical practicum. Presentation at the annual meeting of the American Speech-Language-Hearing Association, Atlanta, GA. [Abstract in *ASHA* 21(9), 748.]

Schram, J. B., Conrad, C. M., & Rector, K. L. (1986). Computer stimulation in the Alzheimer's population: Effectiveness and implications. Presentation at the annual meeting of the American Speech-Language-Hearing Association, Detroit, MI. [Abstract in *Asha*, 28(10), 145.]

Schuldt, M. E. (No Date). *Automated IEP System—Hypernasality Goal Bank* [Computer program]. Orem, Utah: Harding & Harris Behavior Research.

Schuldt, M. E. (No Date). *CDTS—Initial/Final Report* [Computer program]. Orem, Utah: Harding & Harris Behavior Research.

Schuldt, M. E. (1986). Artificial intelligence: Diagnostic applications. In M. L. Grossfeld & C. A. Grossfeld (Eds.), *Microcomputer Applications in Rehabilitation of Communication Disorders*. Rockville, MD: Aspen, 239–256.

Schuldt, M. E., & Harding, D. C. (1985). *The Automated IEP System-Version 4.2* [Computer program]. Orem, UT: Harding & Harris Behavioral Research.

Schultz, S. (1985). *Ship Ahoy/Word Scramble* [Review of computer program]. *Asha*, 27(9), 74.

Schumacher, G. P., & Tasselbring, T. S. (1982). A microcomputer-based feedback system for training speech-language pathologists. Presentation at the annual meeting of the American Speech-Language-Hearing Association, Toronto, Canada. [Abstract in *Asha*, 24(10), 746.]

Schwartz, A. H. (1984a). Evaluating microcomputer software. In A. H. Schwartz (Ed.), *Handbook of Microcomputer Applications in Communication Disorders*. San Diego, CA: College-Hill, pp. 126–146.

Schwartz, A. H. (Ed.). (1984b). *Handbook of Microcomputer Applications in Communication Disorders*. San Diego, CA: College-Hill Press.

Schwartz, A. H. (1985a). Computer Software for the Exceptional Student [Review of computer program]. *Asha*, 27(11), 73–74.

Schwartz, A. H. (1985b). A primer for evaluating clinical software. Presentation at the annual meeting of the American Speech-Language-Hearing Association, Washington, DC. [Abstract in *Asha*, 27(10), 109.]

Schwartz, A. H. (Ed.) (1986a). *Computer Conference Proceedings: Orlando, FL. January 21–25, 1986*. Rockville, MD: American Speech-Language-Hearing Foundation.

Schwartz, A. H. (Ed.) (1986b). *1986 Computer Conference Software Directory for Communication Sciences and Disorders*. Rockville, MD: American Speech-Language-Hearing Foundation.

Schwartz, A. H. (1986c). Microcomputer applications-what changes hath this tool wrought? *Tejas*, 12, 4–9.

Schwartz, A. H. (1988a). Goldojarb Software Classification System (GSCS) [Review of computer program]. *Journal for Computer Users in Speech and Hearing*, 4(1), 54–58.

Schwartz, A. H. (1988b). Microcomputer software availability: An analysis of features. Presentation at the annual meeting of the American Speech-Language-Hearing Association, Boston, MA. [Abstract in *Asha*, 30(10), 166.]

Schwartz, A. H. (1988c). PICApad II: PICA Report Generating Program [Review of computer program]. *Journal for Computer Users in Speech and Hearing*, 4(1), 49–53.

Schwartz, A. H. (1988d). Slow Speech-Rate Drill for Dysarthric Speakers [Review of computer program]. *Journal for Computer Users in Speech and Hearing*, 4(1), 62–63.

Schwartz, A. H. (1989a). A look at the needs for the application of microcomputers in the 1990s. *Journal for Computer Users in Speech and Hearing*, 5(2), 114–124.

Schwartz, A. H. (1989b). Pacer/Tally for Pacing and Tallying Responses [Review of computer program]. *Journal for Computer Users in Speech and Hearing*, 5(1), 40–43.

Schwartz, A. H. (1989c). Words & Concepts [Review of computer program]. *Journal for Computer Users in Speech and Hearing*, 5(2), 135–139.

Schwartz, A. H. (Summer/Spring 1990). Tips for obtaining funding to integrate technology into clinical activities. *Hearsay*, 64–66.

Schwartz, A. H., Brogan, V. M., Emond, G. A., & Oleksiak, J. F. (1993). Technology-enhanced accent modification. *Asha*, 35(8), 44–46, 51.

Schwartz, A. H., & Cohen, C. G. (1989). Decision making in upgrading microcomputers for clinical administrative applications. Presentation at the annual meeting of the American Speech-Language-Hearing Association, St. Louis, MO. [Abstract in *Asha*, 31(10), 100.]

Schwartz, A. H., Clymer, E. W., Larkins, P. G., Olson, J. S., Ruder, K. F., Shearer, W. R., Smaldino, J., & Testut, E. W. (1987). Teaching clinical applications for computer technology. Presentation at the annual meeting of the American Speech-Language-Hearing Association, New Orleans, LA. [Abstract in *Asha*, 29(10), 72.]

Schwartz, A. H., Gelatt, J. P., Lilly, D. J., & Quinn, M. M. (1986). Infusing computer applications: What we have learned. Presentation at the annual meeting of the American Speech-Language-Hearing Association, Detroit, MI. [Abstract in *Asha*, 28(10), 134.]

Schwartz, A. H., Koller, D. E., & Cassidy, R. (1984). The uses of word processing for clinical report writing. Part II: Program features for developing report formats. *Journal of Childhood Communication Disorders*. 8, 23–35.

Schwartz, A. H., Koller, D. E., & Koczot, K. A. (1984). Augmentative applications for microcomputers. Presentation at the annual meeting of the American Speech-Language-Hearing Association, San Francisco, CA. [Abstract in *Asha*, 26(10), 171.]

Schwartz, A. H., Kunicki, E., Del Calzo, P. V., & Brown, V. (1989). Project DISC: Developing and integrating skills with computers. Presentation at the annual meeting of the American Speech-Language-Hearing Association, St. Louis, MO. [Abstract in *Asha*, 31(10), 189.]

Schwartz, A. H., & Rushakoff, G. E. (1986). The Clock Hour Program [Computer program]. *Journal for Computer Users in Speech and Hearing*, 2(1), 38–39.

Schwejda, P., & Vanderheiden, G. C. (1982). Adaptive-firmware card for the Apple II. *Byte*, 7, 276–314.

Scudder, R. R. (1990). SunTool Speech/Language IEP Writer+ [Review of computer program]. *Journal for Computer Users in Speech and Hearing*, 6(1), 71–72.

Seal, B. C., & Filter, M. D. (1990). The use of spreadsheets in assuring accountability in university supervision loads. *Journal for Computer Users in Speech and Hearing*, 6(1), 33–37.

Seal, B. C., Smith, J. E., & Runyan, S. E. (1989). Establishing a rationale for using minicomputers in appraising clinical competence. Presentation at the annual meeting of the American Speech-Language-Hearing Association, St. Louis, MO. [Abstract in *Asha*, 31(10), 132.]

Seaton, W. H. (1983). The statistical analysis system for program management. *Asha*, 25(5).

Seaton, W. H. (1989). Some future considerations for computer users in speech and hearing. *Journal for Computer Users in Speech and Hearing*, 5(1), 19–31.

Seaton, W. H. (1990). *Managing Information in Communication Sciences and Disorders with Appleworks Software* [Computer program]. Hudson, OH: Seaton & Sibs, 5929 Sunset Drive.

Seaton, W. H. (1991a). How to survive the paperwork: Appleworks as an information management tool. Presentation at the annual meeting of the American Speech-Language-Hearing Association, Atlanta, GA. [Abstract in *Asha*, 33(10), 123.]

Seaton, W. H. (1991b). Managing customer/client billing with microsoft works. *Journal for Computer Users in Speech and Hearing*, 7(1), 161–169.

Seaton, W. H. (1991c). A spreadsheet-based payroll management system. *Journal for Computer Users in Speech and Hearing*, 7(1), 170–181.

Seaton, W. H. (1991d). Spreadsheets in communication sciences and disorders: Tutorial and application. *Journal for Computer Users in Speech and Hearing*, 7(1), 149–160.

Seaton, W. H., & McVey, D. E. (1983). Using SAS for displaying data and preparing poster session material. *Asha*, 25(5), 41–42.

Seaton, W. H., Richards, H., & Harter, M. (1985). Integrating computer technology into educational programs: Ohio University's experience. *Journal for Computer Users in Speech and Hearing*, 1(1), 36–44.

Secord, W. A., Pallante, D., & Wiig, E. H. (1994). Team-based problem solving: Designing, implementing, and evaluating classroom interventions. Presentation at the annual meeting of the American Speech-Language-Hearing Association, New Orleans, LA. [Abstract in *Asha*, 36(10), 106.]

Seikel, J. A., Drumright, D. G., Whites, M. M., LaVoi, G., & Kammermeier, M. (1991). Speech science and clinical practice: Bridging the gap. Presentation at the annual meeting of the American Speech-Language-Hearing Association, Atlanta, GA. [Abstract in *Asha*, 33(10), 162.]

Sellers, D. E. (1990). SSW C*I*R [Review of computer program]. *Asha*, 32(8), 70.

Semel, E., Wiig, E. H., & Secord, W. (1990). *CELF-R Scoring Assistant* [Computer program]. San Antonio, TX: Psychological Corporation.

Seron, X., Deloche, G., Moulard, G., & Rousselle, M. (1980). A computer-based therapy for the treatment of aphasic clients with writing disorders. *Brain and Language*, 45–58.

Sevcik, R. A., & Romski, M. A. (1985). Comprehension of synthesized speech by nonspeaking severely retarded persons. Presentation at the annual meeting of the American Speech-Language-Hearing Association, Washington, DC. [Abstract is *Asha*, 27(10), 88.]

Shadden, B. B. (1985). Cognitive Rehabilitation [Review of computer program]. *Asha*, 27(12), 74–75.

Shadden, B. B., & Aslin, L. W. (1992). Facilitating clinical observation skills through interactive computer/laser disk. Presentation at the annual meeting of the American Speech-Language-Hearing Association, San Antonio, TX. [Abstract in *Asha*, 34(10), 161.]

Shane, H. C. (1985). Augmentative communication. Presentation at the American Speech and Hearing Foundation Conference on Microcomputers, New Orleans, LA. [Abstract in the *Journal for Computer Users in Speech and Hearing*, 1(2), 89.]

Shane, H. C. (1990a). *Augmentative Communication Series: Message Maker-Keyboard* [Computer program]. San Antonio, TX: Psychological Corporation.

Shane, H. C. (1990b). *Augmentative Communication Series: Scan and Speak* [Computer program]. San Antonio, TX: Psychological Corporation.

Shane, H. C. (1990c). *Augmentative Communication Series: Touch & Speak* [Computer program]. San Antonio, TX: Psychological Corporation.

Shannon, D. A., Staewen, W. S., Miller, J. T., & Cohen, B. S. (1981). Morse-code-controlled communication aid for the nonvocal quadriplegic. *Medical Instrumentation*, 15(5), 341–343.

Shaw, C. A., & McKenna, K. (1991). Microcomputer activities for attention training. Presentation at the annual meeting of the American Speech-Language-Hearing Association, Atlanta, GA. [Abstract in *Asha*, 33(10), 209.]

Shearer, W. M. (1984). Academic and instructional applications for microcomputers. In A. H. Schwartz (Ed.), *Handbook of Microcomputer Applications in Communication Disorders*. San Diego, CA: College-Hill, pp. 193–218.

Shearer, W. M. (1988). *ASHA Project IMPACT: #3 Assessment for Speech and Language Professionals* [Computer program]. Rockville, MD: American Speech-Language-Hearing Association.

Shearer, W. M. (1992). Programmed evaluation of voice disorders. Presentation at the annual meeting of the American Speech-Language-Hearing Association, San Antonio, TX. [Abstract in *Asha*, 34(10), 212.]

Sheeley, E. C. (1984). Microcomputers: Software directory and selected bibliography. *Ear and Hearing*, 5(6), 371–374.

Sheeley, E. C. (1986). Microcomputers: Software directory and selected bibliography. *Ear and Hearing*, 7, 106–112.

Shewan, C. M. (1988). 1988 omnibus survey: Adaptation and progress in times of change. *Asha*, 30, 27–30.

Shewan, C. M. (February 1989). Computer usage on the rise. *Asha*, 31, 35.

Shortliffe, E. H. (1976). *Computer-based Medical Consultations:MYCIN*. New York: Elsevier.

Shriberg, L. D. (no date). *Computer Graphics for the Photo Articulation Test* [Computer program]. Danville, IL: Interstate Printers and Publishers.

Shriberg, L. D. (1985). Computer assisted phonetic/phonologic/prosodic analyses: Issues and options. Presentation at the American Speech and Hearing Foundation Conference on Microcomputers, New Orleans, LA. [Abstract in the *Journal for Computer Users in Speech and Hearing*, 1(2), 90.]

Shriberg, L. D. (1986). *Programs to Examine Phonetic and Phonologic Evaluation Records (PEPPER)* [Computer program]. Hillsdale, NJ: Lawrence Eribaum.

Shriberg, L. D., & Kwiatkowski, J. (1983). Computer-assisted natural process analysis (NPA): Recent issues and data. *Seminars in Speech & Language*, 4, 389–406.

Shriberg, L. D., & Kwiatkowski, J. (1985). Continuous speech sampling for phonologic analysis of speech-delayed children. *Journal of Speech and Hearing Disorders*, 50, 323–334.

Shriberg, L. D., Kwiatkowski, J., & Snyder, T. (1985). Comparative tests of articulation test administration: Booklet versus microcomputer. Presentation at the annual meeting of the American Speech-Language-Hearing Association, Washington, DC. [Abstract in *Asha*, 27(10), 187.]

Shriberg, L. D., Kwiatkowski, J., & Snyder, T. (1986). Articulation testing by microcomputer. *Journal of Speech and Hearing Disorders*, 51, 309–324.

Shriberg, L. D., Kwiatkowski, J., & Synder, T. (1988). Comparative studies of table-top versus microcomputer-assisted management: Response evocation activities. Presentation at the annual meeting of the American Speech-Language-Hearing Association, Boston, MA. [Abstract in *Asha*, 30(10), 103.]

Shriberg, L. D., Kwiatkowski, J., & Snyder, T. (1989a). *PEPTALK* [Computer program]. Tucson, AZ: Communication Skill Builders.

Shriberg, L. D., Kwiatkowski, J., & Snyder, T. (1989b). Tabletop versus microcomputer-assisted speech management: Stabilization phase. *Journal of Speech and Hearing Disorders*, 54, 233–248.

Shriberg, L. D., Kwiatkowski, J., & Snyder, T. (1990). Tabletop versus microcomputer-assisted speech management: Response evocation phase. *Journal of Speech and Hearing Disorders*, 55, 635–655.

Shuler, J. F., & Konow, C. (1993). Computer Users in Rehabilitation and Education (C.U.R.E.). Presentation at the annual meeting of the American Speech-Language-Hearing Association, Anaheim, CA. [Abstract in *Asha*, 35(10), 171.]

Siegel, L. G., & Yanz, J. (198•). *Pure-Tone Audiometry Simulation* [Computer program]. San Diego, CA: College-Hill.

Silbar, J. C., & Konarska, K. A. (1984). Reports with ease: Word processing for fast and easy reports. Presentation at the annual meeting of the American Speech-Language-Hearing Association, San Francisco, CA. [Abstract in *Asha*, 26(10), 186.]

Silverman, F. H. (1985a). *Clinical Software for Speech-Language Pathology and Audiology.* Greendale, WI: CODI Publications.

Silverman, F. H. (1985b). *StutterExpert* [Computer program]. Greendale, WI: CODI Publications.

Silverman, F. H. (1985c). *Why Is It Being Recommended That My Child Learn Sign Language?* [Computer program]. Greendale, WI: CODI Publications.

Silverman, F. H. (1987). *Microcomputers in Speech-Language Pathology and Audiology: A Primer.* Englewood Cliffs, NJ: Prentice Hall.

Silverman, F. H. (1992a). *Legal-Ethical Considerations, Restrictions, and Obligations for Clinicians Who Treat Communicative Disorders.* Springfield, IL: Charles C. Thomas.

Silverman, F. H. (1992b). *Stuttering and Other Fluency Disorders.* Englewood Cliffs, NJ: Prentice Hall.

Silverman, F. H. (1993a). *Research Design and Evaluation in Speech-Language Pathology and Audiology* (3rd Ed.). Englewood Cliffs, NJ: Prentice Hall.

Silverman, F. H. (1993b). Telecommunication relay services: An option for persons who are severely speech impaired. *Augmentative and Alternative Communication, .*

Silverman, F. H. (1995). *Communication for the Speechless* (3rd Ed.). Englewood Cliffs, NJ: Prentice Hall.

Silverman, F. H. (1996). Stuttering and Other Fluency Disorders (2nd Ed.). Needham Heights, MA: Allyn & Bacon.

Simmons, J. O., & Condon, M. (1992). A survey of microcomputer application in university programs. Paper presented at the annual meeting of the American Speech-Language-Hearing Association, San Antonio.

Simmons, J. O., & Condon, M. (1993). Microcomputer applications used by first-to second-year professionals. Presentation at the annual meeting of the American Speech-Language-Hearing Association, Anaheim, CA. [Abstract in *Asha*, 35(10), 125.]

Simmons, N. N. (1987). SpeechMaster [Review of computer program]. *Asha*, 29(2), 76.

Simpson, D. M., & Puls, B. D. (1984). Computerized program investigating effects of latency on auditory comprehension tasks. Presentation at the annual meeting of the American Speech-Language-Hearing Association, San Francisco, CA. [Abstract in *Asha*, 26(10), 189.]

Simpson, K. O. (1995). MacEuclid: Writing assistance for professionals. Presentation at the annual meeting of the American Speech-Language-Hearing Association, Orlando, FL. [Abstract in *Asha*, 37(10), 79.]

Simpson, K. O., & Sharpe, T. (1995). Data collection and analysis of multiple time-based events. Presentation at the annual meeting of the American Speech-Language-Hearing Association, Orlando, FL. [Abstract in *Asha*, 37(10), 79.]

Simpson, T. H. (1994). Computing HCP performance: As easy as 1–2–3. *Hearing Instruments*, 45(2), 26–30.

Sims, D. G. (1988). Video methods for speechreading instruction. In C. L. De Filippo & D. G. Sims (Eds.), *New Reflections on Speechreading* [Monograph]. *Volta Review*, 90(5), 273–288.

Sims, D. G., & Clymer, E. W. (1986). Computer-assisted instruction for the hearing impaired. In J. L. Northern (Ed.), *The Personal Computer for Speech, Language, and Hearing Professionals.* Boston, MA: Little, Brown, pp. 157–176.

Sims, D. G., & Cronic, B. J. (1979). Computer assisted instructional television for speechreading drill and practice. Presentation at the annual meeting of the American Speech-Language-Hearing Association, Atlanta, GA. [Abstract in *Asha*, 21(9), 718.]

Sims, D. G., Knight, S., & Austin, A. (1992). Macintosh software for revised NAL hearing-aid fitting prescription. *Journal for Computer Users in Speech and Hearing*, 8(1, 2), 8–14.

Sims, D. G., Kopra, L., Dunlop, R., & Kopra, M. (1985). A survey of microcomputer applications in aural rehabilitation. *Journal of the Academy of Rehabilitative Audiology*, 18, 9–26.

Sims, D. G., Scott, L., & Meyers, T. (1982). Past, present, and future computer assisted communication training at the National Technical Institute for the Deaf. *Journal of the Academy of Rehabilitation Audiology*, 15, 103–115.

Sims, D. G., VonFeldt, J., Dowaliby, F., Hutchinson, K., & Meyers, T. (1979). A pilot experiment in computer assisted speechreading instruction utilizing the DAVID. *American Annals of the Deaf*, 124, 616–623.

Slovick, L. (1982). CAI at CSDF: Microcomputer-based authoring systems. *American Annals of the Deaf*, 127, 545–563.

Smaldino, J. J. (1985). Comparing computer-assisted hearing aid selection software. *Hearing Instruments*, 36, 16–21.

Smaldino, J. J., & Carlson, D. L. (1984). Comparison of computerized hearing aid fitting schemes. Presentation at the annual meeting of the American Speech-Language-Hearing Association, San Francisco, CA. [Abstract in *Asha*, 26(10), 119.]

Smaldino, J. J., & Smaldino, S. E. (1991). Hypermedia in the aural rehabilitation process. Presentation at the annual meeting of the American Speech-Language-Hearing Association, Atlanta, GA. [Abstract in *Asha*, 33(10), 135.]

Smaldino, S. E., & Smaldino, J. J. (1985). An evaluation system for software used for therapeutic and educational purposes. Presentation at the American Speech and Hearing Foundation Conference on Microcomputers, New Orleans, LA. [Abstract in the *Journal for Computer Users in Speech and Hearing*, 1(2), 90–91.]

Smaldino, S. E.,. & Smaldino, J. J. (1992). Don't get hyper . . . about hypermedia development. *Journal for Computer Users in Speech and Hearing*, 8(1, 2), 94–99.

Smith, J. B. (1984). *Cognitive Rehabilitation* [Computer program]. Dimondale, MI: Hartley Courseware.

Smith, J. B. (1991). *Memory Challenge! Improving Spatial Memory Skills* [Computer program]. Pacific Grove, CA: Critical Thinking Press and Software, P. O. Box 448.

Smith, J. B., Nancarrow, D. P., & Messner, C. (1986). Clinician authored software: Do-it-yourself clinical materials. Presentation at the annual meeting of the American Speech-Language-Hearing Association, Detroit, MI. [Abstract in *Asha*, 28(10), 158.]

Smith, K. R. (1990). Pure Tone Simulation [Review of computer program]. *Asha*, 32(8), 72.

Smith, M. C., Kneil, T. R., Hodson, B. W., Bernstorf, E. D., & Gladhart, M. A. (1994). A computerized presentation of stimuli for assessing rhyming abilities. Presentation at the annual meeting of the American Speech-Language-Hearing Association, New Orleans, LA. [Abstract in *Asha*, 36(10), 174.]

Snavely, J. (1995). *Picture Identification* [Computer program]. West Bloomfield, MI: Parrot Software.

Snell, K. B. (1989). A personalized videodisk training program for vowel perception. Presentation at the annual meeting of the American Speech-Language-Hearing Association, St. Louis, MO. [Abstract in *Asha*, 31(10), 157.]

Snope, T., & Duran, J. (1980). Developing a comprehensive information system. *Asha*, 22(8), 550–555.

Software review checklist (1985). *Asha*, 27(3), 71.

Sohlberg, M. M., & Mateer, C. A. (1987). Effectiveness of an attention-training program. *Journal of Clinical and Experimental Neuropsychology*, 9, 117–130.

Sohlberg, M. M., & Mateer, C. A. (1989). *Introduction to Cognitive Rehabilitation: Theory and Practice*. New York: Guilford Press.

Sohlberg, M. M., & Mateer, C. A. (1990). The use of computers in cognitive rehabilitation. *Journal for Computer Users in Speech and Hearing*, 6(2), 101–106.

Sokolov, J. L., & Snow, C. E. (1995). *Handbook of Research in Language Development using CHILDES*. Lawrence Erlbaum Associates.

Somers, H. (1979). Using the computer to analyze articulation test data. *British Journal of Disorders of Communication*, 14(3), 231–240.

Sonies, B. C., & Larkins, P. G. (1982). Diagnostic reporting simplified: Use of a computerized assessment system. Presentation at the annual meeting of the American Speech-Language-Hearing Association, Toronto, Canada. [Abstract in *Asha*, 24(10), 728.]

Sosinsky, B. (1991). *Using FileMaker*. Carmel, IN: Que Corporation.

SoundScope [Computer program] (1994). Somerville, MA: GW Instruments. [Advertisement in *Asha*, 36(10), 22.]

Sound Therapy [Computer program] (1994). The Speech Bin. [Advertisement in *Asha*, 36(10), 248.]

Sparks, D. W. (1972). The feasibility of computerized audiometry. *Journal of Audiological Research*, 12, 62–66.

Speech Assessment and Interactive Learning System [Computer program] (1994). London, Ontario, Canada: AVAAZ Innovations. [Advertisement in *Asha*, 36(10), 116.]

SpeechViewer [Computer program] (1988). Atlanta, GA: IBM Support Center for Persons with Disabilities, P.O. Box 2150.

Stach, B. A., & Jerger, J. F. (1983). The application of microcomputer use in audiology. Presentation at the annual meeting of the American Speech-Language-Hearing Association, Cincinnati, OH. [Abstract in *Asha*, 25(10), 61.]

Stach, B. A., & Jerger, J. F. (1986). Microcomputer applications in audiology. In J. L. Northern (Editor), *The Personal Computer for Speech, Language, and Hearing Professionals*. Boston: Little, Brown, pp. 113–134.

Strassen, H. B., Soede, M., & Bakker, H. (1982). The lightspot operated typewriter: A communication aid for severely bodily handicapped patients. *Scandinavian Archives of Physical Medicine and Rehabilitation*, 14, 159–161.

Steelman, J. D., Coleman, P. P., Koppenhaver, D. A., & Yoder, D. E. (1992). Literacy and computer skills: The road to employment. Presentation at the annual meeting of the American Speech-Language-Hearing Association, San Antonio, TX. [Abstract in *Asha*, 34(10), 184.]

Steelman, J. D., Koppenhaver, D. A., Coleman, P. P., & Yoder, D. (1992). Technology, Interaction, Literacy Learning, and Teaching: A tool for everyone. Presentation at the annual meeting of the American Speech-Language-Hearing Association, San Antonio, TX. [Abstract in *Asha*, 34(10), 126.]

Steiner, S., & Larson, V. L. (1991). Integrating microcomputers into language intervention with children. *Topics in Language Disorders*, 11(2), 18–30.

Stevens, G., & Bernstein, J. (1985). Intelligibility and machine recognition of deaf speech. *Proceedings of the 8th Annual Conference on Rehabilitation Engineering*, 308–310.

Stevens, J. C. (1983). Microprocessors in audiology and neurophysiology. *Journal of Medical Engineering and Technology*, 7(6), 307–308.

Stilwell, C. A., Runyan, C. M., & Goebel, M. D. (1988). Speech naturalness ratings of stutterers treated using the CAFET program. Presentation at the annual meeting of the American Speech-Language-Hearing Association, Boston, MA. [Abstract in *Asha*, 30(10), 179.]

Stoker, R. (1983). A computer-assisted diagnostic and prescriptive tool for use in teaching speech to the deaf. *American Annals of the Deaf*, 128, 625–630.

Stokes, N. H., & Soso, V. H. (1985). The transition from theory to clinical application through computer instruction. Presentation at the annual meeting of the American Speech-Language-Hearing Association, Washington, DC. [Abstract in *Asha*, 27(10), 93.]

Stone, M., & Sonies, B. C. (1985). Application of computers in a speech language pathology clinical research program. Presentation at the American Speech and Hearing Foundation Conference on Microcomputers, New Orleans, LA. [Abstract in the *Journal for Computer Users in Speech and Hearing*, 1(2), 91–92.]

Studebaker, G. A., & Matesich, J. S. (1992). A derivation of the modulation transfer function. Paper presented at the annual meeting of the American Speech-Language-Hearing Association, San Antonio.

Studebaker, G. A., Sherbecoe, R. L., & Gilmore, C. (1991). Model predicting average speech recognition performance under circumscribed conditions. Presentation at the annual meeting of the American Speech-Language-Hearing Association, Atlanta, GA. [Abstract in *Asha*, 33(10), 192.]

Stunden, A. A. (1966). Computer simulation of therapy—The client-clinician match. *Asha*, 8(4), 100–104.

Sturner, R., Heller, J., Funk, S., & Feezor, M. (1991). Preschool hearing screening via speech signals. Presentation at the annual meeting of the American Speech-Language-Hearing Association, Atlanta, GA. [Abstract in *Asha*, 33(10), 161.]

Sullivan, J. A., Levitt, H., & Hwang, J. Y. (1985). The Chameleon: A computerized hearing-aid measurement and simulation system. Presentation at the annual meeting of the American Speech-Language-Hearing Association, Washington, DC. [Abstract in *Asha*, 27(10), 185.]

Sun, I. (1990). SunTool. *Speech/Language IEP Writer* [Computer program]. Columbia, MO: Author, 2304 Mission Court.

Swank, P. R., & Carrow-Woolfolk, E. (1986). COMPUSCORE: A computerized scoring program for the TACL-R. Presentation at the annual meeting of the American Speech-Language-Hearing Association, Detroit, MI. [Abstract in *Asha*, 28(10), 133.]

Swanson, T. J., & Griffin, R. F. (1984). Computer translated IEPs. Presentation at the annual meeting of the American Speech-Language-Hearing Association, San Francisco, CA. [Abstract in *Asha*, 26(10), 186.]

Swartz, B. L. (1990). A caution regarding computer-programmed determination of temporal features of speech. *Journal for Computer Users in Speech and Hearing*, 6(2), 88–99.

Swenson, C., & Associates (no date). *Hearing Aid Client Management System* [Computer program]. Watertown, MA: Swenson Associates, Inc., Riverbend Office Park, Nine Galen Street.

Symposium on research and utilization of educational media for teaching the deaf. Computer assisted research and instruction for the hearing impaired. National Conference. Lincoln, Nebraska (1983). *American Annals for the Deaf*, 128(5), 507–782.

Symposium on research and utilization of educational media for teaching the deaf: Microcomputers in education of the hearing impaired. National Conference. Lincoln, Nebraska (1982). *American Annals for the Deaf*, 127(5), 463–716.

Szablewski, J. B., Fisher, C. A., & Speake, J. A. (1985). Implementing computer assisted habilitation: An administrator's flowchart for success. Presentation at the annual meeting of the American Speech-Language-Hearing Association, Washington, DC. [Abstract in *Asha*, 27(10), 89.]

Talk:About [Computer program] (1994). Lake Zurich, IL: Don Johnston, Inc.

Tanenhaus, J. B. (1989). Bypassing the keyboard: Alternate options for computer access. Presentation at the annual meeting of the American Speech-Language-Hearing Association, St. Louis, MO. [Abstract in *Asha*, 31(10), 59.]

Tatchell, R. H., Letson, J. A., Zlotolow, S., & DeLauro, G. (1993). Multimedia learning module for diagnosis of unilateral vocal fold paralysis. Presentation at the annual meeting of the American Speech-Language-Hearing Association, Anaheim, CA. [Abstract in *Asha*, 35(10), 120.]

Telage, K. (1980). Computerized place-manner distinctive feature program for articulation analysis. *Journal of Speech and Hearing Disorders*, 45, 481–494.

Terrell, S. L. (1989). Effect of media types upon children's acquisition of novel vocabulary. Presentation at the annual meeting of the American Speech-Language-Hearing Association, St. Louis.

Terrell, S. L. (1991). Effectiveness of machine and human mediums upon novel word learning. Presentation at the annual meeting of the American Speech-Language-Hearing Association, Atlanta, GA. [Abstract in *Asha*, 33(10), 121.]

Terrio, L., & Oshrin, S. (1990). *Computerized Masking Procedure Analysis (COMPASS)* [Computer program]. Hattiesburg, MS: Diversified Educational Management Systems, Inc., Software Products Division, 123 South 25th Avenue.

Testut, E. W., Van Son, G., Seidman, S. A., & Ryan, W. J. (1988). *ASHA Project IMPACT: #1 Overview of Microcomputer Applications for Speech, Language, and Hearing Professionals* [Computer program]. Rockville, MD: American Speech-Language-Hearing Association.

Thomas-Stonell, N. L., Johnson, P., Jutal, J., & Schuller, R. (1993). Assessment and training of cognitive-communication skills following head injury. Presentation at the annual meeting of the American Speech-Language-Hearing Association, Anaheim, CA. [Abstract in *Asha*, 35(10), 126.]

Thomas-Stonell, N. L., Leeper, H. A., & Young, P. I. (1993). Stepping stones software: Rate modification and perception in dysarthric children. Presentation at the annual meeting of the American Speech-Language-Hearing Association, Anaheim, CA. [Abstract in *Asha*, 35(10), 178.]

Thompson, D. J. (1990a). Dynamic Acoustics [Review of computer program]. *Asha*, 32(8), 73–74.

Thompson, D. J. (1990b). Understanding Decibels [Review of computer program]. *Asha*, 32(8), 72–73.

Thompson, D. J., & Raffin, M. J. M. (1986). Occupational Hearing Conservation Management on the Kaypro 10 and IBM-PC/XT [Review of computer program]. *Asha*, 28(3), 75–76.

Thompson, D. J., & Robinette, L. N. (1981). System for automated collection of aural acoustic immittance. Presentation at the annual meeting of the American Speech-Language-Hearing Association, Los Angeles, CA. [Abstract in *Asha*, 23(10), 807–808.]

Thornton, A., Han, Y., Halpin, C., & Hou, Z. (1992). Development of expert systems: Audiometry. Presentation at the annual meeting of the American Speech-Language-Hearing Association, San Antonio, TX. [Abstract in *Asha*, 34(10), 148.]

Till, J. A. (1990). Computer-assisted evaluation of speech disorders: Rationale and directions for future development. *Journal for Computer Users in Speech and Hearing*, 6(2), 134–148.

Till, J. A., & Stivers, D. K. (1981). Instrumentation and validity for direct-readout voice onset time measurement. *Journal of Communication Disorders*, 14, 507–512.

Tiller, P. L., McGuire, R. A., & Nelson, L. K. (1992). Microcomputer-assisted biofeedback in the treatment of disordered speech sounds. Presentation at the annual meeting of the American Speech-Language-Hearing Association, San Antonio, TX. [Abstract in *Asha*, 34(10), 145.]

Titze, I. R., Wong, D., Milder, M. A., Hensley, S. R., & Ramig, L. O. (1995). Comparison between clinician-assisted and fully automated procedures for obtaining a voice range profile. *Journal of Speech and Hearing Research*, 38, 526–535.

Tobin, H., Baquet, G. M., & Tishman, A. (1991). The development of a computerized audiologic habilitation program: Using the Nonsense Syllable Test. Presentation at the annual meeting of the American Speech-Language-Hearing Association, Atlanta, GA. [Abstract in *Asha*, 33(10), 161.]

Tomblin, J. B., & Hurtig, R. R. (1980). A computer assisted language analysis system. Scientific exhibit presented at the annual meeting of the American Speech-Language-Hearing Association, Detroit, MI.

Tonkovich, J. D., Horowitz, D. M., Kawahigashi, J. N., Krainen, G. H., & Kronick, D. (1991). An application of voice recognition technology for clinical documentation. Presentation at the annual meeting of the American Speech-Language-Hearing Association, Atlanta, GA. [Abstract in *Asha*, 33(10), 188.]

Torng, P. (1995). Interactive Software for Learning Phonetics (ISLP). Presentation at the annual meeting of the American Speech-Language-Hearing Association, Orlando, FL. [Abstract in *Asha*, 37(10), 101.]

Townsend, T. H. (1989a). *Dynamic Acoustics* [Computer program]. West Bloomfield, MI: Parrot Software.

Townsend, T. H. (1989b). *Pure Tone Simulation* [Computer program]. West Bloomfield, MI: Parrot Software.

Townsend, T. H. (1991). *Auditory Anatomy* [Computer program]. West Bloomfield, MI: Parrot Software.

Townsend, T. H. (1995). *Audiogram Generator* [Computer program]. West Bloomfield, MI: Parrot Software.

Townsend, T. H., & Olson, C. C. (1995a). *Electroacoustic Immittance Generator* [Computer program]. West Bloomfield, MI: Parrot Software.

Townsend, T. H., & Olson, C. C. (1995b). *Electroacoustic Immittance Simulation* [Computer program]. West Bloomfield, MI: Parrot Software.

Townsend, T. H., & Weiss, M. S. (1989). *Understanding Decibels* [Computer program]. West Bloomfield, MI: Parrot Software.

Traynor, R. M., et al. (1985). High technology in aural rehabilitation. Presentation at the annual meeting of the American Speech-Language-Hearing Association, Washington, DC. [Abstract in *Asha*, 27(10), 106.]

Trujillo, C. D. (1983). A microcomputer-based teaching module for central auditory processing testing. Unpublished master's thesis, New Mexico State University, Las Cruces, New Mexico.

Turner, R. G. (1986). *Audio-PC Version 2.0* [Computer program]. Birmingham, MI: Varanus Technical Services, 31760 Verona South.

Tye-Murray, N. (1991). Repair strategy usage by hearing-impaired adults and changes following instruction. *Journal of Speech and Hearing Research*, 23, 921–928.

Tye-Murray, N. (1992). Laser videodisc technology in the aural rehabilitaion setting: Good news for people with severe and profound hearing impairments. *American Journal of Audiology*, 1(2), 33–36.

Tye-Murray, N., & Tyler, R. S. (1988). Using laser videodisc technology to train speechreading and assertive listening. Presentation at the annual meeting of the American Speech-Language-Hearing Association, Boston, MA. [Abstract in *Asha*, 30(10), 171.]

Tye-Murray, N., Tyler, R. S., Bong, B., & Nares, T. (1988). Using laser videodisc technology to train speechreading and assertive listening skills. *Journal of the Academy of Rehabilitative Audiology*, 21, 143–152.

Tye-Murray, N., Tyler, R. S., & Lowder, M. (1987). Laser videodisc tests of sentence and consonant recognition. Presentation at the annual meeting of the American Speech-Language-Hearing Association, New Orleans, LA. [Abstract in *Asha*, 29(10), 122.]

Tyler, R. S. (1982). Minicomputers and the assessment of hearing loss and tinnitus. In J. Raviv (Ed.), *Uses of Computers in Aiding the Disabled*. Amsterdam: North-Holland.

Tyler, R. S., Preece, J. P., & Tye-Murray, N. (1986). *The Iowa Phoneme and Sentence Tests*. Iowa City, IA: University of Iowa Hospitals and Clinics.

Uryase, M. C., & McLennon, B. (1991). Increasing critical thinking skills for assessment and diagnosis. Presentation at the annual meeting of the American Speech-Language-Hearing Association, Atlanta, GA. [Abstract in *Asha*, 33(10), 122.]

Valentine, D. (1995a). Database program to facilitate scheduling in a clinic-based program. Presentation at the annual meeting of the American Speech-Language-Hearing Association, Orlando, FL. [Abstract in *Asha*, 37(10), 59.]

Valentine, D. (1995b). QuickTime video clips and their use in language treatment. Presentation at the annual meeting of the American Speech-Language-Hearing Association, Orlando, FL. [Abstract in *Asha*, 37(10), 59.]

Van Meter, A., Lee, K. J., Kett, R. L., & Levine, S. P. (1986). Audio scan alternative communication system for a visually impaired quadriplegic. Presentation at the annual meeting of the American Speech-Language-Hearing Association, Detroit, MI. [Abstract in *Asha*, 28(10), 161.]

Van Vliet, L. (1995). Use of E-mail to enhance learning. Presentation at the annual meeting of the American Speech-Language-Hearing Association, Orlando, FL. [Abstract in *Asha*, 37(10), 71.]

Van Vliet, L., & Henchey, C. E. (1983). Computer usage to enhance initiation of communication in a group. Presentation at the annual meeting of the American Speech-Language-Hearing Association, Cincinnati, OH. [Abstract in *Asha*, 25(10), 117.]

Vanderheiden, G. C. (1990). The use of Hyper-text to create user-accessible databases. *Augmentative and Alternative Communication*, 6, 116.

Vanderheiden, G. C., Snyder, T., & Kelso, D. (1992). Development of a ussr-friendly directly consumer accessible database service. *Augmentative and Alternative Communication*, 8, 175.

Vanderheiden, G. C., & Walstead, L. (Eds.) (1982). *Trace Center International Software/Hardware Registry*. Madison, WI: University of Wisconsin Trace Center.

Vekovius, G. T. (1995). Managed care 101. *Asha*, 37(9), 44–47.

Venable, G. P. (1987a). Moptown Hotel [Review of computer program]. *Asha*, 29(11), 67.

Venable, G. P. (1987b). Moptown Parade [Review of computer program]. *Asha*, 29(11), 66–67.

Venable, G. P. (1988). Writer Rabbit [Review of computer program]. *Asha*, 30(8), 58–59.

Venkatagiri, H. S. (1988). Public domain software: A resource guide for speech-language pathologists. *Journal for Computer Users in Speech and Hearing*, 4(2), 90–99.

Venkatagiri, H. S. (1989a). *The Messenger* [Computer program]. Ames, IA: SAGA Software, 626 Meadow Place.

Venkatagiri, H. S. (1989b). Computer Aided Stuttering Treatment (CAST). Presentation at the annual meeting of the American Speech-Language-Hearing Association, St. Louis, MO. [Abstract in *Asha*, 31(10), 165.]

Venkatagiri, H. S. (1992). The Messenger, an AAC program. Presentation at the annual meeting of the American Speech-Language-Hearing Association, San Antonio, TX. [Abstract in *Asha*, 34(10), 161.]

Venkatagiri, H. S. (1994). Efficient keyboard layouts for AAC. Presentation at the annual meeting of the American Speech-Language-Hearing Association, New Orleans, LA. [Abstract in *Asha*, 36(10), 75.]

Video Voice Speech Training System [Computer program] (1994). Ann Arbor, MI: Micro Video, P. O. Box 7357. [Description in *Asha*, 36(10), 9.]

Vigil, M. (1983). The validity and versatility of a microcomputer program to tabulate language sample analysis data. Unpublished master's thesis, New Mexico State University, Las Cruces.

Vince, J. (1995). *Virtual Reality Systems*. Reading, MA: Addison-Wesley.

Voeks, S. (1977). Computerized PICA scoring. Presentation at the annual meeting of the American Speech-Language-Hearing Association, Chicago, IL.

Vogel, D. (1988). Aphasia V: Vocabulary by Sentence Completion [Review of Computer Program]. *Asha*, 30(2), 70.

Vogen, C. S. (1985). Computerized records of speech-language pathology and audiology services. Presentation at the annual meeting of the American Speech-Language-Hearing Association, Washington, DC. [Abstract in *Asha*, 27(10),89.]

Volin, R. A. (1986a). Considerations in the design and programming of clinical software. In M. L. Grossfeld & C. A. Grossfeld (Eds), *Microcomputer Applications in Rehabilitation of Communication Disorders*. Rockville, MD: Aspen, pp. 25–42.

Volin, R. A. (1986b). Frenchay Dysarthria Assessment Computer Differential Analysis [Review of computer program]. *Asha*, 28(7), 78–79.

Volin, R. A. (1989). On to 1999: The computer as an integral component in the clinic. *Journal for Computer Users in Speech and Hearing*, 5(2), 89–92.

Volin, R. A. (1991a). Biofeedback for speech in the microcomputer age. Presentation at the annual meeting of the American Speech-Language-Hearing Association, Atlanta, GA. [Abstract in *Asha*, 33(10), 209.]

Volin, R. A. (1991b). Microcomputer-based systems providing biofeedback of voice and speech production. *Topics in Language Disorders*, 11, 65–79.

Volin, R. A. (1993a). Computer technology: Clinical applications of biofeedback. *Asha*, 35(8), 43–44, 51.

Volin, R. A. (1993b). Talking Nouns I, Talking Nouns II, Talking Verbs [Review of computer programs]. *Asha*, 35(2), 71.

Volin, R. A., & Groher, M. E. (1986a). *Language Stimulation Software #1, Sentence Completion: Semantics* [Computer program]. Rockville, MD: Aspen Systems Corporation, 1600 Research Bouldvard..

Volin, R. A., & Groher, M. E. (1986b). *Language Stimulation Software #2, Rebuilding Sentences: Syntax* [Computer program]. Rockville, MD: Aspen Systems Corporation, 1600 Research Boulevard.

Volin, R. A., & Groher, M. E. (1986c). *Language Stimulation Software #4, Associative Naming: Mixed Cues* [Computer program]. Rockville, MD: Aspen Systems Corporation, 1600 Research Boulevard.

Volin, R. A., & Groher, M. E. (1986d). *Language Stimulation Software #6, Selecting Modifiers: Semantics* [Computer program]. Rockville, MD: Aspen Systems Corporation, 1600 Research Boulevard.

Wagner, R. (1992). Hypermedia: Your personal solution to individual needs. Presentation at the annual meeting of the American Speech-Language-Hearing Association, San Antonio, TX. [Abstract in *Asha*, 34(10), 149–150.]

Walence, W. W. (1985). Apple Macintosh with MacPaint for forms generation. *Journal for Computer Users in Speech and Hearing*, 1(2), 144–145.

Walker, J. C. (1987). *The Ear* [Computer program]. Winston-Salem, NC: Bio-Psych Educational Tools, P.O. Box 6436.

Walker-Batson, D., Barnes, L. A., & Lauka, L. L. (1985). Use of computer assisted productive language analysis in aphasia. Presentation at the annual meeting of the American Speech-Language-Hearing Association, Washington, DC. [Abstract in *Asha*, 27(10), 86.]

Waryas, C. L., & Waryas, P. A. (1984). Utilizing "notebook" microcomputers in clinical applications in speech and hearing. Presentation at the annual meeting of the American Speech-Language-Hearing Association, San Francisco, CA. [Abstract in *Asha*, 26(10), 185.]

Waryas, P. A. (1986). Computer-assisted instruction (CAI) in audiology practicum. Presentation at the annual meeting of the American Speech-Language-Hearing Association, Detroit, MI. [Abstract in *Asha*, 28(10), 84.]

Watanabe, H., Shin, T., Matsuo, K., Oda, M., & Fukaura, J. (1986). A new computer analyzing system for clinical use with a strobo-videoscope. *Archives of Otolaryngology, Head, and Neck Surgery*, 112, 978–981.

Watson, C., & Kewley-Port, D. (1989). Advances in computer-based speech training: Aids for the profoundly hearing impaired. In N. McGarr (Ed.), *Research on the Use of Sensory*

Aids for Hearing-Impaired People. Washington, DC.: Alexander Graham Bell Association for the Deaf, pp. 29–45. [May be in Volta Review, 91, 29–45.]

Watson, C., Reed, D., Kewley-Port, D., & Maki, D. (1989). The Indiana speech training aid (ISTRA) I: Comparisons between human and computer-based evaluation of speech quality. *Journal of Speech and Hearing Research*, 32, 245–251.

Weiner, F. F. (1982). *Phonological Analysis and Treatment* [Computer program]. State College, PA: Parrot Software.

Weiner, F. F. (1983). Computer animation techniques for use in speech and language software. Presentation at the annual meeting of the American Speech-Language-Hearing Association, Cincinnati, OH. [Abstract in *Asha*, 25(10), 60.]

Weiner, F. F. (Ed.) (1986). *Computer Review for Apple Users in Speech and Hearing* (Volume 1). State College, PA: Snavely, Vidmar, and Associates.

Weiner, F. F. (1995a). *Aphasia 1: Noun Association Enhanced* [Computer program]. West Bloomfield, MI: Parrot Software.

Weiner, F. F. (1995b). *Aphasia 2: Opposites and Similarities* [Computer program]. West Bloomfield, MI: Parrot Software.

Weiner, F. F. (1995c). *Aphasia 3: Categories* [Computer program]. West Bloomfield, MI: Parrot Software.

Weiner, F. F. (1995d). *Aphasia 5: Sentence Completion* [Computer program]. West Bloomfield, MI: Parrot Software.

Weiner, F. F. (1995e). *Aphasia 6: Definitions* [Computer program]. West Bloomfield, MI: Parrot Software.

Weiner, F. F. (1995f). *Aphasia 7: Picture Identification* [Computer program]. West Bloomfield, MI: Parrot Software.

Weiner, F. F. (1995g). *Aphasia 8: Picture Naming* [Computer program]. West Bloomfield, MI: Parrot Software.

Weiner, F. F. (1995h). *Aphasia 11: Understanding Attributes* [Computer program]. West Bloomfield, MI: Parrot Software.

Weiner, F. F. (1995i). *Attention, Perception, and Discrimination* [Computer program]. West Bloomfield, MI: Parrot Software.

Weiner, F. F. (1995j). *Auditory and Visual Instructions* [Computer program]. West Bloomfield, MI: Parrot Software.

Weiner, F. F. (1995k). *Auditory and Visual Picture Recognition* [Computer program]. West Bloomfield, MI: Parrot Software.

Weiner, F. F. (1995l). *Automatic Articulation Analysis* [Computer program]. West Bloomfield, MI: Parrot Software.

Weiner, F. F. (1995m). *Categorization, Association, and Sequencing* [Computer program]. West Bloomfield, MI: Parrot Software.

Weiner, F. F. (1995n). *Categories Plus* [Computer program]. West Bloomfield, MI: Parrot Software.

Weiner, F. F. (1995o). *Cognitive Disorders 5: Making Change for Money* [Computer program]. West Bloomfield, MI: Parrot Software.

Weiner, F. F. (1995p). *Cognitive Disorders 7: Word Order in Sentences* [Computer program]. West Bloomfield, MI: Parrot Software.

Weiner, F. F. (1995q). *Cognitive Disorders 9: Sorting by Category* [Computer program]. West Bloomfield, MI: Parrot Software.

Weiner, F. F. (1995r). *Cognitive Disorders 10: Categories: Completion from Partial Information* [Computer program]. West Bloomfield, MI: Parrot Software.

Weiner, F. F. (1995s). *Cognitive Disorders 16: Math Story Problems Using a Calculator* [Computer program]. West Bloomfield, MI: Parrot Software.

Weiner, F. F. (1995t). *Cognitive Disorders 17: Reading Comprehension and Picture Association* [Computer program]. West Bloomfield, MI: Parrot Software.

Weiner, F. F. (1995u). *Compensatory Memory Strategies: Chunking* [Computer program]. West Bloomfield, MI: Parrot Software.

Weiner, F. F. (1995v). *Compensatory Memory Strategies: Loci* [Computer program]. West Bloomfield, MI: Parrot Software.

Weiner, F. F. (1995w). *Completion from Partial Information* [Computer program]. West Bloomfield, MI: Parrot Software.

Weiner, F. F. (1995x). *Conditional Statements* [Computer program]. West Bloomfield, MI: Parrot Software.

Weiner, F. F. (1995y). *Deductive Reasoning* [Computer program]. West Bloomfield, MI: Parrot Software.

Weiner, F. F. (1995z). *Definitions* [Computer program]. West Bloomfield, MI: Parrot Software.

Weiner, F. F. (1995aa). *Diagnostic Report Writer* [Computer program]. West Bloomfield, MI: Parrot Software.

Weiner, F. F. (1995bb). *Functional Vocabulary* [Computer program]. West Bloomfield, MI: Parrot Software.

Weiner, F. F. (1995cc). *Inferential Naming* [Computer program]. West Bloomfield, MI: Parrot Software.

Weiner, F. F. (1995dd). *Listening Skills* [Computer program]. West Bloomfield, MI: Parrot Software.

Weiner, F. F. (1995ee). *Memory for Animated Sequences* [Computer program]. West Bloomfield, MI: Parrot Software.

Weiner, F. F. (1995ff). *Memory for Directions* [Computer program]. West Bloomfield, MI: Parrot Software.

Weiner, F. F. (1995gg). *Minimal Contrast Therapy* [Computer program]. West Bloomfield, MI: Parrot Software.

Weiner, F. F. (1995hh). *Opposites and Similarities* [Computer program]. West Bloomfield, MI: Parrot Software.

Weiner, F. F. (1995ii). *Parrot Easy Language Sample Analysis* [Computer program]. West Bloomfield, MI: Parrot Software.

Weiner, F. F. (1995jj). *Perception of Environmental Sounds* [Computer program]. West Bloomfield, MI: Parrot Software.

Weiner, F. F. (1995kk). *Picture Categories* [Computer program]. West Bloomfield, MI: Parrot Software.

Weiner, F. F. (1995ll). *Picture Naming* [Computer program]. West Bloomfield, MI: Parrot Software.

Weiner, F. F. (1995mm). *Real Live Video* [Computer program]. West Bloomfield, MI: Parrot Software.

Weiner, F. F. (1995nn). *Remembering Names* [Computer program]. West Bloomfield, MI: Parrot Software.

Weiner, F. F. (1995oo). *Sentence Completion* [Computer program]. West Bloomfield, MI: Parrot Software.

Weiner, F. F. (1995pp). *Sorting by Category* [Computer program]. West Bloomfield, MI: Parrot Software.

Weiner, F. F. (1995qq). *Traffic Signs* [Computer program]. West Bloomfield, MI: Parrot Software.

Weiner, F. F. (1995rr). *Verbal Analogies* [Computer program]. West Bloomfield, MI: Parrot Software.

Weiner, F. F. (1995ss). *Visual and Auditory Memory Span* [Computer program]. West Bloomfield, MI: Parrot Software.

Weiner, F. F. (1995tt). *Visual Memory* [Computer program]. West Bloomfield, MI: Parrot Software.

Weiner, F. F. (1995uu). *Visual Pattern Memory* [Computer program]. West Bloomfield, MI: Parrot Software.

Weiner, F. F. (1995vv). *Word Association* [Computer program]. West Bloomfield, MI: Parrot Software.

Weiner, F. F. (1995ww). *Word Order* [Computer program]. West Bloomfield, MI: Parrot Software.

Weiner, F. F., & Dillon, L. H. (1995). *Real Life Pictures for Use With Windows Versions of Visual Confrontational Naming and Functional Vocabulary* [Computer programs]. West Bloomfield, MI: Parrot Software.

Weiner, F. F., Polackoff, B., & Provenzano, N. (1995). *Instant IEP and Report Writer* [Computer program]. West Bloomfield, MI: Parrot Software.

Weiner, F. F., & Weiner, C. E. (1995). *Multimedia Reading Comprehension* [Computer program]. West Bloomfield, MI: Parrot Software.

Weiner, F. F., & Young, E. C. (1984). *Function Pictures* [Computer program]. State College, PA: Parrot Software.

Weiner, M. (1995). *Cognitive Disorders 11: Semantic Development Using Code Breaking Strategies* [Computer program]. West Bloomfield, MI: Parrot Software.

Weiner, M., & Weiner, F. F. (1995). *Cognitive Disorders 6: Verbal Analogies* [Computer program]. West Bloomfield, MI: Parrot Software.

Weinreb, G. (1986). *MacSpeech Lab 2.0* [Computer program]. Cambridge, Ma: GW Instruments.

Weiss, C. J. (1987a). Reading Recognition Programs [Review of computer programs]. *Asha*, 29(8), 60.

Weiss, C. J. (1987b). Verbal Reasoning [Review of computer program]. *Asha*, 29(8), 60–61.

Wertz, F. C. (1983). Blissymbol instruction with the Apple II computer. Presentation at the annual meeting of the American Speech-Language-Hearing Association, Cincinnati, OH. [Abstract in *Asha*, 25(10), 80.]

Wertz, R. T., Katz, R. C., & Loverso, F. L. (1991). Extending our reach or extending our grasp: Microcomputers and aphasia. Presentation at the annual meeting of the American Speech-Language-Hearing Association, Atlanta, GA. [Abstract in *Asha*, 33(10), 83–84.]

Weston, A. D., Schriberg, L. D., & Miller, J. F. (1989). Analysis of language-speech samples with SALT and PEPPER. *Journal of Speech and Hearing Research*, 32, 755–766.

White, R. A., Platzman, K. A., & Millen, C. E. (1981). Computer-based symbol acquisition: A feasibility study. Presentation at the annual meeting of the American Speech-Language-Hearing Association, Los Angeles, CA. [Abstract in *Asha*, 23(10), 720.]

Whiteside, J. D., Larson, L. C., Nelson, P. B., & Rainbolt, H. R. (1983). Bits and bytes in supervision. Presentation at the annual meeting of the American Speech-Language-Hearing Association, Cincinnati, OH. [Abstract in *Asha*, 25(10), 103.]

Whiteside, J. D., & Whiteside, H. C. (1986). Linking-up aphasics with microcomputers. Videotape presented at the annual meeting of the American Speech-Language-Hearing Association, Detroit, MI. [Abstract in *Asha*, 28(10), 122.]

Widen, J. E., & Bull, D. H. (1984). Clinical application of an automated version of visual reinforcement audiometry. Presentation at the annual meeting of the American Speech-Language-Hearing Association, San Francisco, CA. [Abstract in *Asha*, 26(10), 155.]

Wiepsuj, V. M., Xue, A., & Savage, H. (1992). Voice disorders HyperCard guidance system. Presentation at the annual meeting of the American Speech-Language-Hearing Association, San Antonio, TX. [Abstract in *Asha*, 34(10), 121.]

Wier, C. C. (1987). Applied artificial intelligence: Expert system technology. *Journal for Computer Users in Speech and Hearing*, 3(1), 69–85.

Wier, C. C. (1989). Research and diagnostic workstations. *Journal for Computer Users in Speech and Hearing*, 5(2), 93–96.

Wiig, E. H., & Wiig, E. D. (1994). Assessment of aspects of word knowledge with TOWK-CB. Presentation at the annual meeting of the American Speech-Language-Hearing Association, New Orleans, LA. [Abstract in *Asha*, 36(10), 246–247.]

Wiig, E. H., & Wiig, E. D. (1995a). *Semantique 1: Antonyms, Synonyms, and Multiple Meanings* [Computer program]. West Bloomfield, MI: Parrot Software.

Wiig, E. H., & Wiig, E. D. (1995b). *Semantique 2: Know Your Root Words* [Computer program]. West Bloomfield, MI: Parrot Software.

Wilkins, W. R. (1984). Informational resources, systems, and services. In A. H. Schwartz (Ed.), *Handbook of Microcomputer Applications in Communication Disorders*. San Diego, CA: College-Hill, pp. 53–78.

Wilkinson, K. M., Sevcik, R. A., Adamson, L. B., & Romski, M. A. (1989). Comparative orthography of SALT, CHAT, and LINGQUEST1 transcription features. Presentation at the annual meeting of the American Speech-Language-Hearing Association, St. Louis, MO. [Abstract in *Asha*, 31(10), 89.]

Williams, C. K., & Watt, B. (1993). Turn commercially available children's software into powerful clinical tools for speech-language pathologists. Presentation at the annual meeting of the American Speech-Language-Hearing Association, Anaheim, CA. [Abstract in *Asha*, 35(10), 178.]

Williams, R. (1990). *The Mac Is Not a Typewriter*. Berkeley, CA: Peachpit press.

Williams, R. (1994). *The Non-designer's Design Book: Design and Typographic Principles for the Visual Novice*. Berkeley, CA: Peachpit press.

Wilson, K. W. (1984). Issues and controversies in the use of microcomputers. In A. H. Schwartz (Ed.), *Handbook of Microcomputer Applications in Communication Disorders*. San Diego, CA: College-Hill, pp. 247–258.

Wilson, M. S., & Fox, B. J. (1980). Computer managed language diagnosis and treatment. Scientific exhibit presented at the annual meeting of the American Speech-Language-Hearing Association, Detroit, MI.

Wilson, M. S., & Fox, B. J. (1981a). The bilingual computer: Promise of the eighties. *Asha*, 23(9), 651.

Wilson, M. S., & Fox, B. J. (1981b). Microcomputer software development: The challenge of the eighties. Presentation at the annual meeting of the American Speech-Language-Hearing Association, Los Angeles, CA. [Abstract in *Asha*, 23(10), 737.]

Wilson, M. S. & Fox, B. J. (1983). Microcomputers: A clinical aid. In H. Winitz (Ed.), *For Clinicians, by Clinicians*. Baltimore, MD: University Park Press.

Wilson, M. S., & Fox, B. J. (1984). *Microcomputer Language Assessment and Development System (Micro-LADS)* [Computer program]. Winooski, VT: Laureate Learning Systems.

Wilson, M. S., & Fox, B. J. (1986). Microcomputer language assessment, intervention, and enhancement. In J. L. Northern (Ed.), *The Personal Computer for Speech, Language,and Hearing Professionals*. Boston, MA: Little, Brown, pp. 101–112.

Wilson, M. S., & Fox, B. J. (1987a). *Words & Concepts* [Computer program]. Winooski, VT: Laureate Learning Systems.

Wilson, M. S., & Fox, B. J. (1987b). *Words & Concepts II* [Computer program]. Winooski, VT: Laureate Learning Systems.

Wilson, M. S., & Fox, B. J. (1987c). *Words & Concepts III* [Computer program]. Winooski, VT: Laureate Learning Systems.

Wilson, M. S., & Fox, B. J. (1988). *Twenty Categories* [Computer program]. Winooski, VT: Laureate Learning Systems.

Wilson, M. S., & Fox, B. J. (1989). *Concentrate! on Words and Concepts Series* [Computer programs]. Winooski, VT: Laureate Learning Systems.

Wilson, M. S., & Fox, B. J. (1990). *Early Emerging Rules* [Computer program]. Winooski, VT: Laureate Learning Systems.

Wilson, M. S., & Fox, B. J. (1991a). *First Categories* [Computer program]. Winooski, VT: Laureate Learning Systems.

Wilson, M. S., & Fox, B. J. (1991b). *First Words* [Computer program]. Winooski, VT: Laureate Learning Systems.

Wilson, M. S., & Fox, B. J. (1991c). *First Words II* [Computer program]. Winooski, VT: Laureate Learning Systems.

Wilson, M. S., & Fox, B. J. (1991d). *First Verbs* [Computer program]. Winooski, VT: Laureate Learning Systems.

Wilson, M. S., & Fox, B. J. (1991e). From the banks of the Winooski: Clinicians and publishers . . . Ever the twain shall meet. *Journal for Computer Users in Speech and Hearing*, 7(1), 128–131.

Wilson, M. S., & Fox, B. J. (1991f). Sequential software for early language intervention. Presentation at the annual meeting of the American Speech-Language-Hearing Association, Atlanta, GA. [Abstract in *Asha*, 33(10), 218.]

Wilson, M. S., & Fox, B. J. (1991g). *Talking Nouns* [Computer program]. Winooski, VT: Laureate Learning Systems.

Wilson, M. S., & Fox, B. J. (1992a). *First Categories: IBM Compatible Version* [Computer program]. Winooski, VT: Laureate Learning Systems.

Wilson, M. S., & Fox, B. J. (1992b). *Talking Nouns I* [Computer program]. Winooski, VT: Laureate Learning Systems.

Wilson, M. S., & Fox, B. J. (1992c). *Talking Nouns II* [Computer program]. Winooski, VT: Laureate Learning Systems.

Wilson, M. S., & Fox, B. J. (1992d). *Talking Verbs* [Computer program]. Winooski, VT: Laureate Learning Systems.

Wilson, M. S., & Fox, B. J. (1993). Emerging technology meets universal grammar. *Asha*, 35(8), 37–38.

Wilson, P. B. (1983). Software selection and use in language and cognitive retraining. *Cognitive Rehabilitation*, 1, 1.

Wilson, R. H., Cambron, N. K., Marshall, L., & Requejo, R. (1991). A simple computerized up-down tracking procedure (Békésy). Presentation at the annual meeting of the American Speech-Language-Hearing Association, Atlanta, GA. [Abstract in *Asha*, 33(10), 192–193.]

Winkler, D., & Kamins, S. (1990). *HyperTalk 2.0: The Book*. New York, NY: Bantam Books.

Winkler, D., & Knaster, S. (1990). *Cooking with HyperTalk 2.0*. New York, NY: Bantam Books.

Woessner, G. L. (1985). Level of independence for computer assisted speech/language treatment in rehabilitation hospital patients. Presentation at the American Speech and Hearing Foundation Conference on Microcomputers, New Orleans, LA. [Abstract in the *Journal for Computer Users in Speech and Hearing*, 1(2), 93.]

Wohl, C. B., & Schwartz, A. H. (1986). Assessing members' needs for instructional materials in applied computer technology. Presentation at the annual meeting of the American Speech-Language-Hearing Association, Detroit, MI. [Abstract in *Asha*, 28(10), 167.]

Wolfman, W. J., & Silverman, F. H. (1985). Microcomputer usage by speech-language pathologists. *Asha*, 27(10), 9.

Wolpe, J. (1958). *Psychotherapy by Reciprocal Inhibition*. Stanford, CA: Stanford University Press.

Wood, T. J., Wittich, W. W., & Mahaffey, R. B. (1973). Computerized pure-tone audiometric procedures. *Journal of Speech and Hearing Research*, 16, 676–684.

Wrench, A. A., Jackson, M. S., Beck, J. M., & Robertson, G. A. (1994). Objective assessment and rehabilitation of intraoral cancer patients: Voiceless fricatives. Presentation at the annual meeting of the American Speech-Language-Hearing Association, New Orleans, LA. [Abstract in *Asha*, 36(10), 247.]

Wynne, M. K. (1987). PEPPER: A review [Review of computer program]. *Journal for Computer Users in Speech and Hearing*, 3(2), 148–158.

Wynne, M. K. (1991). Editorial: Competencies for the new era of speech-language pathology and audiology. *Journal for Computer Users in Speech and Hearing*, 7(1), 6–9.

Wynne, M. K. (1992a). Editorial: Don't box in your thinking. *Journal for Computer Users in Speech and Hearing*, 8(1, 2). 6–7.

Wynne, M. K. (1992b). Voice Conservation Index [Review of computer program]. *Journal for Computer Users in Speech and Hearing*, 8(1,2), 157–160.

Wynne, M. K. (1992c). Voice Conservation Index [Review of computer program]. *Asha*, 34(8), 101.

Wynne, M. K., & Allen, R. L. (1991). Expert system technology: Applications in communicative disorders. Presentation at the annual meeting of the American Speech-Language-Hearing Association, Atlanta, GA. [Abstract in *Asha*, 33(10), 219.]

Wynne, M. K., Allen, R. L., Kampe, S. D., & Piatz, K. K. (1992). Software applications in hearing aid office management. Presentation at the annual meeting of the American Speech-Language-Hearing Association, San Antonio, TX. [Abstract in *Asha*, 34(10), 212.]

Wynne, M. K., Allen, R. L., & Seaton, W. H. (1991). Alphabet soup: What DOS the audiologist need to know? Presentation at the annual meeting of the American Speech-Language-Hearing Association, Atlanta, GA. [Abstract in *Asha*, 33(10), 171.]

Wynne, M. K., Allen, R. L., Seaton, W. H., Felder, H. M., & Pugh, C. M. (1992). Demystifying DOS. Presentation at the annual meeting of the American Speech-Language-Hearing Association, San Antonio, TX. [Abstract in *Asha*, 34(10), 133.]

Wynne, M. K., Culpepper, B., Mendel, L. L., Grote, M. J., & Seewald, R. (1995). Computer-assisted implementation of the Desired Sensation Level (DSL Version 3.1). Presentation at the annual meeting of the American Speech-Language-Hearing Association, Orlando, FL. [Abstract in *Asha*, 37(10), 105.]

Wynne, M. K., Diefendorf, A. O., Whitelaw, G. M., & Grote, M. J. (1994). Exploring shareware and public domain software alternatives for speech-language pathologists and audiologists. Presentation at the annual meeting of the American Speech-Language-Hearing Association, New Orleans, LA. [Abstract in *Asha*, 36(10), 176.]

Wynne, M. K., Friedman, P., Friedman, K., & Mendel, L. L. (1994). So much data—so little time: Computer aided statistics and graphics for clinicians. Presentation at the annual meeting of the American Speech-Language-Hearing Association, New Orleans, LA. [Abstract in *Asha*, 36(10), 176.]

Wynne, M. K., Friedman, P., Friedman, K., & Renshaw, J. J. (1993). Computer aided statistics and graphics: It's not just for statisticians. Presentation at the annual meeting of the American Speech-Language-Hearing Association, Anaheim, CA. [Abstract in *Asha*, 35(10), 195.]

Wynne, M. K., Mahaffey, R. B., & Renshaw, J. J. (1993). Introduction to OS/2. Presentation at the annual meeting of the American Speech-Language-Hearing Association, Anaheim, CA. [Abstract in *Asha*, 35(10), 227.]

Wynne, M. K., Martin, D., & Matt, B. M. (1995). Hypertext modules used for patient education on tinnitis. Presentation at the annual meeting of the American Speech-Language-Hearing Association, Orlando, FL. [Abstract in *Asha*, 37(10), 105.]

Wynne, M. K., Reynolds, B. R., & Murrell, O. B. (1988). Clinic information managment system using dBASE III+. Presentation at the annual meeting of the American Speech-Language-Hearing Association, Boston, MA. [Abstract in *Asha*, 30(10), 149.]

Wynne, M. K., & Richardson, S. (1990). Five year summary of the *Journal for Computer Users in Speech and Hearing*. *Journal for Computer Users in Speech and Hearing*, 6(1), 8–21.

Wynne, M. K., Seaton, W. H., & Allen, R. L. (1993). Computer technology: Office management. *Asha*, 35(8), 50–51.

Wynne, M. K., Whitelaw, , G. M., Diefendorf, A. O., & Grote, M. J. (1995). Exploring shareware and public domain software alternatives for speech-language pathologists and audiologists. Presentation at the annual meeting of the American Speech-Language-Hearing Association, Orlando, FL. [Abstract in *Asha*, 37(10), 105.]

Yanz, J. L., Birck, J. D., & Stach, B. A. (1987). Computerized audiological technology: Bridging the gap between developer and consumer. Presentation at the annual meeting of the American Speech-Language-Hearing Association, New Orleans, LA. [Abstract in *Asha*, 29(10), 67.]

Yanz, J. L., & Siegel, L. G. (1985). Pure Tone Audiometry Simulation [Computer program]. San Diego, CA: College-Hill Press.

Yaruss, J. S. (1994). Measuring rate, accuracy, and fluency of children's diadochokinetic productions. Presentation at the annual meeting of the American Speech-Language-Hearing Association, New Orleans, LA. [Abstract in *Asha*, 36(10), 174.]

Yonovitz, A. (1988). Voice identification. Presentation at the annual meeting of the American Speech-Language-Hearing Association, Boston, MA. [Abstract in *Asha*, 30(10), 74.]

Yorkstron, K. Beukelman, D., & Traynor, C. (1984). *Computerized Assessment of Intelligibility of Dysarthric Speech* [Computer program]. Tigard, OR: C. C. Publications.

Young, E. C., & Weiner, F. F. (1995). *Function Pictures, Association Pictures, and Rhyming Pictures* [Computer programs]. West Bloomfield, MI: Parrot Software.

Zara, C. V. (1993). IBM SpeechViewer: Creative modifications for speech, language, and listening. Presentation at the annual meeting of the American Speech-Language-Hearing Association, Anaheim, CA. [Abstract in *Asha*, 35(10), 138.]

Zarrella, S. (1995). EEG-based brain-computer interface may enable communication in ALS and stroke. *Advance for Speech-Language Pathologists and Audiologists*, 5(15), 6.

Zemmol, C. (1985). The Automated IEP System-Version 4.2 [Review of computer program]. *Journal for Computer Users in Speech and Hearing*, 1(2), 153–154.

Zimmerman, R. (1992). Cognitive Drill Set 1: Visual Tasks [Review of computer program]. *Asha*, 34(2), 80.

Zuckerman, D. (1984). Use of personal computing technology by deaf-blind individuals. *Journal of Medical Systems*, 8(5), 431–436.

Author Index

Subject Index